Data-Centric AI Solutions and Emerging Technologies in the Healthcare Ecosystem

This book offers insight into the healthcare system by exploring emerging technologies and AI-based applications and implementation strategies. It includes current developments for future directions as well as covering the concept of the healthcare system along with its ecosystem.

Data-Centric AI Solutions and Emerging Technologies in the Healthcare Ecosystem focuses on the mechanisms of proposing and incorporating solutions along with architectural concepts, design principles, smart solutions, decision-making process, and intelligent predictions. It offers state-of-the-art approaches for overall innovations, developments, and implementation of the smart healthcare ecosystem and highlights medical signal and image processing algorithms, healthcare-based computer vision systems, and discusses explainable AI (XAI) techniques for healthcare.

This book will be useful to researchers involved in AI, IoT, data, and emerging technologies in the medical industry. It is also suitable as supporting material for undergraduate and graduate-level courses in related engineering disciplines.

Data-Centric AI Solutions and Emerging Technologies in the Healthcare Ecosystem

Edited by
Alex Khang
Geeta Rana
R. K. Tailor
Vugar Abdullayev

CRC Press
Taylor & Francis Group
Boca Raton London New York

CRC Press is an imprint of the
Taylor & Francis Group, an **informa** business

Designed cover image: Shutterstock

MATLAB® is a trademark of The MathWorks, Inc. and is used with permission. The MathWorks does not warrant the accuracy of the text or exercises in this book. This book's use or discussion of MATLAB® software or related products does not constitute endorsement or sponsorship by The MathWorks of a particular pedagogical approach or particular use of the MATLAB® software.

First edition published 2024
by CRC Press
2385 Executive Center Drive, Suite 320, Boca Raton, FL 33431

and by CRC Press
4 Park Square, Milton Park, Abingdon, Oxon, OX14 4RN

CRC Press is an imprint of Taylor & Francis Group, LLC

© 2024 selection and editorial matter, Alex Khang, Geeta Rana, R. K. Tailor, Vugar Abdullayev; individual chapters, the contributors

Library of Congress Cataloguing-in-Publication Data
Names: Khang, Alex, editor. I Rana, Geeta, editor. I Tailor, R. K., editor. I Abdullayev, Vugar, editor.
Title: Data-centric AI solutions and emerging technologies in the healthcare ecosystem / edited by Alex Khang, Geeta Rana, R.K. Tailor, Vugar Abdullayev.
Other titles: Data-centric artificial intelligence solutions and emerging technologies in the healthcare ecosystem
Description: First edition. I Boca Raton : CRC Press, 2024. I Includes bibliographical references and index.
Identifiers: LCCN 2023008181 (print) I LCCN 2023008182 (ebook) I ISBN 9781032398570 (hardback) I
ISBN 9781032410869 (paperback) I ISBN 9781003356189 (ebook)
Subjects: MESH: Artificial Intelligence I Medical Informatics Applications I Internet of Things I Data Science I
Biomedical Technology--trends
Classification: LCC R859 (print) I LCC R859 (ebook) I NLM W 26.55.A7 I DDC 610.285--dc23/eng/20230615
LC record available at https://lccn.loc.gov/2023008181
LC ebook record available at https://lccn.loc.gov/2023008182

ISBN: 978-1-032-39857-0 (hbk)
ISBN: 978-1-032-41086-9 (pbk)
ISBN: 978-1-003-35618-9 (ebk)

DOI: 10.1201/9781003356189

Typeset in Times
by MPS Limited, Dehradun

Contents

Preface

Nowadays, we are seeing a host of powerful artificial intelligence (AI) algorithms, big data, and Internet of Things (IoT) technologies aimed at replicating or replacing the human brain capabilities in computing and communication devices. Therefore, humans are eager to leverage the most multi-faceted AI-based solutions and emerging technologies to develop, deploy, and deliver next-generation medical and healthcare systems.

Most resource-intensive accessories, gadgets, machines, instruments, appliances, devices, equipment, and networks spread across a variety of ecosystems (including cities, buildings, apartments, homes, hotels, hospitals, etc.) are meticulously empowered with the competencies of AI and smart technologies.

Strictly speaking, the convergence of AI, IoT, computer vision (CV), data, and emerging technologies are being touted as a compound of the emerging technology to design and implement a bevy of smart medical ecosystems that could be delivered all kinds of connected healthcare products and/or individually enabled to be more intelligent in their treatment, diagnosis, surgery, dissection, etc.

In spite of available challenges and particular concerns being associated with the big adoption of the smart systems in the complex infrastructure of the medical ecosystem, if these systems are AI-integrated with full functionality to support the decision-making process, then we need to articulate how we design and implement their models and techniques in not only healthcare ecosystems but also in another industries.

This book brings insight into the healthcare ecosystem and offers emerging technologies and AI-based applications and implementation strategies. It includes current developments and future directions and covers the concept of the healthcare systems along with its ecosystem.

This book focuses on the mechanisms of proposing solutions along with architectural concepts, design principles, smart solutions, intelligent predictions, and case studies with visualization simulation for the healthcare systems.

This book is also useful to researchers involved in AI, IoT, data, and emerging technologies in the medical industry and can be a reference for future research. It is also suitable for supporting material for undergraduate and graduate-level courses in related engineering disciplines.

Happy reading!

Editorial team:
Alex Khang
Geeta Rana
R. K. Tailor
Vugar Abdullayev

Preface

Acknowledgments

This book is based on the design and implementation of artificial intelligence (AI), data science, Internet of Things (IoT), Internet of Medical Things (IoMT), blockchain technology, and emerging technologies in the healthcare 4.0 ecosystem. Building a book outline to introduce to readers across the globe is the passion and noble goal of the editorial team. To be able to make ideas a reality and the success of this book, the biggest reward belongs to the efforts, experiences, enthusiasm, and trust of the contributors.

To all the reviewers with whom we have had the opportunity to collaborate and monitor their hard work remotely, we acknowledge their tremendous support and valuable comments not only for the book but also for future book projects.

We also express our deep gratitude for all the pieces of advice, support, motivation, sharing, and inspiration we received from our faculty, educators, professors, scientists, doctors, and academic colleagues.

And last but not least, we are really grateful to our publisher, CRC Press (Taylor & Francis Group), for the wonderful support in the timely processing of the manuscript and bringing out this book to the readers quickly.

Thank you, everyone.

Editorial Team:
Alex Khang, Geeta Rana, R. K. Tailor, Vugar Abdullayev

Biography of Editors

Dr. Alex Khang is a professor in information technology at the Universities of Science and Technology in Vietnam, India, and United States; AI and data scientist, software industry expert, and the chief of technology officer (AI and Data Science Research Center) at the Global Research Institute of Technology and Engineering, North Carolina, United States. He has more than 28 years of teaching and research experience in information technology (Software Development, Database Technology, AI Engineering, Data Engineering, Data Science, Data Analytics, IoT-based Technologies, and Cloud Computing) at the Universities of Science and Technology in Vietnam, India, and USA. He has been the chair session for 20 conferences; keynote speaker for more than 25 international conclaves; an expert tech speaker for over 100 seminars and webinars; an international technical board member for 10 international organizations; an editorial board member for more than 5 ISSNs; an international reviewer and evaluator for more than 100 journal papers; and an international examiner and evaluator for more than 15 PhD theses in the computer science field. He has been contributing to various research activities in the fields of AI and data science while publishing many international articles in renowned journals and conference proceedings. He has published 52 authored books (in computer science between 2000–2010), 2 authored books (software development), 10 book chapters, published 9 edited books, and 10 edited books (calling for book chapters) in the fields of AI ecosystem (AI, ML, DL, robotics, data science, big data, and IoT), smart city ecosystem, healthcare ecosystem, fintech technology, and blockchain technology (since 2020). He has over 28 years of nonstop work as a software product manager; data engineer; AI engineer; cloud computing architect; solution architect; software architect; database expert in the foreign corporations of Germany, Sweden, the United States, and Singapore; and multinationals (former CEO, former CTO, former engineering director, product manager, and senior software production consultant).

Dr. Geeta Rana is an associate professor at the Himalayan School of Management Studies in Swami Rama Himalayan University, Jolly Grant, Dehradun. She received her PhD in management from Indian Institute of Technology (IIT, Roorkee). She has also done certification courses in HR analytics from Indian Institute of Management Rohtak (IIMR). She is engaged in teaching, research, and consultancy assignments. She has more than 15 years of experience in teaching and in handling various administrative as well as academic positions. She has to her credit over 50 papers published in refereed journals of Emerald, Sage, Springer, Taylor & Francis, Elsevier, and InderScience publishers. She also presented several research papers in national and international conferences. She has contributed several chapters in different books published by Cambridge UK, Springer IGI Global, and Palgrave Macmillan. She has authored 12 editor biographies in a book titled *Counseling Skills for Managers* published by New Age Publications. She has conducted and attended various workshops, faculty development programs (FDPs), and management development programs (MDPs). She is recipient of many awards. Her research interests include data analytics, Human

Resource Management 4.0, knowledge management, managerial effectiveness, justice, values, employer branding, and innovation.

Dr. R. K. Tailor is a senior associate professor in the Department of Business Administration, Manipal University Jaipur, Rajasthan, India. He is an expert in robotic process automation and robotic accounting in India for the last 10 years and developed more than 10 patents and served as a consultant in many education institutions, universities, and business houses for the application and adoption of robotic process automation. He has more than 16 years of experience in teaching and research. He has published more than 60 books on the different areas of commerce and management and more than 60 research papers in reputed national and international journals. He is also actively associated with the Indian Commerce Association and Indian Accounting Association as an EC Member and has served as associate editor in the *Indian Journal of Accounting*. He is also associated with high-ranked International reputed publication houses as an editor, reviewer, and advisory board member such as Taylor & Francis, Springer, Elsevier, CRC Publications, IGI GLobal, Scientific Publications, etc. He has also chaired more than 50 national and international conferences as chief guest, chairperson, and key note speaker and resource person. He has also delivered his speech on robotic process automation at the international level in Romania, Malaysia, Nepal, Dubai, Spain, Turkey, Poland, Hungary, and Ireland. He has achieved many awards and accolades from many national and international organizations.

Dr. Vugar Abdullayev is a doctor of technical sciences and an associate professor at Azerbaijan State Oil and Industry University. Baku, Azerbaijan. He has completed his PhD in computer science in 2005. He is currently an associate professor of the Computer Engineering Department at the Azerbaijan State Oil and Industry University, Baku, Azerbaijan. He is an author of 61 scientific papers. His research is related to the study of the cyber physical systems, IoT, big data, smart city, and information technologies.

Contributors

Ragimova Nazila Ali
Azerbaijan State Oil and Industry
    University
Baku, Azerbaijan

P. T. N. Anh
ChoRay Hospital
Ho Chi Minh City
Vietnam

Abuzarova Vusala Alyar
Azerbaijan State Oil and Industry
    University
Baku, Azerbaijan

Vivek AR
Thiagarajar College of Engineering
Madurai, India

Temitayo Balogun
Ekiti State Polytechnic
Isan-Ekiti, Nigeria

Avijit Kumar Chaudhuri
Techno Engineering College Banipur
Kolkata, India

Ritik Chaurasia
Amity University
Lucknow Campus, India

Svetlana Chumachenko
Kharkov National University of Radio
    Electronics
Ukraine

Sulekha Das
Techno Engineering College Banipur
Kolkata, India

Samuel Faluyi
Ekiti State Polytechnic
Isan-Ekiti, Nigeria

Kofoworola Fapohunda
Louisiana Tech University
United States

Rashmi Gujrati
KC Group of Institutions
Nawanshahr, Punjab, India

Vladimir Hahanov
Kharkiv National University of Radio
    Electronics
Ukraine

Abdullayev Vugar Hajimahmud
Azerbaijan State Oil and Industry
    University
Baku, Azerbaijan

Aravindaguru I.
Sri Ramakrishna Engineering College
Coimbatore, Tamil Nadu, India

Babasaheb Jadhav
D. Y. Patil Vidyapeeth (deemed to be
    university)
Global Business School & Research
    Centre
Pune, India

Biranchi Jena
D. Y. Patil Vidyapeeth (deemed to be
    university)
Global Business School and Research
    Centre
Pune, India

Srinivasan K.
Sri Ramakrishna Engineering College
Coimbatore, Tamil Nadu, India

Surya K
Thiagarajar College of Engineering
Madurai, India

P Karthikeyan
Thiagarajar College of Engineering
Madurai, India

A. R. Kavitha
Chennai Institute of Technology
Chennai, Tamil Nadu, India

Satish Khalikar
Tata Trusts, India

Alex Khang
Universities of Science & Technology
Vietnam & United States and Global
    Research Institute of Technology &
    Engineering
North Carolina, United States

Narendra Kumar
Shakuntala Misra National
    Rehabilitation University
Lucknow, India

Divvela Vishnu Sai Kumar
Amity University
Lucknow Campus, India

Anchal Kumari
Lovely Professional University
Jalandhar, Punjab, India

Eugenia Litvinova
Kharkov National University of Radio
    Electronics
Ukraine

Monika Mathur
Manipal University Jaipur
Jaipur, Rajasthan, India

Anuradha Misra
Amity University Uttar Pradesh
Lucknow Campus, India

Praveen Kumar Misra
Shakuntala Misra National
    Rehabilitation University
Lucknow, India

Apeksha Nagawade
Global Business School and Research
    Centre
Dr. D. Y. Patil Vidyapeeth
Pune, India

Arpita Nayak
KIIT University
Bhubaneswar, Odisha, India

Olufunke Oluwabusayo
Ekiti State Polytechnic
Isan-Ekiti, Nigeria

Veeramani P.
Sri Ramakrishna Engineering College
Coimbatore, Tamil Nadu, India

B. C. M. Patnaik
Kalinga Institute of Industrial
    Technology (KIIT)
Bhubaneswar, Odisha, India

Rahul Gowtham Poola
SRM University
Amaravati, Andhra Pradesh, India

M. Ramya
Chennai Institute of Technology
Chennai, Tamil Nadu, India

Punam Rattan
Lovely Professional University
Jalandhar, Punjab, India

Arkadip Ray
Government College of Engineering &
    Ceramic Technology
West Bengal, India

Sakthi S
Thiagarajar College of Engineering
Madurai, India

Vibishanan S
Thiagarajar College of Engineering
Madurai, India

Ipseeta Satpathy
Kalinga Institute of Industrial
    Technology (KIIT)
Bhubaneswar, Odisha, India

Vrushank Shah
Indus University
Ahmedabad, Gujarat, India

Ankita Sharma
Manipal University Jaipur
Jaipur, Rajasthan, India

Muskan Singh
Amity University
Lucknow Campus, India

Vidhi Thakkar
Indus University and GLS University
Ahmedabad, Gujarat, India

Triwiyanto
Poltekkes Kemenkes Surabaya
Indonesia

Hayri Uygun
Recep Tayyip Erdogan University
Rize, Turkey

Radhika V.
Sri Ramakrishna Engineering College
Coimbatore, Tamil Nadu, India

Uday Sankar V.
SRM University
Amaravati, Andhra Pradesh, India

Siva Sankar Y.
SRM University
Amaravati, Andhra Pradesh, India

1 Electronic Health Records Security and Privacy Enhancement Using Blockchain Technology

Vidhi Thakkar, Vrushank Shah, and Alex Khang

CONTENTS

1.1 INTRODUCTION

An electronic health record (EHR) is a digital record of a patient's medical history that is kept by the healthcare practitioner over time. More and more hospitals are employing EHR systems to share patient records. Integrated health records are more advantageous than standalone ones as they ensure the mobility of the records.

The pandemic had a tremendous impact on the healthcare system all over the world, and healthcare data is being generated at an alarming rate in today's society. This massive surge in patient records from various sources necessitates the use of reliable and secure data storage and exchange solutions. In current times, the healthcare organizations store their data on cloud servers but, this raises concerns about data protection, duplication, and fine-grained access control (Khang et al., 2023a).

DOI: 10.1201/9781003356189-1

There are also many other drawbacks with centralized EHR systems, including issues with healthcare data breaches, a single point of failure, challenges with the privacy of sensitive and private information, and difficulty with interoperability across various systems/data sources. As a result, blockchain technology is being investigated and used for EHR management and sharing (Agbo et al., 2019).

Blockchain technology is taking the world by storm and has been described as a technological revolution. Blockchain has the power to completely transform how businesses operate. Blockchain ensures immutability, decentralization, and security of the data through a consensus mechanism. This technology is becoming increasingly popular across a number of industries, including automotive supply chains, healthcare, logistics, banking, and more (Rana et al., 2021).

Blockchain allows users to access and share data securely across multiple blocks without the need for a mediator or any centralized authority (Hölbl et al., 2018). However, the use case is tricky for the healthcare industry where patient privacy and medical data protection are crucial.

There are two types of blockchains: public and permissioned blockchains. The most widely used public blockchain is Ethereum, and permissioned blockchain is a Hyperledger Fabric framework. Ethereum does not restrict network membership. Any node can join the network, send transactions, and generate blocks (Khanh & Khang, 2021).

In the Ethereum blockchain, consensus protocol requires cryptocurrency to be spent on smart contract execution and this can increase risks and attacks during crypto mining operations (Hussain et al., 2022). On the other hand, Hyperledger Fabric allows only permissioned businesses that have been invited to the network to join. Here, the identities of all participating nodes are known (Khang et al., 2022b).

Hyperledger Fabric is a distributed ledger technology that offers companies a robust way of dealing with their concerns about data privacy. Hyperledger Fabric has been gaining popularity in a number of industries, including the Internet of Things (IoT), supply chain management, finance, and healthcare. It is the most deployable permissioned blockchain solution, supporting modular architecture and providing simple APIs that businesses may adjust to improve specific activities (Hajimahmud et al., 2022).

Nodes in a Fabric network do not need to observe or authenticate the update; therefore, reducing the time taken to conduct a transaction. A permissioned blockchain has an influence on healthcare services because it enhances performance, and guarantees trust, traceability, privacy, and security (Khang et al., 2023b).

Many studies have been published on using a Hyperledger Fabric permissioned blockchain framework for secure EHR sharing and management. However, current research still raises questions about data privacy and data confidentiality during transaction consensus.

This chapter proposes a permissioned EHR with Fabric's privacy preservation techniques as well as the few but crucial developments that are required to further protect patients' and healthcare organizations' privacy.

The remainder of the chapter is organized as follows.

- **Section** 1.2 discusses contribution.
- **Section** 1.3 provides a background on the Hyperledger Fabric.

- The related literature is discussed in Section 1.4.
- In **Section** 1.5, Hyperledger Fabric–enabled blockchain architecture for EHR sharing system is presented.
- **Section** 1.6 presents the tools used for the implementation of the proposed blockchain based framework.
- **Section** 1.7 shows the comparison of proposed methods against other Fabric-based EHR studies.
- Finally, **Section** 1.8 summarizes our conclusions.

1.2 CONTRIBUTION

Healthcare organizations face a difficult challenge: finding the right balance between improving healthcare quality while protecting the patients' privacy. Hyperledger Fabric, a permissioned blockchain technology, has emerged as a viable solution for these concerns. This permissioned blockchain system uses multiple access control mechanisms to protect data privacy and confidentiality and allows only authorized participants to join the permissioned system—thus allowing them to transact with each other privately (Khang et al., 2022c).

Hyperledger Fabric allows peers to communicate in a way that ensures their privacy by using channels, private data collections, and transient fields.

Here is a summary of the major contributions: The proposed architecture was created using Hyperledger Fabric to meet security requirements and boost performance. The use of permissioned blockchain technology ensures EHR sharing, access control, data integrity, interoperability, and data privacy (Khang et al., 2023c).

The use of Fabric's privacy preservation techniques is to make transactions private to some members and not visible to other network members. The use of IPFS with Arweave decentralized databases minimizes the risks associated with centralized storage and guarantees system scalability as well as permanence.

1.3 BACKGROUND

1.3.1 HYPERLEDGER FABRIC

Hyperledger is an open-source project that aims to provide enterprise solutions by combining several tools. It includes Fabric, Sawtooth, Iroha, and Cello among others. Among these, Hyperledger Fabric is the most popular since it can execute multiple transactions simultaneously while improving the system's performance (Tailor et al., 2022).

Fabric facilitates the creation of smart contracts using a number of widely used programming languages. The Fabric enables the sending of private transactions (private data collections and transient fields) or the development of parallel and independent lightweight channels to share data with only a portion of the nodes of the blockchain system.

Raft, Kafka (deprecated in the latest version), and Solo (deprecated in the latest version) are three CFT consensus algorithms that Fabric supports. The Fabric reduces the computer power by committing a transaction with multiple endorsers rather than the entire network solving a cryptographic puzzle.

Because it is permissioned and has a modular design, this allows for scalability and confidentiality. The Fabric involves channels, peers, assets, identity, membership, transactions, chain code, ledgers, and consensus procedures as part of the network. Participants essentially sign up through a reputable membership service provider (MSP) that keeps a list of permissioned identities made by certificate authorities (CAs). Fabric CA, a private root CA provider, is in fact in charge of generating digital identities.

1.3.2 STEPS

Transactions are processed by the Fabric in the following three steps:

- **Execute:** First a client submits a transaction to the peers who are endorsing it. Which of the peers will carry out a specific transaction is determined by the endorsement policy. The endorsing peers execute the transaction and store the results in the world state database without making any changes to their version of the ledger. After that, they return signed transactions to the client that needs to be delivered to the orderers.
- **Order:** By arranging the received endorsed transactions into blocks, orderers generate blocks. A block is broadcast to all channel peers once it has been formed.
- **Validate:** Each peer validates the accuracy of each transaction contained in the received block before updating its own copy of the ledger. Transactions are invalidated if they have a read or write conflict with an earlier transaction of the same block.

1.4 RELATED WORK

In this section, we examine Hyperledger Fabric's most recent research on EHR systems sharing and management.

A secure EHR sharing system called Medbloc was proposed by Huang et al., (2019) using Hyperledger Fabric. It was targeted at the New Zealand healthcare industry. The PBFT (Practical Byzantine Fault Tolerant) consensus mechanism and Hyperledger Fabric version 1.1 were used in the development of the system.

The healthcare records were encrypted and stored on the blockchain using a smart contract–based access control scheme. Their system offered a number of advantages, including availability, efficiency, and security.

In order to efficiently preserve patient records in terms of privacy, security, scalability, and availability, Mahore et al., (2019) proposed a permissioned blockchain model. This method addresses the blockchain's scalability issues by keeping patients' sensitive data on an off-chain cloud server and keeping only the hash of the data in a blockchain record (Khang et al., 2022a).

In order to send encrypted data from the patient to the provider, they have also used a proxy re-encryption technique. They used the PBFT consensus algorithm, the solo ordering service, and Hyperledger Fabric version V1.4 to develop their solution.

Using the Hyperledger Caliper, they have also analyzed their approach statistically to see how well it performs.

A number of research studies conducted later in 2020 focused on developing scalable and secure EHR-sharing solutions using the Hyperledger Fabric. An ACTION-EHR was presented by Dubovitskaya et al., (2020) for handling the medical records of cancer patients. The Hyperledger Fabric architecture is used to build the prototype, which will allow researchers and healthcare providers to exchange EMR data. The medical data of patients is encrypted using public-key cryptography and stored on off-chain servers. The system ensures granular access control, data confidentiality, and availability of EMR data.

The Member Ship Service, orderer, cloud server, Hyperledger Fabric v1.4 SDK, and CouchDB for on-chain metadata management and permissions are used in the construction of the ACTION-EHR blockchain network.

In order to build a distributed solution for integrating existing EHRs, Tith et al. (Tith et al., 2020) employed consortium blockchain with Hyperledger Fabric. Encrypted data is transferred from the patient to the doctor through a proxy re-encryption method on a centralized server.

To avoid transactions tracing on the ledger, the eID has been hashed using salt. They were able to accomplish scalability, transparency, traceability, availability, and reliability with their method using Hyperledger Fabric and Hyperledger Composer, Khang et al. (2022d) created a framework for securing electronic health records using permissioned blockchain technology. While huge EHRs were kept on distributed IPFS, the blockchain only contained encrypted hashes of the records. The new paradigm has resulted in a better assurance of data integrity, scalability, privacy, and interoperability.

The system was developed using the Fabric's MSP, CA, PBFT consensus, CouchDB, and chain code components. Their study has made it possible to increase scalability while ensuring a high level of security and privacy. PREHEALTH, a privacy-preserving EHR management solution utilizing Hyperledger Fabric, was introduced by (Stamatellis et al., 2020). Identity Mixer is discussed in the solution to guarantee transaction anonymity and unlinkability.

The solution adheres to GDPR and focuses on Hyperledger Fabric's privacy-preserving capabilities. However, they have not disclosed Hyperledger Fabric's configuration information. PCHDM, a patient-centered healthcare data management solution, was introduced by (Mani et al., 2021). Their approach also uses off-chain and on-chain technologies to maintain health records.

The IPFS technology securely stores encrypted health data together with hashes of medical records. Smart contracts are deployed within secure containers, making use of Byzantine Fault Tolerance (BFT) consensus. This allows for high levels of security, privacy, and scalability. Performance is evaluated using Hyperledger Caliper benchmarks for transaction latency, throughput, and resource usage.

This study's findings suggest that permissioned blockchain technology can be used to enhance the performance, privacy, and interoperability of healthcare data administration.

1.5 HYPERLEDGER FABRIC–ENABLED BLOCKCHAIN ARCHITECTURE

In this section, we will propose a hyperledger fabric–enabled blockchain architecture for an EHR sharing system, as shown in figure 1.1. The Hyperledger Fabric permissioned blockchain framework has been implemented for secure data storage and sharing of electronic health records. Privacy-preserving mechanisms of the Hyperledger Fabric are implemented to preserve data privacy, security, and integrity (Private data, 2020 & Using Private Data in Fabric, 2022).

In our system, the patient has ownership of their healthcare data. The study offers effective access control between patients and doctors, through encryption techniques. A working prototype based on Hyperledger Fabric and IPFS with Arweave data storage system (Arweave + IPFS bridge system) is made to illustrate the system's viability (Khang et al., 2023c).

The approach is a tamper-resistant mechanism as only metadata (hashed data, data reference URLs, and permissions) will be stored as hash values for every healthcare transaction in the blockchain. If an attempt is made to modify the off-chain database, this hash will be recorded onto the consultation blockchain.

All the information will be encrypted using AES before storing to the database and keys will be encrypted using ECC (elliptical curve cryptography) for fetching information. IPFS is a well-known P2P network for decentralized data exchange, but it is missing one essential component: permanence.

The information can be permanently lost if no one hosts it. Utilizing Arweave blockchain, files can be stored and pinned onto IPFS, and they will always be accessible through IPFS hash. The latter makes use of the file-sharing protocol IPFS and is a distributed database. IPFS creates the hash of each block that is stored when storing the data.

Arweave (CRYPTO: AR) is a Web3 protocol that offers data storage on a decentralized network of devices. Like other storage coin projects, it matches people who need storage with users who have extra space available.

1.5.1 EXPLANATION

In our system, when the doctor wants to add a prescription for a patient, he would ask the permission of the patient. After the patient approves the transaction, patient ID, date of visit, disease, etc. are as shown in figure 1.1.

Information will be stored on the private data collection of that organization and permission list on the peer's CouchDB and heavy files such as reports would be stored on IPFS with Arweave data storage and hashes of the transaction would be stored on the blockchain (Bhambri et al., 2022).

1. The client submits transactions with encrypted input data. Data such as patient name, doctor name, and organization name are passed through the transient field for privacy preservation purposes. Suppose a patient wants to give data access consent to another doctor; that request is submitted.

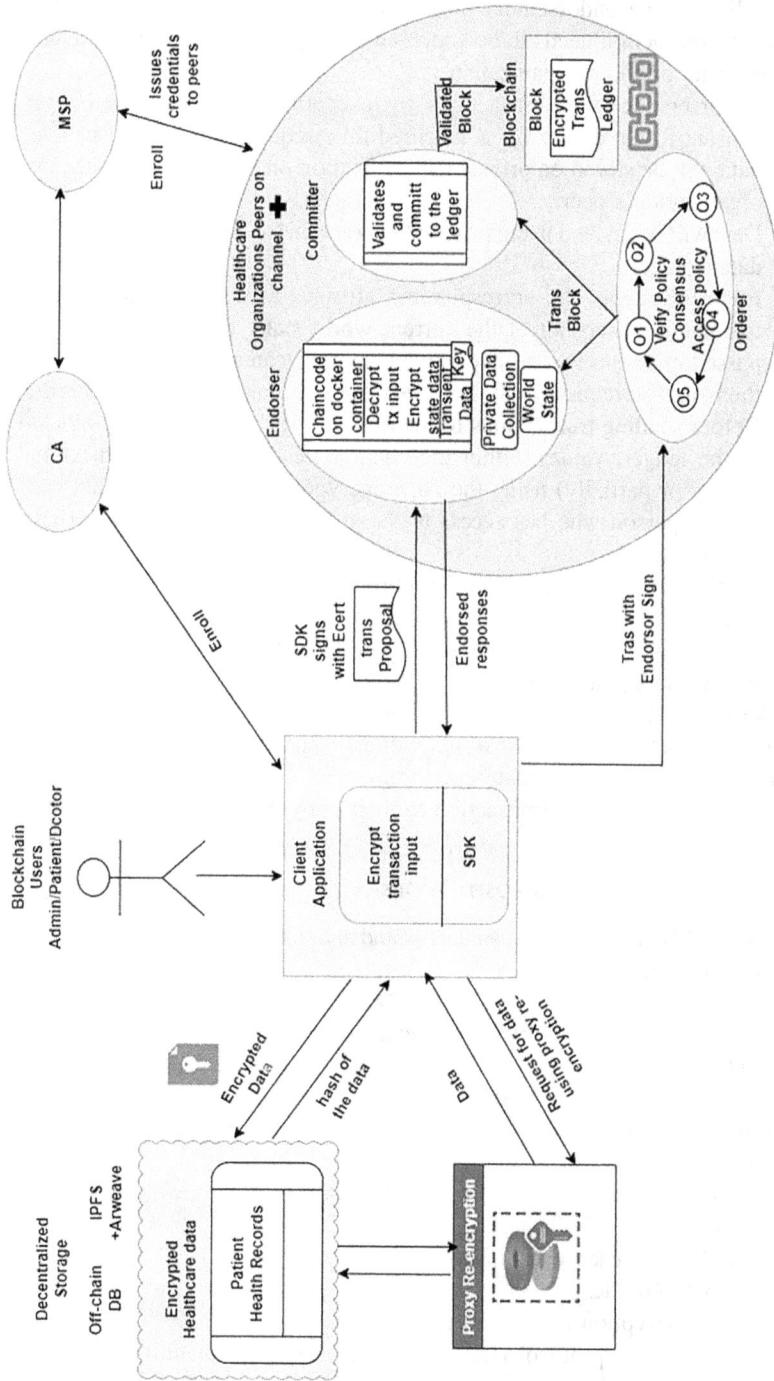

FIGURE 1.1 Hyperledger Fabric–integrated blockchain architecture for secure EHR sharing system.

Source: Author's owner.

2. This transaction would be passed to the identified endorsers and endorsed according to the endorsement policy. The endorsement policy specifies that this transaction needs to be endorsed by the doctors' organization and patient data provider organization.

   a. Endorsers endorse transactions by executing chain code and give consent to the doctor for a specified time request and fetched patient data will be stored on private data collection on a particular healthcare organization's peer.

   b. Data will be fetched using proxy re-encryption from IPFS with Arweave data storage.

   c. Endorsers apply the corresponding changes to a state database that maintains a snapshot of the current world state. If transient data are passed in a transaction, then only chain code can access them, decrypt them, and store them to the private data collection of the organizations.

   d. Before sending transactions to the ordering service and adding blocks to the ledger, values within the chain code can be encrypted (completely or partially) using the AES encryption to protect the data.

   e. Only a person who has access to the appropriate key can decrypt encrypted data.

3. After endorsement, this signed transaction will be submitted to the client's application.

4. Then the client submits this transaction to the ordering service with read/write sets and signature from the endorsers.

5. Ordering service after checking the endorsement policy puts the transaction into blocks and sends it to the validator nodes.

6. Validator/committers validate each transaction in the block and commit the block and store the transaction to their copy of the blockchain.

1.5.2 FEATURES OF OUR PROPOSED WORK

Patients and healthcare providers can access and share health records in a usable yet privacy-preserving manner.

- Longitudinal view of the patient's health story.
- Patients give or withdraw consent for regulating access to their records.
- User privacy will not be disclosed to any nodes on the channel.
- An encryption mechanism and enforcing a smart contract–based access control mechanism for regulating access.
- Docker-based chain code execution and passing secret keys through the transient field.
- Private data for each organization can be stored using PDC and is compatible with GDPR.
- Proxy Rr-encryption for better performance.
- IPFS + Arweave protocol (Off-chain database) for scalability and EHR permanence.

TABLE 1.1

Tools Used for the Implementation of the Proposed Blockchain

System	Ubuntu 18.4
Hyperledger Fabric SDK	Fabric-JavaScript-SDK v2.3.1
No. of healthcare organizations	5 organizations
No. of peer per organization	2–3
Consensus	Raft
World state DB	CouchDB
Concept	Docker-based
Chain code language	Node.js
Front End:	HTML, CSS, JavaScript
Other integration	Hyperledger Explorer and Caliper
Data storage	IPFS + Arweave Data Storage
Access control	It is used to restrict access to smart contract transactions based on role.
CA and MSP	X.509 certificates
Transient filed	For passing the symmetric key to chain code through the docker as well as all the input parameters of the transaction will be passed through the transient field only.
Private data collection	For each organization as well as between OrgA and OrgB OrgB and OrgC
Chain code	Create medical record Save data Update medical record Allow doctor write Update ownership/patient gives consent to another doctor doctor fetches patient data Public key encryption is made possible by using elliptical curve cryptography (ECC)

Source: Author's owner.

The configuration files are **start.sh, scripts.sh, configtx.yaml, crypto-config.yaml**, and **docker-compose.yaml**. The tool dumps and parses these five configuration files as a network configuration based on their intended uses.

1.5.3 Tools

Tools used for the implementation of the proposed blockchain-based framework are shown in table 1.1.

Table 1.1 depicts the list of tools that used for the implementation of the proposed blockchain in this chapter (Khanh & Khang, 2021).

TABLE 1.2

Comparison of the Proposed Against Existing Fabric-Based EHR Sharing Systems

Reference and Year	Fabric Version	Storage	Consensus/ Ordering Service	Immutability	Performance and Scalability	Utilized Fabric Privacy Preservation Mechanisms
Huang et al., 2019	Hyperledger Fabric (V1.1)	On-chain	PBFT	Y	Low	N
Mahore et al., 2019	Hyperledger Fabric (V1.4)	Cloud	–	N	High	N
Dubovitskaya et al., 2020	Hyperledger Fabric (V1.4)	Cloud	PBFT Solo	N	High	N
Chenthara et al., 2020	Hyperledger and Fabric Composer (Deprecated) Hyperledger and Fabric (V1.3)	IPFS	PBFT Kafka	Y	High	N
Tith et al., 2020	Hyperledger Fabric	Cloud	BFT	N	HIgh	N
Stamatellis et al., 2020	Hyperledger Fabric	–	–	–	–	Y
Mani et al., 2021	Hyperledger Fabric	orbitDB+ IPFS	BFT	Y	High	N
Proposed Privacy Preserved EHR System	Hyperledger Fabric (V2.X)	IPFS+Arweave	Raft	Y	High	Y

Source: Author's owner.

1.6 COMPARISON

Comparison of the proposed method against other Fabric-based EHR studies. Table 1.2 presents a comparison of features/functions between the proposed Fabric-based EHR system and other Fabric-integrated healthcare systems already studied in the related works section.

This comparison shows that they have not utilized Fabric's privacy preservation techniques such as private data collections and transient field to preserve data privacy inside the fabric network. Many studies were published using the Hyperledger Fabric permissioned blockchain framework to secure EHR sharing and management.

However, they have utilized a lower Fabric version, deprecated the consensus mechanism, and not utilized the Fabric's privacy preservation techniques to preserve sensitive data inside the network. The Fabric includes privacy-protection techniques that are more robust in preventing data breaches and attacks than those used by the existing studies (Rani et al., 2021).

1.7 CONCLUSION

In this chapter, we presented Hyperledger Fabric–integrated blockchain architecture for a secure EHR sharing system. The use of the Hyperledger Fabric blockchain network to enhance consent transparency, privacy, and traceability in clinical trials has been discussed within this work (Morris et al., 2023).

Transactions can be conducted in a private subnet of communication between defined network members called channels (Rani et al., 2022).

Healthcare data are preserved using the Fabric's privacy preservation mechanisms, ensuring that no unauthorized parties have access to them, and they cannot be altered by any other applications on the system. Heavy data are stored on IPFS with Arweave data storage for the better permeance and scalability of the network (Misra et al., 2023).

REFERENCES

Agbo, C.C., Mahmoud, Q.H., & Eklund, J.M. (2019, April). Blockchain technology in healthcare: A systematic review. *In Healthcare*, 7(2), 56. *MDPI*. https://www.mdpi.com/440052

Bhambri, P., Rani, S., Gupta, G., & Khang, A. (2022). Cloud and fog computing platforms for Internet of Things, ISBN: 978-1-032-101507, CRC Press. 10.1201/9781003213888

Chenthara, S., Ahmed, K., Wang, H., Whittaker, F., & Chen, Z. (2020). Healthchain: A novel framework on privacy preservation of electronic health records using blockchain technology. *Plos One*, 15(12), e0243043. https://journals.plos.org/plosone/article?id=10.1371/journal.pone.0243043

Dubovitskaya, A., Baig, F., Xu, Z., Shukla, R., Zambani, P.S., Swaminathan, A. & Wang, F. (2020). ACTION-EHR: Patient-centric blockchain-based electronic health record data management for cancer care. *Journal of Medical Internet Research*, 22(8), e13598. https://www.jmir.org/2020/8/e13598/

Hajimahmud, V.A., Khang, A., Hahanov, V., Litvinova, E., Chumachenko, S., & Alyar, A.V. (2022). Autonomous robots for smart city: Closer to augmented humanity. *AI-Centric Smart City Ecosystems: Technologies, Design and Implementation* (1st Ed.). 7(12), CRC Press. 10.1201/9781003252542-7

Hölbl, M., Kompara, M., Kamišalić, A., & Nemec Zlatolas, L. (2018). A systematic review of the use of blockchain in healthcare. *Symmetry*, 10(10), 470. https://www.mdpi.com/349208

Huang, J., Qi, Y.W., Asghar, M.R., Meads, A., & Tu, Y.C. (2019, August). MedBloc: A blockchain-based secure EHR system for sharing and accessing medical data. *In 2019 18th IEEE International Conference on Trust, Security and Privacy in Computing and Communications/13th IEEE International Conference on Big Data Science and Engineering (TrustCom/BigDataSE)* (pp. 594–601). IEEE. https://ieeexplore.ieee.org/abstract/document/8887337/

Hussain, S.H., Sivakumar, T.B., & Khang, A. (Eds.). (2022). Cryptocurrency methodologies and techniques. *The Data-Driven Blockchain Ecosystem: Fundamentals, Applications, and Emerging Technologies* (1st ed.), pp: 149–164. CRC Press. 10.1201/9781003269281-2

Khang, A., Chowdhury, S., & Sharma, S. (Eds.). (2022a). *The Data-Driven Blockchain Ecosystem: Fundamentals, Applications, and Emerging Technologies* (1st ed.). CRC Press. 10.1201/9781003269281

Khang, A., Gupta, S.K., Rani, S., & Karras, D.A., (Eds.). (2023a). *Smart Cities: IoT Technologies, Big Data Solutions, Cloud Platforms, and Cybersecurity Techniques* (1st Ed.). CRC Press. 10.1201/9781003376064

Khang, A., Hahanov, V., Abbas, G.L., & Hajimahmud, V.A. (2022b). Cyber-physical-social system and incident management. *AI-Centric Smart City Ecosystems: Technologies, Design and Implementation* (1st Ed.). 2(15), CRC Press. 10.1201/9781003252542-2

Khang, A., Hahanov, V., Litvinova, E., Chumachenko, S., Hajimahmud, V.A., & Alyar, A.V. (2022c). The key assistant of smart city – Sensors and tools. *AI-Centric Smart City Ecosystems: Technologies, Design and Implementation* (1st ed.). 17(10), CRC Press. 10.1201/9781003252542-17

Khang, A., Ragimova, N.A., Hajimahmud, V.A., & Alyar, A.V. (2022d). Advanced Technologies and data management in the smart healthcare system. *AI-Centric Smart City Ecosystems: Technologies, Design and Implementation* (1st Ed.). 16(10), CRC Press. 10.1201/9781003252542-16

Khang, A., Rana, G., Tailor, R.K., & Hajimahmud, V.A., (Eds.). (2023b). *Data-Centric AI Solutions and Emerging Technologies in the Healthcare Ecosystem* (1st Ed.). CRC Press. 10.1201/9781003356189

Khang, A., Rani, S., Gujrati, R., Uygun, H., Gupta, S.K., (Eds.). (2023c). *Designing Workforce Management Systems for Industry 4.0: Data-Centric and AI-Enabled Approaches* (1st Ed.). CRC Press. 10.1201/99781003357070

Khanh, H.H., & Khang, A. (2021). The role of artificial intelligence in blockchain applications. *Reinventing Manufacturing and Business Processes through Artificial Intelligence*. 2(20), pp. 20–40, CRC Press. 10.1201/9781003145011-2.

Mahore, V., Aggarwal, P., Andola, N., & Venkatesan, S. (2019, December). Secure and privacy focused electronic health record management system using permissioned blockchain. *In 2019 IEEE Conference on Information and Communication Technology* (pp. 1–6). IEEE. https://ieeexplore.ieee.org/abstract/document/9066204/

Mani, V., Manickam, P., Alotaibi, Y., Alghamdi, S., & Khalaf, O.I. (2021). Hyperledger healthchain: Patient-centric IPFS-based storage of health records. *Electronics*, 10(23), 3003. https://www.mdpi.com/1386886

Misra, A., Khang, A., Gupta, S.K., & Shah, V., (Eds.). (2023). *AI-aided IoT Technologies and Applications in the Smart Business and Production* (1st Ed.). CRC Press. 10.1201/9781003392224

Morris, G., Babasaheb, J., Khang, A., Gupta, S.K., & Hajimahmud, V.A. (2023). *AI-Centric Modelling and Analytics: Concepts, Designs, Technologies, and Applications* (1st Ed.). CRC Press. 10.1201/9781003400110

Private data. (2020). Hyperledger-Fabric.Readthedocs.i. Retrieved May 2022, from https:// hyperledger-fabric.readthedocs.io/en/release-2.0/private-data/private-data.html

Rana, G., Khang, A., Sharma, R., Goel, A.K., & Dubey, A.K. (2021). Reinventing manufacturing and business processes through artificial intelligence, (Eds.). CRC Press. 10.1201/9781003145011

Rani, S., Bhambri, P., Kataria, A., & Khang, A. (2022). Smart city ecosystem: Concept, sustainability, design principles and technologies. *AI-Centric Smart City Ecosystems: Technologies, Design and Implementation* (1st Ed.). 1(20), CRC Press. 10.1201/9781 003252542-1

Rani, S., Chauhan, M., Kataria, A., & Khang, A. (2021). IoT equipped intelligent distributed framework for smart healthcare systems. *Networking and Internet Architecture*, (Eds.). 2, p. 30. CRC Press. 10.48550/arXiv.2110.04997

Stamatellis, C., Papadopoulos, P., Pitropakis, N., Katsikas, S., & Buchanan, W.J. (2020). A privacy-preserving healthcare framework using hyperledger fabric. *Sensors*, 20(22), 6587. https://www.mdpi.com/893880

Tailor, R.K., Pareek, R., & Khang, A., (Eds.). (2022). Robot process automation in blockchain. *The Data-Driven Blockchain Ecosystem: Fundamentals, Applications, and Emerging Technologies* (1st ed.), pp: 149–164. CRC Press. 10.1201/9781003269281-8

Using Private Data in Fabric. (2022). Https://Hyperledger-Fabric.Readthedocs.Io/. Retrieved May 2022, from https://hyperledger-fabric.readthedocs.io/en/latest/private_data _tutorial.html/

Tith, D., Lee, J.S., Suzuki, H., Wijesundara, W.M.A.B., Taira, N., Obi, T., & Ohyama, N. (2020). Application of blockchain to maintaining patient records in electronic health record for enhanced privacy, scalability, and availability. *Healthcare Informatics Research*, 26(1), 3–12. https://synapse.koreamed.org/articles/1142058

2 Internet of Medical Things (IoMT) Driving the Digital Transformation of the Healthcare Sector

Vrushank Shah and Alex Khang

CONTENTS

DOI: 10.1201/9781003356189-2

2.1   INTRODUCTION

The Internet of Medical Things (IoMT) collects data from smart devices and sensors in one location using modern software. Data analysis is where machines excel. The Internet of Things (IoT) automates data and tracking processes, which is crucial for healthcare.

How will the Internet of Medical Things transform the industry? By integrating IoT with medical, we may remotely manage the storage temperature while carrying vaccinations and meds, follow illness signs without doctor visits, take prescriptions appropriately and most efficiently, and more (Rani et al., 2021).

The IoT in healthcare is promising (Koonin et al., 2020). This technique can revolutionize to support and solve most the issues in the fields of medicine and healthcare.

IoMT has improved remote patient monitoring. Connecting patients to their doctors and transferring health data via a secure network saves hospital visits and healthcare system strain. Healthcare personnel may remotely access patient data, monitor important biometrics in real time, and follow prospective difficulties to prevent future complications (Khang et al., 2023c).

IoMT allows patients to communicate health data to clinicians, improving diagnosis, reducing errors, and lowering expenses. Due to the COVID-19 epidemic, in-person medical visits have decreased, preventing its spread.

IoMT's improved remote patient monitoring (RPM) monitors patients' vital indicators including heart rate and glucose levels and alerts clinicians when needed (Koonin et al., 2020). IoMT can stimulate emergency reactions and manage chronic disorders. Wearables can track glucose and heart rate.

Smart gadgets may exchange activity tracker data with remote health providers to seek medical advice. IoMT transformed healthcare procedures. According to *Forbes*, "The Internet of Medical Things (IoMT) is set to alter how we keep people safe and healthy especially as the need for solutions to cut healthcare expenses rise in the future years".

The IoMT may enhance diagnosis, efficiency, patient care, and cost. It can monitor, notify, and offer healthcare practitioners particular data to identify concerns before they become serious (Liaqat, 2020). The IoMT helps insurers examine patient data faster and process claims more accurately. The IoMT improves patient care; thus, all stakeholders—pharmaceuticals and insurance companies—benefit.

The IoMT is a subset of the IoT that includes smart devices like wearables and medical or vital monitors for health monitoring. Some smart wearables can monitor a user's physiological characteristics, such as oxygen saturation (pulse oximeter), blood glucose levels, heart rate, electrocardiogram (ECG) patterns, cardiac pacemaker electrical activity, etc., in real time and send the data to the doctor (Liaqat, 2020).

It may be worn at home, at clinics, or hospitals. In the Internet of Medical Things, "Things" might include infusion pumps, heart monitoring implants, and other devices that administer pre-programmed fluids to patients.

Insulin pumps, cochlear implants, and pacemakers are other devices. Internet-connected gadgets send data to healthcare practitioners. It lets doctors remotely monitor patients. Instead of waiting for patients to visit the doctor, they may quickly address difficulties (Khan et al., 2020).

For instance, a smart health watch that measures heart rate and sleeping pattern utilizes Bluetooth technology to tabulate the findings on an iPhone and exchange the data with a doctor over Wi-Fi. The IoMT also connects medical data-collecting software to hospital IT systems through internet computer networks.

2.2 BENEFITS OF INTERNET OF MEDICAL THINGS

Despite ongoing improvement, the global healthcare system still faces huge issues with catastrophic repercussions. It's about miscommunication, human error in symptom identification and monitoring, routines, and uncovering new research prospects, as well as curing new and incurable diseases (Singh et al., 2020). Following are a few of the benefits of the IoMT.

2.2.1 TELEMEDICINE

The IoT allows physicians to monitor their patients' health and patients to seek treatment anytime, anyplace. It's about convenience, emergency treatment, and improving medical access (Khang et al., 2023a).

2.2.2 IMMUNIZATION

Preventing sickness is preferable. Healthcare IoT solutions include tracking and monitoring tools to assist customers monitor their health, change their behaviors, enhance their lifestyle, and discover early symptoms of health concerns (Khang et al., 2022a).

2.2.3 LESS EXPENDITURE AND BETTER APPOINTMENTS

IoT-powered medical gadgets and sensors allow patients self-monitor and reduce doctor visits. IoT healthcare apps provide clinicians with a lot of data, making these visits more efficient (Rani et al., 2023).

2.2.4 MEDICAL RECORDS

People used to visit laboratories, doctors, or use a variety of gadgets at home to assess blood pressure, heart rate, glucose, and blood oxygen levels. Amazingly, tiny IoMT devices can track all of these routinely and provide clear individual information in your health app (Khang et al., 2023b).

2.2.5 DIAGNOSTICS

IoT healthcare devices can track almost everything about your health, making it simpler to spot irregularities and symptoms. This lets doctors assess your health and detect potential diseases sooner and more correctly.

2.2.6   HEALTHCARE MANAGEMENT

The IoT in healthcare may benefit individuals, institutions, and the system as a whole. Medical IoT can assess the condition and efficacy of unique equipment or provide worldwide illness information (Vrushank et al., 2023).

2.2.7   BETTER PHARMACOLOGICAL TREATMENT

Medication therapy is vital to treatment; therefore, patients must take it frequently and effectively. IoT health monitoring systems optimize medicine therapy.

2.2.8   CONSULTATION

The IoMT collects infinite reliable medical data for studies. Instead of manually collecting, compiling, and analyzing this data, scientists may focus on more difficult tasks.

2.3   IOMT ARCHITECTURE

The architecture for IoMT consists of three layers: The first layer is the things layer, followed by the cloud layer and then the fog layer (Bhambri et al., 2022).

In this design, medical professionals are also able to connect directly with one another through the router that is located between the thing layer and the fog layer as well as through the local processing servers that are located at the fog layer (Joyia et al., 2017). Each layer is explained in more detail below.

2.3.1   THE THINGS LAYER

The things layer includes components such as patient monitoring devices, sensors, actuators, medical records, pharmacy controls, and a diet regimen generator, among other things (Khang et al., 2022b).

- This layer has immediate communication with the people who make use of the ecosystem.
- This layer is responsible for collecting the data that is generated by elements such as wearables, patient monitoring data, and remote care data.
- In order to maintain the reliability of the data that is acquired, the apparatus that is utilized here should be stored in a safe location. Connecting these devices to the fog layer is the responsibility of the local routers that are spread across the ecosystem.
- Additional processing of the data takes place both at the fog layer and at the cloud layer in order to provide relevant information.
- Additionally, in order to cut down on the amount of time wasted waiting for information, the healthcare specialists may access the patient data through this router.

2.3.2   THE FOG LAYER

The fog layer operates between the cloud and the things layer.

- This layer consists of local servers and gateway devices for a sparsely distributed fog net-working framework.
- The local processing power is harnessed by the lower layer devices for real-time response to their users. These servers are also used to manage and administer the security and integrity of the system.
- The gateway devices at this layer are responsible for redirecting this data from these servers to the cloud layer for further processing.
- Further, in order to reduce the delay, the healthcare experts can get the patient data through this router.

2.3.3   THE CLOUD LAYER

The cloud layer is comprised of data storage and computing resources, allowing for the aforementioned data to be analyzed and the corresponding decision-making systems to be derived from them.

- The cloud also provides a large reach that may easily encompass enormous medical and healthcare systems so that they can manage their day-to-day operations.
- This layer is made up of cloud resources, and it is where the data that is produced by the medical infrastructure will be kept, and where analytical work might be carried out in the future if it is judged required.

2.4   IoMT Communication Technologies

Personal area networks (PANs), local area networks (LANs), and wide area networks (WANs) are the three types of networks that are most frequently used for Internet of Things (IoT) application technologies.

Each variety of network utilizes a diverse collection of wireless protocols. Following this, we will present specific information on the architectures of the IoMT communication environment (Bharati et al., 2021).

There are a number of well-known communication technologies, including WiFi, ZigBee, Bluetooth, Li-Fi, and LTE; however, there are also a number of new networking choices that are becoming available.

The application, as well as aspects such as range, data needs, security, power demands, and battery life of the device, all play a role in determining which communication technologies, alone or in combination, should be used in IoMT.

2.5   IOMT APPLICATIONS

Nowadays, Internet of Things (IoT) technology is a very fast-growing field of computing, and it is really applicable to almost all human endeavors in the real world, as shown in figure 2.1.

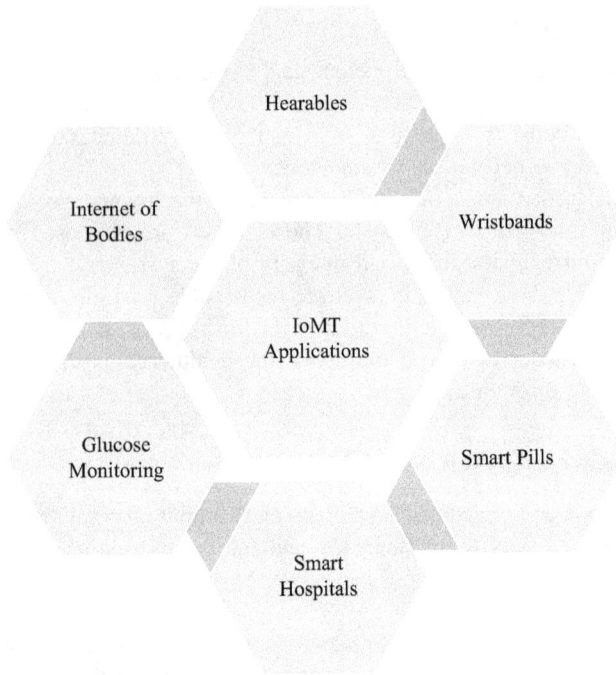

FIGURE 2.1   Application of IoMT technology.

Source: Author's owner.

The application of IoT into the fields of medicine and healthcare brought IoT that so-called Internet of Medical Things (IoMT) and has really reshaped the smart healthcare ecosystem globally, despite some apprehension to security threats, and especially risks in prediction activities for the field of medicine. Major IoMT applications are as listed follows.

2.5.1   INTERNET OF BODIES (IoBs)

The Internet of Bodies uses human bodies to collect medical and fitness data. IoB devices capture biometric, physiological, or behavioral data, which is exchanged over IoT system networks, stored and processed by back-end infrastructure, and provided to the end user through a mobile app (Khan et al., 2019).

The Internet of Bodies may bring to mind wearable smart fitness gear. However, it encompasses biometric identification, implants, prosthetics, artificial organs, pill dispensers, and almost any technology you may wear, implant, or consume. This technology helps clinicians identify, monitor, and support chronic patients, as shown in figure 2.2.

2.5.2   WRISTBANDS

The most common IoT healthcare technologies are smartwatches and bands. They can be used for exercise, medicine, and accessories. Wristbands can display time,

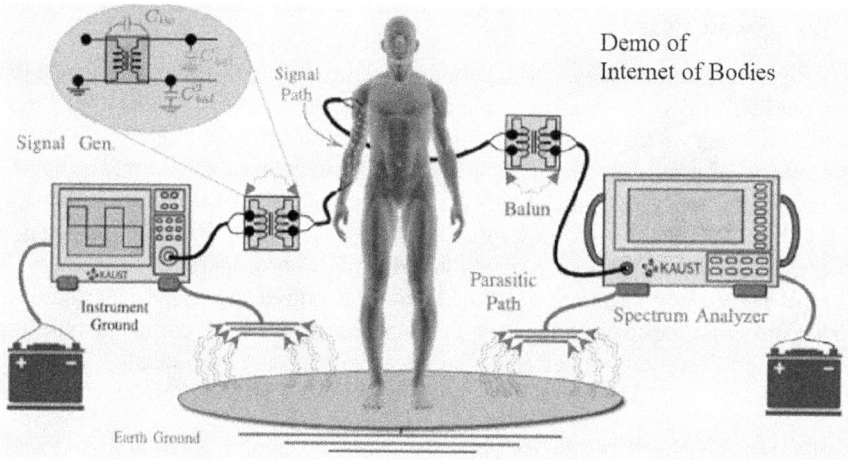

FIGURE 2.2 Illustration of Internet of Bodies.

Source: Author's redrawn.

weather, messages, and call contacts. This type of smart gadget tracks sleep, heart rate, and steps.

IoMT devices from Apple, Samsung, Huawei, Garmin, Fitbit, and others are available. The latter launched the Fitbit Charge 5 fitness and health tracker. This gadget also tracks mood, breathing rate, heart rhythm abnormalities, oxygen saturation, skin temperature, and menstrual cycle.

2.5.3 Hearables

Intelligent hearing aids are now in development. Cutting-edge technology have been integrated into the design of the next generation of hearing aids to make a real difference for those who suffer from hearing loss. Modern hearables link with other devices through Bluetooth, letting you modify the external soundscape from your phone. Among the best instances of Internet of Medical Things products, the Whisper Hearing System is a must-have for anyone with hearing impairments.

The company's hearing aids monitor and optimize environmental sound, providing the greatest possible listening experience, by combining the most cutting-edge IoT in healthcare technology with AI (Khang et al., 2022c). Indeed, the system is rather intelligent, growing in sophistication with each new update thanks to its capacity for learning and adaptation. Intelligent hearing aids are now in development.

Cutting-edge technology have been integrated into the design of the next generation of hearing aids to make a real difference for those who suffer from hearing loss. Modern hearables link with other devices through Bluetooth, letting you modify the external soundscape from your phone.

2.5.4 SMART PILLS

Scientists and engineers are working on the development of a pill-sized capsule that can house full-fledged medical equipment. In spite of the fact that these trials provide a touch of science fiction to the field of medical technology, such sensors are capable of providing the most precise diagnoses that are now conceivable.

In the past ten years, researchers at the Massachusetts Institute of Technology (MIT) have been hard at work developing ingestible sensors that have the potential to completely supplant more conventional diagnostic procedures.

One of their contributions was the creation of a tiny capsule that, instead of an endoscopy, may be used to identify gastrointestinal issues, in particular bleeding. The capsule is stuffed with sensors and bacteria that have been created in a lab.

2.5.5 GLUCOSE MONITORING

Diabetes is a condition that is quite widespread around the globe. Only in the United States of America does this diagnosis affect more than 11% of the population, and close to 40% of individuals have prediabetes.

Due to these eye-opening numbers, glucose monitoring medical gadgets are more important than they have ever been. Certain businesses are always working on developing new ways to improve glucose monitoring technologies.

For example, Abbott has developed a suite of Internet of Things (IoT) health-care solutions for people with diabetes called FreeStyle Libre. These solutions include non-invasive sensors that keep an eye on your glucose level round the clock and notify you via a mobile app if there are any warning deviations from the normal range.

2.5.6 HYGIENE MONITORING

The COVID-19 outbreak has highlighted the significance of practising proper hand hygiene. Washing one's hands is now an essential step in everyone's daily routine and cannot be skipped. In addition, it has long been a fundamental prerequisite for doctors and other medical professionals to work in hospitals.

The firm Biovigil provides assistance to medical facilities and institutions in maintaining compliance with hand hygiene standards at all times. The hospital as a whole may monitor the level of compliance with hygiene standards thanks to the IoMT badge, which also serves as a reminder for personnel to sanitize their hands. Patients may have complete confidence that whatever procedure they undergo will be carried out in a risk-free manner thanks to this system.

2.5.7 MOODABLES

Do you think it's possible that in the future there will be intelligent medical gadgets that may directly affect patients' mental health? In any case, in addition to traditional psychotherapy or medicine, people are already able to enhance both their mood and their cognitive capacities via the use of Medtech.

FeelZing has crammed the power of neuro stimulation into discreet and convenient patches that may be worn throughout the day to increase one's productivity and sense of well-being.

The patches generate waveforms that have an effect on your nerve system, resulting in improved mental clarity and calmness. Over 30,000 investigations have conclusively demonstrated that the procedure is both risk-free and effective.

2.5.8 SMART HOSPITALS

The Internet of Medical Things gives hospitals additional power, enabling their employees to do their jobs in a more coordinated and effective manner. It helps to build fruitful cooperation between medical care experts and technical employees, which in turn allows for the provision of quality service to patients and the extension of the useful life of medical equipment and gadgets (Razdan & Sharma, 2021).

2.5.9 SMART LABS

Research is the primary focus of lab labor, although the work itself is less thrilling and more routine. Colleagues in the laboratory manage enormous volumes of scientific data and frequently use various pieces of laboratory equipment. It can rather frequently result in tiredness as well as mistakes that arise spontaneously (Kumar et al., 2023).

Because of this, scientists are always looking for new ways to automate labor-intensive processes that take up a lot of time and resources. The Internet of Medical devices also becomes relevant at this point.

2.5.10 REHABILITATION

The phase of therapy known as rehabilitation typically comes at the end of several different types of treatment. Nevertheless, this critical phase may continue for a considerable amount of time, and patients require ongoing assistance and direction. Medical Internet of Things devices can help patients recover more quickly and safely (Khang et al., 2022c).

The ReHub system developed by DyCare is one illustration of the Internet of Things being used in the medical field for the purpose of rehabilitation (Vishnu, Ramson & Jegan, 2020). It is a platform that allows medical professionals to communicate with their patients and monitor the progress of their recovery with the use of artificial intelligence and the Internet of Things (IoT).

2.5.11 ROBOTIC SURGERY

The most accomplished surgeons in the world, in collaboration with robotics engineers and software developers, are teaching advanced surgical techniques to robots so that these machines may do even the most intricate operations with pinpoint precision. Therefore, in today's world, automated instruments driven by the Internet of Things (IoT) may conduct certain surgical procedures even more effectively than human workers (Hajimahmud et al., 2022).

In particular, it has been demonstrated that robotic surgery is quicker, more accurate, less intrusive, and less painful, results in fewer scars for patients, reduces the risk of infection, and shortens the amount of time needed for rehabilitation. This is true for the majority of the common types of surgical procedures.

Therefore, in addition to general surgery, surgeons rely on robots for procedures involving the heart, spine, digestive tract, thoracic region, and gynecologic and urologic procedures (Das et al., 2019).

2.6 CONCLUSION

IoMT technology, in its most basic form, makes it possible to bring about improvements in the ways in which patients' states are monitored and in which medical personnel, such as physicians, nurses, and others, are alerted in the case of an emergency.

It has resulted in a significant improvement in the monitoring of distant patients remotely. The Internet of Medical Things (IoMT) is an initiative with the goals of enabling connected medical equipment and sensors to continuously gather and evaluate patient health data in real time, track the progression of a patient's condition, and improve the accuracy of a physician's diagnoses. It has the capacity to connect vast networks of medical equipment located all over the world (Mathad & Khang, 2023).

We provide details about the Internet of Medical Things (IoMT) and presented an architecture for IoMTs, benefits of IoMT, and major applications of IoMT. The present problems that affect the nation's healthcare systems include a severe lack of key medical personnel, excessively lengthy wait times, an increase in the number of people who require treatment, and budgetary limits (Khanh & Khang, 2021).

IoMT might be helpful in alleviating some limitations by reducing the amount of time healthcare professionals that spend on repetitive chores (by utilizing AI approaches), which would free up their time to concentrate on other tasks, such as visiting more patients (Rana et al., 2021).

REFERENCES

Bhambri, P., Rani, S., Gupta, G., Khang, A., "Cloud and fog computing platforms for Internet of Things," ISBN: 978-1-032-101507, (2022), CRC Press. 10.1201/9781003213888

Bharati, S., et al., "Applications and challenges of cloud integrated IoMT." *Cognitive Internet of Medical Things for Smart Healthcare* (2021): 67–85. https://link.springer.com/chapter/10.1007/978-3-030-55833-8_4

Das, P. K., et al., "Smart medical healthcare of Internet of medical things (IOMT): application of non-contact sensing." *2019 14th IEEE Conference on Industrial Electronics and Applications (ICIEA)*. IEEE, (2019). https://ieeexplore.ieee.org/abstract/document/8833992/

Hajimahmud, V. A., Khang, A., Hahanov, V., Litvinova, E., Chumachenko, S., Alyar, A. V., "Autonomous robots for smart city: Closer to augmented humanity," *AI-Centric Smart City Ecosystems: Technologies, Design and Implementation* (1st Ed.), (2022), CRC Press. 7(12). 10.1201/9781003252542-7

Joyia, Gulraiz J., et al., "Internet of medical things (IoMT): Applications, benefits and future challenges in healthcare domain." *J. Commun.* 12.4 (2017): 240–247. http://www.jocm.us/uploadfile/2017/0428/20170428025024260.pdf

Khan, S. R., et al., "IoMT-based computational approach for detecting brain tumor." *Future Generation Computer Systems* 109 (2020): 360–367. https://www.sciencedirect.com/science/article/pii/S0167739X20307688

Khan, S. U., et al., "An e-Health care services framework for the detection and classification of breast cancer in breast cytology images as an IoMT application." *Future Generation Computer Systems* 98 (2019): 286–296. https://www.sciencedirect.com/science/article/pii/S0167739X18325536

Khang, A., Gupta, S. K., Hajimahmud, V. A., Babasaheb, J., Morris, G., *AI-Centric Modelling and Analytics: Concepts, Designs, Technologies, and Applications* (1st Ed.), (2023a), CRC Press. 10.1201/9781003400110

Khang, A., Gupta, S. K., Rani, S., Karras, D. A., (Eds.), *Smart Cities: IoT Technologies, Big Data Solutions, Cloud Platforms, and Cybersecurity Techniques* (1st Ed.), (2023b), CRC Press. 10.1201/9781003376064

Khang, A., Gupta, S. K., Shah, V., Misra A., (Eds.), *AI-aided IoT Technologies and Applications in the Smart Business and Production* (1st Ed.), (2023c), CRC Press. 10.1201/9781003392224

Khang, A., Hahanov, V., Abbas, G. L., Hajimahmud, V. A., "Cyber-physical-social system and incident management," *AI-Centric Smart City Ecosystems: Technologies, Design and Implementation* (1st Ed.), (2022a), CRC Press. 10.1201/9781003252542-2

Khang, A., Hahanov, V., Litvinova, E., Chumachenko, S., Hajimahmud, V. A., Alyar, A. V., "The key assistant of smart city – Sensors and tools," *AI-Centric Smart City Ecosystems: Technologies, Design and Implementation* (1st ed.) (2022b), CRC Press. 10.1201/9781003252542-17

Khang, A., Rani, S., Sivaraman, A. K., *AI-Centric Smart City Ecosystems: Technologies, Design and Implementation* (1st Ed., (2022c), CRC Press. 10.1201/9781003252542

Khanh, H. H., Khang, A., "The role of artificial intelligence in blockchain applications," *Reinventing Manufacturing and Business Processes through Artificial Intelligence*, pp. 20–40, (2021), CRC Press. 10.1201/9781003145011-2

Koonin, Lisa M., et al., "Trends in the use of telehealth during the emergence of the COVID-19 pandemic—United States, January–March 2020." *Morbidity and Mortality Weekly Report* 69.43 (2020): 1595. https://www.ncbi.nlm.nih.gov/pmc/articles/PMC7641006/

Kumar, D. V. S., Chaurasia, R., Misra, A., Misra, P. K., Khang, A., "Heart disease and liver disease prediction using machine learning," *Data-Centric AI Solutions and Emerging Technologies in the Healthcare Ecosystem* (1st ed.), p. 4, (2023), CRC Press. 10.1201/9781003356189-13

Liaqat, S., et al., "SDN orchestration to combat evolving cyber threats in Internet of Medical Things (IoMT)." *Computer Communications* 160 (2020): 697–705. https://www.sciencedirect.com/science/article/pii/S0140366420312044

Mathad, K., Khang, A., "Hospital 4.0: Capitalization of health and healthcare in Industry 4.0 economy," *Data-Centric AI Solutions and Emerging Technologies in the Healthcare Ecosystem* (1st ed.), p. 4, (2023), CRC Press. 10.1201/9781003356189-19

Rana, G., Khang, A., Sharma, R., Goel, A. K., Dubey, A. K., "Reinventing manufacturing and business processes through artificial intelligence", (Eds.). (2021). CRC Press. 10.1201/9781003145011

Rani, S., Bhambri, P., Kataria, A., Khang A., Sivaraman, A. K. (Eds.), *Big Data, Cloud Computing and IoT: Tools and Applications* (1st Ed.), (2023), Chapman and Hall/CRC. 10.1201/9781003298335

Rani, S., Chauhan, M., Kataria, A., Khang, A., "IoT equipped intelligent distributed framework for smart healthcare systems," *Networking and Internet Architecture*, (Eds.). (2021). CRC Press. 10.48550/arXiv.2110.04997

Razdan, S., Sharma, S., "Internet of Medical Things (IoMT): Overview, emerging technologies, and case studies." *IETE Technical Review* (2021): 1–14. https://www.tandfonline.com/doi/abs/10.1080/02564602.2021.1927863

Singh, R. P., et al., "Internet of Medical Things (IoMT) for orthopaedic in COVID-19 pandemic: Roles, challenges, and applications." *Journal of Clinical Orthopaedics and Trauma* 11.4 (2020): 713–717. https://www.sciencedirect.com/science/article/pii/S097656622030179X

Vishnu, S., Jino Ramson, S. R., Jegan, R., "Internet of medical things (IoMT)-An overview." 2020 *5th International Conference on Devices, Circuits and Systems* (ICDCS). IEEE, (2020). https://ieeexplore.ieee.org/abstract/document/9075733/

Vrushank, S., Vidhi, T., Khang, A., "Electronic health records security and privacy enhancement using blockchain technology," *Data-Centric AI Solutions and Emerging Technologies in the Healthcare Ecosystem.* (1st ed.), p. 1, (2023), CRC Press. 10.1201/9781003356189-1

3 AI-Enabled Solution

A Game Changer for Private Healthcare Providers

Rashmi Gujrati, B. C. M. Patnaik, and Ipseeta Satpathy

CONTENTS

3.1 INTRODUCTION

Information technology (IT) innovations in healthcare are highly anticipated by policymakers, authorities, and healthcare providers in many high-income countries because they will contribute to better healthcare efficiency and quality, as well as increased diagnostic efficiency (Alhashmi et al., 2020).

Artificial intelligence (AI) is a significant IT innovation that is becoming increasingly prominent in healthcare and has the potential to reduce overall costs for businesses (Barlow et al., 2006).

In contrast, AI in healthcare is still at an early stage of development, as is the case with most IT innovations (Batalden et al., 2016). The implementation of new technology in healthcare is often quite challenging, despite numerous examples of successful implementation (Beil et al., 2019).

Although implementation science has provided insights into the barriers to implementing such innovations and outlined strategies for overcoming them, this knowledge has not yet been applied to the understanding and support of AI implementation in healthcare (Choudhury et al., 2020).

DOI: 10.1201/9781003356189-3

Even with the extensive and still increasing research on AI in healthcare, there is a huge knowledge gap regarding how to successfully tackle implementation challenges and how to increase the likelihood of sustainable adoption (Eldh et al., 2017).

Most research on AI in healthcare has focused on developing algorithms; evaluating proofs-of-concept; and exploring technical, legal, and ethical issues (Fernandes et al., 2020). Oncology, neurology, radiology, and cardiology are the primary clinical specialties in which research is conducted (Eldh et al., 2017).

It is also important to keep in mind the challenges and aspects to be considered when developing and implementing AI in healthcare, as well as the potential of this technology. The main problem with such articles is that they are based on undeveloped evidence bases. As such, they are less useful for guiding implementation initiatives (Khang & Sivaraman, 2022a).

Most of the research literature relevant to implementation-related issues has been conducted in the form of systematic reviews; morals; medical and patient results (Vrushank, Vidhi & Khang, 2023); and economic impact. Studying AI implementation in real-world clinical settings is essential as a result of these studies.

Researchers have studied the effects of AI technology in practice using robust methodologies, such as randomized controlled trials, and found that AI can improve real-time data, save time and resources, and reduce physician workloads, but How AI can be translated into daily healthcare practices does not have specific AI implementation theories, models, or frameworks (Rana et al., 2021).

Data security and accelerated drug development are benefits of artificial intelligence. Recently, artificial intelligence has been used in surgical procedures and remote monitoring (Khang et al., 2022b). Also, it facilitates health insurance with smart risk prediction. Location tracking and alerts were made possible by these is (Reed et al., 2018). Health accessibility is improved and healthcare risks can be predicted early with AI technology innovation (Misra et al., 2023).

We will investigate AI's relevance to private healthcare providers, as well as the opinions of different stakeholder groups. An innovative healthcare hub in eastern India will be the focus of this study. Among the hospitals in this region will be top super specialty hospitals (Khang & Hajimahmud, 2022b).

Data and scenario for this chapter is the hospitals in India country include Kalinga Institute of Medical Science (KIMS), Kalinga Hospital, Care Hospital, Utkal Hospital, Appolo Hospital, AMRI Hospital, SUM Ultimate Medicare, AIIMS Hospital, Sparsh Hospital & Critical Care and Aditya Aswin Hospital and Aswin Hospital, and LV Prasad Eye Hospital (Rani et al., 2021).

3.2   RESEARCH DESIGN

The present study was undertaken by reviewing various earlier studies and after that, 8 core group discussions were made by consisting of 5 members each consisting of different stakeholders after that questionnaire was prepared for the pilot study consisting of 46 respondents. Initially, 21 questions were there but after the pilot study, 16 attributes were finalized for collecting the data (Rani et al., 2023).

The data was collected by adopting simple random sampling and 216 samples were collected out of 263 questionnaires distributed for the survey in various

TABLE 3.1

Sampling Frame of Category of Respondents

Category of Respondents	Male	Female	Total
Patients	20	14	34
Attendants of the patients	14	34	48
Nursing staff	24	32	56
Lab technicians	28	14	42
Doctors	21	15	36
Total	107	109	216

Source: Author's owner.

hospitals. The respondents include patients, attendees of patients, nursing staff, lab technicians, and doctors (Morris et al., 2023).

3.3 SAMPLE SIZE DETERMINATION

"In the present study, the sample size was calculated in the ratio range of 1:4 to 1:10". A minimum sample size of four items should be used, while a maximum of ten items should be used, as shown in table 3.1.

In this study, 16 items were collected, so both 64 and 160 samples would be needed. However, during the data collection 239 responses were received, out of which 216 were in the proper and complete form so we included all the data (Bhambri et al., 2022) for better representation, as in table 3.2 and table 3.3.

OP – Opinion of patients, OAT – Opinion of attendants' patients, ONS – Opinion of nursing staff, OLT – Opinion of lab technicians, and OD – Opinion of doctors

3.4 RESULTS AND DISCUSSION

Analytics uses sample data from Tables 3.4–3.10.

3.4.1 BASED ON SERVICE EFFICIENCY

In responding to the questions, the total perception score for the OP, OAP, ONS, OLT, and OD were 1086, 1612, 1962, 1510, and 1289, respectively. It represents 79.85%, 83.96%, 87.59%, 89.88%, and 89.51%, respectively, of the maximum possible scores. The average scores were 86.16%. This shows that the various attributes considered for the present study have a significant impact on healthcare services.

3.4.2 BASED ON COST AND EFFICIENCY

The total score of OP, OAP, ONS, OLT, and OD were 527, 786, 1003, 755, and 620, respectively. This shows that percentages of actual scores to the maximum possible score were 77.5%, 81.88%, 89.55%, 89.88%, and 86.11%, respectively.

TABLE 3.2
Computation of Maximum Possible Weight and Least Possible Score

Category	Based on Service Efficiency	Based on Cost and Time Efficiency	Based on Transparency
Opinion of patients			
Maximum possible Score	34 × 8 × 5 = 1360	34 × 4 × 5 = 680	34 × 4 × 5 = 680
Least possible score	34 × 8 × 1 = 272	34 × 4 × 1 = 136	34 × 4 × 1 = 136
Opinion of attendants of patients			
Maximum possible Score	48 × 5 × 8 = 1920	48 × 4 × 5 = 960	48 × 4 × 5 = 960
Least possible score	48 × 1 × 8 = 384	48 × 4 × 1 = 192	48 × 4 × 1 = 192
Opinion of nursing staff			
Maximum possible Score	56 × 8 × 5 = 2240	56 × 4 × 5 = 1120	56 × 5 × 4 = 1120
Least possible score	56 × 8 × 1 = 448	56 × 4 × 1 = 224	56 × 5 × 1 = 224
Opinion of lab technicians			
Maximum possible Score	42 × 8 × 5 = 1680	42 × 4 × 5 = 840	42 × 4 × 5 = 840
Least possible score	42 × 8 × 1 = 336	42 × 4 × 1 = 168	42 × 4 × 1 = 168
Opinion of doctors			
Maximum possible Score	36 × 8 × 5 = 1440	36 × 4 × 5 = 720	36 × 4 × 5 = 720
Least possible score	36 × 8 × 1 = 288	36 × 4 × 1 = 144	36 × 4 × 1 = 144

Source: Own compilation.

TABLE 3.3
Analysis of Data

Variables	OP	OAP	ONS	OLT	OD
Based on service efficiency					
Increased efficiency of the diagnostic process	138	205	253	183	167
May reduce physician stress	129	214	249	187	160
Accelerating drug development	135	200	240	180	164
Improving patient experience	140	191	243	193	170
Robot-assisted surgery	142	192	247	189	155
Risk prediction	128	204	245	197	159
Smart health insurance	138	201	242	186	155
Prediction of healthcare risks early	136	205	243	195	159
Total score	1086	1612	1962	1510	1289
Maximum score	1360	1920	2240	1680	1440
Least score	272	384	448	336	288
% of the total score to the maximum possible score	79.85	83.96	87.59	89.88	89.51
Average score			86.16%		
Based on cost and time efficiency					
Reduced overall costs of running the business	133	193	251	185	154

TABLE 3.3 (Continued)
Analysis of Data

Variables	OP	OAP	ONS	OLT	OD
Provides real-time data	133	197	255	189	155
Streamlines tasks	132	195	242	190	155
Saves time and resources	129	201	255	191	156
Total score	527	786	1003	755	620
Maximum score	680	960	1120	840	720
Least score	136	192	224	168	144
% of the total score to the maximum possible score	77.5	81.88	89.55	89.88	86.11
Average score			**84.98%**		
Based on transparency					
Data security	138	205	256	201	164
Remote monitoring	119	192	250	196	154
Location tracking and alerts (LTA)	125	188	241	192	155
Healthcare accessibility	142	201	244	184	164
Total score	524	786	991	773	637
Maximum score	680	960	1120	840	720
Least score	136	192	224	168	144
% of the total score to the maximum possible score	77.06	81.88	88.48	92.09	88.47
Average score			**85.60%**		

Source: Annexure A, B, C, D, and E.

The average score for the same was 84.98%. This justifies that AR and VR made a lot of impact on the delivery of the healthcare system. It helped considerably increase efficiency and reduction of costs at the same time (Tailor et al., 2022).

3.4.3 BASED ON TRANSPARENCY

The actual scores for the OP, OAP, ONS, OLT, and OD were 524, 786, 991, 773, and 637, respectively. "The percentage of actual score to the maximum possible score" was 77.06%, 81.88%, 88.48%, 92.09%, and 88.47%, respectively. The average score was 85.60%. This concludes that the role of AR and VR is a game changer for the transparency and overall healthcare services in Odisha city.

3.5 CONCLUSION

There is no doubt that artificial intelligence can improve healthcare systems. Clinical schedules can be freed up by automating tedious tasks, which allows clinicians to devote more time to patient interaction. Providing healthcare professionals with better access to data assists them in preventing illness (Hajimahmud et al., 2022).

The use of real-time data can help speed up and improve the diagnostic process. Using artificial intelligence, administrative errors can be reduced and resources can be saved. In terms of AI development, SMEs are becoming more involved, which makes the technology more accessible to more people (Khanh & Khang, 2021).

Increasingly, artificial intelligence is being applied to healthcare, and challenges and limits are being faced. There are still some limitations to AI, such as the need to include social variables, the lack of information regarding the population, and its vulnerability to increasingly sophisticated cyberattacks (Khang et al., 2022d).

It is evident that AI will prove to be a valuable tool in the medical field in spite of some of the challenges and limitations it faces. It is AI that is improving the lives of patients and physicians alike (Khang et al., 2023).

3.6   SOURCE PRIMARY DATA

TABLE 3.4

Annexure-A: Opinion of Patients (OP)-34 Respondents

Attributes	CA	A	N	DA	CDA	Score
	5	4	3	2	1	
Based on service efficiency						
Increased efficiency of the diagnostic process	18	7	4	3	2	138
May reduce physician stress	17	6	3	3	5	129
Accelerating drug development	19	5	4	2	4	135
Improving patient experience	21	4	3	4	2	140
Robot-assisted surgery	22	3	3	5	1	142
Risk prediction	18	5	2	4	4	128
Smart health insurance	22	2	2	6	2	138
Prediction of healthcare risks early	21	4	2	2	5	136
Based on cost and time efficiency						
Reduced overall costs of running the business	19	4	4	3	4	133
Provides real-time data	20	3	2	6	3	133
Streamlines tasks	18	6	2	4	4	132
Saves time and resources	17	5	3	6	3	129
Based on transparency						
Data security	21	4	3	2	4	138
Remote monitoring	19	3	2	6	4	119
Location tracking and alerts (LTA)	17	4	2	7	4	125
Healthcare accessibility	22	3	4	3	2	142

Source: Primary data of Annexure-A: Opinion of patients (OP) – 34 respondents.

TABLE 3.5
Annexure-B: Opinion of Attendants of Patients (OAP)-48 Respondents

Attributes	CA	A	N	DA	CDA	Score
	5	4	3	2	1	
Based on service efficiency						
Increased efficiency of the diagnostic process	32	6	3	5	2	205
May reduce physician stress	36	5	2	3	2	214
Accelerating drug development	31	6	3	4	4	200
Improving patient experience	30	4	1	8	6	191
Robot-assisted surgery	29	5	3	7	4	192
Risk prediction	32	6	4	2	4	204
Smart health insurance	33	4	3	3	5	201
Prediction of healthcare risks early	34	5	2	2	5	205
Based on cost and time efficiency						
Reduced overall costs of running the business	31	3	4	4	6	193
Provides real-time data	32	4	3	3	6	197
Streamlines tasks	30	5	5	2	6	195
Saves time and resources	33	4	3	3	5	201
Based on transparency						
Data security	34	3	3	6	2	205
Remote monitoring	31	4	2	4	7	192
Location tracking and alerts (LTA)	30	3	4	3	8	188
Healthcare accessibility	32	4	5	3	4	201

Source: Primary data of Annexure-B: Opinion of attendants of patients (OAP) – 48 respondents.

TABLE 3.6
Annexure-C: Opinion of Nursing Staff-(ONS)-56 Respondents

Attributes	CA	A	N	DA	CDA	Score
	5	4	3	2	1	
Based on service efficiency						
Increased efficiency of the diagnostic process	41	7	4	4	0	253
May reduce physician stress	43	4	3	3	3	249
Accelerating drug development	40	3	4	7	2	240
Improving patient experience	39	6	5	4	2	243
Robot-assisted surgery	44	2	3	3	4	247
Risk prediction	41	5	4	2	4	245
Smart health insurance	43	2	3	2	6	242
Prediction of healthcare risks early	41	4	4	3	4	243
Based on cost and time efficiency						
Reduced overall costs of running the business	42	6	3	3	2	251
Provides real-time data	44	3	5	4	0	255

(*Continued*)

TABLE 3.6 (Continued)
Annexure-C: Opinion of Nursing Staff-(ONS)-56 Respondents

Attributes	CA	A	N	DA	CDA	Score
	5	4	3	2	1	
Streamlines tasks	40	4	4	6	2	242
Saves time and resources	43	5	4	3	1	255
Based on transparency						
Data security	45	4	3	2	2	256
Remote monitoring	42	6	3	2	3	250
Location tracking and alerts (LTA)	41	5	2	2	6	241
Healthcare accessibility	42	4	2	4	4	244

Source: Primary data of Annexure-C: Opinion of Nursing staff- (ONS) – 56 respondents.

TABLE 3.7
Annexure-D: Opinion of Lab Technicians (OLT)-42 Respondents

Attributes	CA	A	N	DA	CDA	Score
	5	4	3	2	1	
Based on service efficiency						
Increased efficiency of the diagnostic process	30	4	3	3	2	183
May reduce physician stress	32	3	2	4	1	187
Accelerating drug development	29	4	3	4	2	180
Improving patient experience	33	3	4	2	0	193
Robot-assisted surgery	31	5	2	4	0	189
Risk prediction	34	4	3	1	0	197
Smart health insurance	32	2	5	0	3	186
Prediction of healthcare risks early	34	3	3	2	0	195
Based on cost and time efficiency						
Reduced overall costs of running the business	31	3	4	2	2	185
Provides real-time data	32	4	2	3	1	189
Streamlines tasks	33	2	3	4	0	190
Saves time and resources	32	3	5	2	0	191
Based on transparency						
Data security	36	3	3	0	0	201
Remote monitoring	34	3	4	1	0	196
Location tracking and alerts (LTA)	33	4	3	0	2	192
Healthcare accessibility	31	3	3	3	2	184

Source: Primary data of Annexure-D: Opinion of lab technicians (OLT) – 42 respondents.

TABLE 3.8

Annexure-E: Opinion of Doctors (OD)-36 Respondents

Attributes	CA	A	N	DA	CDA	Score
	5	4	3	2	1	
Based on service efficiency						
Increased efficiency of the diagnostic process	29	3	2	2	0	167
May reduce physician stress	28	2	2	2	2	160
Accelerating drug development	27	4	3	2	0	164
Improving patient experience	30	3	2	1	0	170
Robot-assisted surgery	26	3	1	4	2	155
Risk prediction	27	2	2	4	1	159
Smart health insurance	26	4	0	3	3	155
Prediction of healthcare risks early	27	3	2	2	2	159
Based on cost and time efficiency						
Reduced overall costs of running the business	26	3	1	3	3	154
Provides real-time data	25	4	2	3	2	155
Streamlines tasks	24	5	2	4	1	155
Saves time and resources	26	3	2	3	2	156
Based on transparency						
Data security	28	3	2	3	0	164
Remote monitoring	27	2	1	2	4	154
Location tracking and alerts (LTA)	26	3	2	2	3	155
Healthcare accessibility	28	4	0	4	0	164

Source: Primary data of Annexure-E: Opinion of doctors (OD) – 36 respondents.

REFERENCES

Alhashmi S., Alshurideh M., Kurdi B., Salloum S. "A systematic review of the factors affecting the artificial intelligence implementation in the health care sector," *April 8–9, 2020; Cairo, Egypt. Cham, Switzerland: Springer.* 2020. pp. 37–49. https://link.springer.com/chapter/10.1007/978-3-030-44289-7_4

Barlow J., Bayer S., Curry R. "Implementing complex innovations in fluid multi-stakeholder environments: Experiences of 'telecare' Technovation," 2006 Mar; 26(3): 396–406. doi: 10.1016/j.technovation.2005.06.010

Batalden M., Batalden P., Margolis P., Seid M., Armstrong G., Opipari-Arrigan L., Hartung H. "Coproduction of healthcare service," *BMJ Qual Saf.* 2016 Jul; 25(7): 509–517. doi: 10.1136/bmjqs-2015-004315

Beil M., Proft I., van Heerden D., Sviri S., van Heerden P. V. "Ethical considerations about artificial intelligence for prognostication in intensive care," *Intensive Care Med Exp.* 2019 Dec 10; 7(1): 70. doi: 10.1186/s40635-019-0286-6. http://europepmc.org/abstract/MED/31823128.10.1186/s40635-019-0286-6

Bhambri P., Rani S., Gupta G., Khang A. "Cloud and fog computing platforms for Internet of Things," ISBN: 978-1-032-101507, 2022, CRC Press. 10.1201/9781003213888

Choudhury A., Asan O. "Role of artificial intelligence in patient safety outcomes: Systematic literature review," *JMIR Med Inform.* 2020 Jul 24; 8(7): e18599. doi: 10.2196/18599. https://medinform.jmir.org/2020/7/e18599/v8i7e18599

De Nigris S., Craglia M., Nepelski D., Hradec J., Gomez-Gonzales E., Gomez Gutierrez E., Vazquez-Prada Baillet M., Righi R., De Prato G., Lopez Cobo M., Samoili S., Cardona M. *AI Watch: AI Uptake in Health and Healthcare 2020, EUR 30478 EN.* https://publications.jrc.ec.europa.eu/repository/handle/JRC122675

Eldh A. C., Almost J., DeCorby-Watson K., Gifford W., Harvey G., Hasson H., Kenny D., Moodie S., Wallin L., Yost J. "Clinical interventions, implementation interventions, and the potential greyness in between: A discussion paper," *BMC Health Serv Res.* 2017 Jan 07; 17(1): 16. doi: 10.1186/s12913-016-1958-5

Fernandes M., Vieira S. M., Leite F., Palos C., Finkelstein S., Sousa J. M. "Clinical decision support systems for triage in the emergency department using intelligent systems: A review," *Artif Intell Med.* 2020 Jan; 102:101762. doi: 10.1016/j.artmed.2019.101762. S0933-3657(19)30126-5

Hajimahmud V. A., Khang A., Hahanov V., Litvinova E., Chumachenko S., Alyar A. V. "Autonomous robots for smart city: Closer to augmented humanity," *AI-Centric Smart City Ecosystems: Technologies, Design and Implementation* (1st Ed.), 2022. CRC Press. 10.1201/9781003252542-7

Khang A., Hahanov V., AbbasG. L., Hajimahmud V. A. "Cyber-physical-social system and incident management," *AI-Centric Smart City Ecosystems: Technologies, Design and Implementation* (1st Ed.), 2022a. CRC Press. 10.1201/9781003252542-2

Khang A., Hahanov V., Litvinova E., Chumachenko S., Hajimahmud V. A., Alyar A. V. "The key assistant of smart city – Sensors and tools," *AI-Centric Smart City Ecosystems: Technologies, Design and Implementation* (1st ed.), 2022b. CRC Press. 10.1201/9781003252542-17

Khang A., Ragimova N. A., Hajimahmud V. A., Alyar A. V. "Advanced technologies and data management in the smart healthcare system," *AI-Centric Smart City Ecosystems: Technologies, Design and Implementation* (1st Ed.), 2022c. CRC Press. 10.1201/9781003252542-16

Khang A., Rana G., Tailor R. K., Hajimahmud V. A., (Eds.). *Data-Centric AI Solutions and Emerging Technologies in the Healthcare Ecosystem* (1st Ed.), 2023. CRC Press. 10.1201/9781003356189

Khang A., Rani S., Sivaraman A. K. *AI-Centric Smart City Ecosystems: Technologies, Design and Implementation* (1st Ed.), 2022d. CRC Press. 10.1201/9781003252542

Khanh H. H., Khang A. "The role of artificial intelligence in blockchain applications," *Reinventing Manufacturing and Business Processes through Artificial Intelligence,* pp. 20–40, 2021, CRC Press. 10.1201/9781003145011-2

Misra A., Shah V., Khang A., Gupta S. K., (Eds.). *AI-aided IoT Technologies and Applications in the Smart Business and Production* (1st Ed.), 2023. CRC Press. 10.1201/9781003392224

Morris G., Babasaheb J., Khang A., Gupta S. K., Hajimahmud V. A., (1 Ed.). *AI-Centric Modelling and Analytics: Concepts, Designs, Technologies, and Applications* (1st Ed.), 2023. CRC Press. 10.1201/9781003400110

Rana G., Khang A., Sharma R., Goel A. K., Dubey A. K. "Reinventing manufacturing and business processes through artificial intelligence", (Eds.), 2021. CRC Press. 10.1201/9781003145011

Rani S., Bhambri P., Kataria A., Khang A., Sivaraman A. K. (Eds.). *Big Data, Cloud Computing and IoT: Tools and Applications* (1st Ed.), 2023. Chapman and Hall/CRC. 10.1201/9781003298335

Rani S., Chauhan M., Kataria A., Khang A. "IoT equipped intelligent distributed framework for smart healthcare systems," *Networking and Internet Architecture*, (Eds.), 2021. CRC Press. 10.48550/arXiv.2110.04997

Reed J. E., Howe C., Doyle C., Bell D. "Simple rules for evidence translation in complex systems: A qualitative study," *BMC Med.* 2018 Jun 20; 16(1): 92. doi: 10.1186/s1291 6-018-1076-9. https://bmcmedicine.biomedcentral.com/articles/10.1186/s12916-018-1076-9

Tailor R. K., Pareek R., Khang A., (Eds.). "Robot process automation in blockchain," *The Data-Driven Blockchain Ecosystem: Fundamentals, Applications, and Emerging Technologies* (1st ed.), pp. 149–164, 2022. CRC Press. 10.1201/9781003269281-8

Vrushank S., Vidhi T., Khang, A. "Electronic health records security and privacy enhancement using blockchain technology," *Data-Centric AI Solutions and Emerging Technologies in the Healthcare Ecosystem.* (1st ed.), p. 1, (2023), CRC Press. 10.1201/9781003356189-1

4 The Analytics of Hospitality of Hospitals in a Healthcare Ecosystem

*Alex Khang, Vladimir Hahanov, Eugenia Litvinova,
Svetlana Chumachenko, Triwiyanto,
Abdullayev Vugar Hajimahmud,
Ragimova Nazila Ali, Abuzarova Vusala Alyar, and
P. T. N. Anh*

CONTENTS

DOI: 10.1201/9781003356189-4

4.1   INTRODUCTION

Although today's healthcare is more developed than in the last century, or even in previous years, the dangers to people's lives are also increasing in parallel. We can mention hundreds of concepts that can be considered dangerous for human life: diseases, natural or man-made accidents, etc. (Vrushank, Vidhi & Khang, 2023).

Today, certain diseases are at the top of the problems that concern the healthcare world the most. One of the biggest threats facing the world's health is COVID-19, which is still ongoing and is considered a pandemic. Before COVID, the World Health was faced with the Ebola virus, which occurred in the nearest time interval and was considered as an epidemic.

The World Health Organization (WHO) has warned people about the possibility of new pandemics. At this point, the main issue is whether healthcare is strong enough to withstand the next pandemic.

It is known that the COVID-19 pandemic is now more under control than in the early days. This is proof that healthcare can cope with pandemics like COVID-19. But let's also take into account that the COVID-19 pandemic is still ongoing. So, healthcare has not yet fully coped with COVID. And the next pandemics may be more dangerous than COVID-19.

The modern healthcare system is constantly evolving with innovations to have a strong resistance against potential threats (diseases) that may occur next.

We can look at the *1Modern-, *2Modern, and *3Modern+ healthcare eco-system in the following directions:

1. *1Modern- (old healthcare system)
2. *2Modern (current healthcare system)
3. *3Modern+ (future healthcare system)
   - Infrastructure
   - Modern Healthcare
   - Technological "Care"
   - Applications
   - Data exchange
   - The Future of Healthcare: Modern+

4.2   INFRASTRUCTURE

Healthcare infrastructure is a system that includes individuals, healthcare facilities, and "all" connections between them. Healthcare infrastructure are shown in figure 4.1.

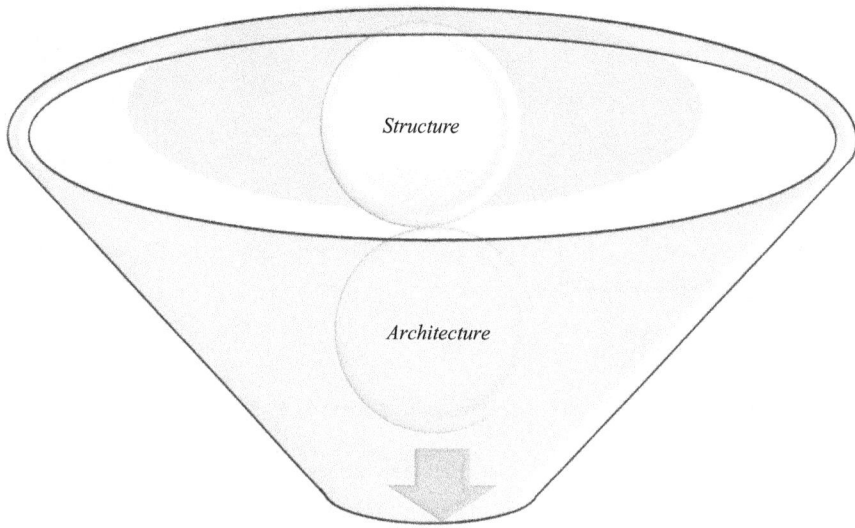

FIGURE 4.1 Infrastructure = Structure + Architecture. Figure 4.1 presents the infrastructure of system.

Source: Author's owner.

4.2.1 STRUCTURE

The concept of structure generally refers to objects and the relationship between them. Architecture implies the relationship between these objects.

Structure is the main central part of healthcare infrastructure: it represents people, healthcare facilities, and all the relationships between them. Today, the basis of these relations is the data exchange.

With the help of a common database, it is possible to make a specific diagnosis for a specific patient. Even today, one of the most demanded technologies in the field of healthcare is big data technology.

Today, the role of this technology in healthcare is irreplaceable. Even some experts point out that it is possible to treat some dangerous diseases with the help of this technology; for example, cancer. The main benefit of big data is briefly this:

> Thus, the information got during the treatment of some patients is stored in a common database and used for other patients if appropriate. Or, by collecting that information, it analyzes (analyzes) and a common denominator is got. With this, any disease is treated.

4.2.2 ARCHITECTURE

Although it may sound a little strange, the main "customers" of hospitals are patients. Hospitals operate for patients. Research hospitals also serve patients indirectly.

In this respect, the structure and design of hospitals should be in a form that can "comfort" patients so patients should feel at home. So, the place where a person

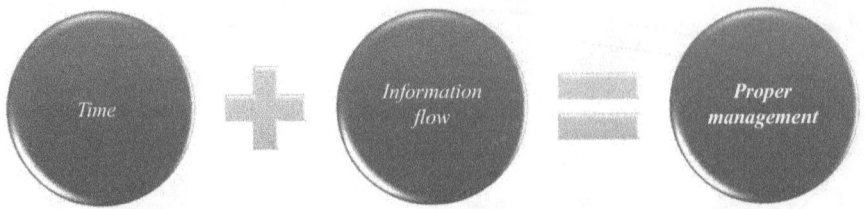

FIGURE 4.2 Time + information flow = proper management. Figure 4.2 presents the components of proper management.

Source: Author's owner.

feels the most comfortable is his home. In this regard, hospitals should be a second home for patients.

The architecture of hospitals exists between the same and three main elements as structure: People, objects, and relationships between them.

We will look at architecture, design, and principles here: The proper service of a modern hospital is also related to its interior design. Hospitals that promise a comfortable place will have a good effect on a person psychologically.

Comfortable rooms, friendly staff, correct information flow – in short, correct management – will have a positive effect even for people with the most serious diseases. Psychological comfort will help a person feel in a higher mood. One of the main influences on this is space.

A modern hospital design should include several principles:

1. Patient satisfaction
2. High level and on-site service
3. Correct management (continuity of information flow)
4. Ensuring a high level of personnel training (moral and physical)
5. High technological accessibility
6. Proper time management (making the right diagnosis in time)
7. High hygienic conditions
8. Home fresh space, etc.

Note: In general, time is very important for any field. Proper time management, timely access to information, and proper flow of information are the main steps in making the right decisions. For the hospital, it is the main stages in making the right diagnosis for the patient, as shown in figure 4.2.

4.2.2.1 Design and Principles

According to the principles mentioned above, experts recommend the following hospital designs (Ragimova et al., 2021), as shown in figure 4.3.

4.2.2.2 Avoiding Overcrowding

Having a large room for the patient is one of the ideal options to make him feel comfortable. Even individual and several-person rooms should be large enough to

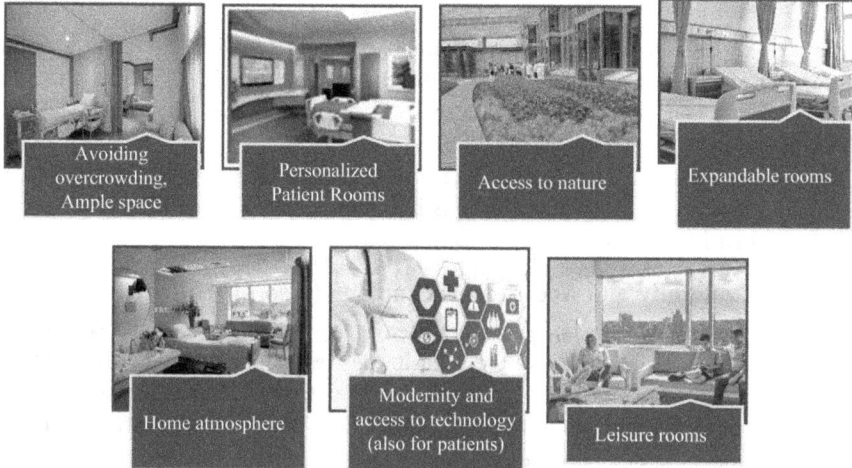

FIGURE 4.3 Design for hospitals. Figure 4.3 presents the designs advised by experts.

Source: Author's owner.

determine the patient's own space. A spacious room is quite eye-catching, both in terms of ventilation and design. For the patient's inner comfort, it is important that the surrounding environment is comfortable enough.

Personalized rooms: In hospitals, we see several patients staying in one room. Of course, this happens in terms of the internal structure of the hospital. However, regardless of the patient's illness, receiving treatment in private rooms will have a positive effect on the patient himself.

Features such as patient communication boards and customizable digital boards with the patient's name, family photos, weather forecasts, etc. are being incorporated into healthcare facilities (Ragimova et al., 2021).

This allows you to create a home environment for the patient. And it prioritizes patient comfort.

4.2.2.3 Accessibility to Nature

Interacting with nature is important for both sick and healthy people. However, for patients treated in a hospital setting – imagine spending months in a room with four walls. This is such a boring situation for a healthy person – it is even more important to constantly interact with nature. It is more appropriate for hospitals to be located in a position where the patient will always have access to nature. It is important to have greenery around the hospital, a closed area, and plenty of trees. Psychologically, being in constant interaction with nature helps to quickly eliminate the disease.

4.2.2.4 Expandable Rooms

Because patients may have more than one visitor at a time, hybrid products such as sofa beds and recliners should ensure that caregivers and visitors have the space they need without crowding the room (Ragimova et al., 2021).

4.2.2.5 Home Atmosphere

In other words, it is intended as a personalized room function. Creating a home atmosphere in the hospital will help the patient feel comfortable. For example, the patient's room can be designed like a room in his own home. That is, it does not mean changing the color of the room, etc.

As we mentioned above, family photos or things he uses, drawing tools if he is into painting, musical instruments if he is into music, or toys if he likes to play, etc. can be placed in the room.

4.2.2.6 Modernity and Access to Technology (Also for Patients)

In modern times, smart technologies are used in any sector. The health sector also belongs here. Smart technologies are used in the treatment of patients. In addition, there are a number of smart technologies that serve patients. Like robot assistants, etc.

The use of technology should be accessible not only to hospital staff, but also to patients. Patients should not be satisfied with receiving information about their health only from doctors. At the same time, they should monitor their own health progress.

It is true that it can have both positive and negative effects. However, the patient's awareness of his health will help him to be more confident in his recovery.

4.2.2.7 Leisure Rooms

Patients should not spend their time only in their rooms or in the garden around the hospital. There should be rest rooms for patients and they should play different games, interact with each other, talk, and socialize in these rooms.

One of the main problems in sick people is that they try to regulate themselves from the outside. Unfortunately, this causes the patient to psychologically surrender himself to the arms of the disease. However, if the patient tries to live a social life on the contrary, it will have a positive effect on him.

Leisure rooms can also be mobile in nature. That is, certain social activities should be implemented for bedridden people.

4.3 MODERN HEALTHCARE

Modern healthcare provides modern services. Many of these services are implemented with technologies, especially with smart technologies. The modern services provided by healthcare include robotic medical assistants – patient caregivers, implementation of virtual operations with AR and VR technologies, telemedicine services, analysis of diagnoses, analysis of treatments, creation of common treatment methods with the analysis of successful treatments and their application on other patients, and with the help of this the possibility of faster recovery of other patients occurs.

The position of healthcare today is quite heartening. However, in terms of the ongoing pandemic, it should be recognized that there are still certain gaps (problems) in healthcare. Taking into account that pandemics and epidemics may occur in the future, it is important to allocate sufficient funds for the development of the country's healthcare.

With the application of technology to healthcare, the era of technological "care" has begun.

4.4 TECHNOLOGICAL "CARE"

The era of technological "care" began with the integration of technology into healthcare. Today, patient care is not only provided by doctors. Technologies are also involved in the care process.

As an example of this, we can show the robot nurses that we mentioned at the beginning.

Today, thousands of people are being treated for various diseases in hundreds of hospitals around the world. These people belong to different age groups. The number of personnel to deal with so many patients is sometimes not enough. We saw this most clearly when the COVID-19 pandemic reached its peak. The lack of staff in hospitals was particularly evident. Robot assistants were needed both daily and during a certain pandemic.

In everyday situations, robotic medical assistants take care of patients and monitor their condition. It takes into account his wishes. At the same time, within the framework of certain decision-making, it reminds patients of medication times and assists patients in taking medications. Of course, all of these are implemented through the interaction of artificial intelligence and databases.

However, given the above considerations, it may be somewhat risky for robotic medical assistants to perform decision-making on their own, because when robotic medical assistants offer the patient to take medicine, the patient can refuse it. And this refusal may not be meaningful.

When the patient refuses for certain reasons (for example, the patient takes this drug, feels sick, etc.), robotic medical assistants can be programmed to force the patient to take the drug. And this can be dangerous for the patient. It is precisely in this respect that it is wrong for robotic medical assistants to act independently. They must be controlled, as in figure 4.4 (Yeung et al., 2020).

During a pandemic, the presence of robotic medical assistants is more appropriate from the point of view of the health of medical workers. One of the main countries that used robots in the fight against the COVID-19 pandemic was China. So, the China government used the help of robots in many fields, not only in healthcare, as shown in figure 4.5.

Other countries have also started to learn from China's epidemic prevention experience. China's telemedicine robots, delivery robots, disinfection robots, and patrol drones have provided support functions for medical treatment and epidemic prevention and control, and their models have been copied by many countries.

However, robotic medical assistants are currently among the most "caregiving" technologies. For example, by 2050, the number of people aged 65+ is predicted to increase [U.S. reports], and robotic medical assistants are specifically designed to deal with this group of people. Today, more research in this field continues to be conducted in Japan. Several advanced robots are already operating in Japanese hospitals.

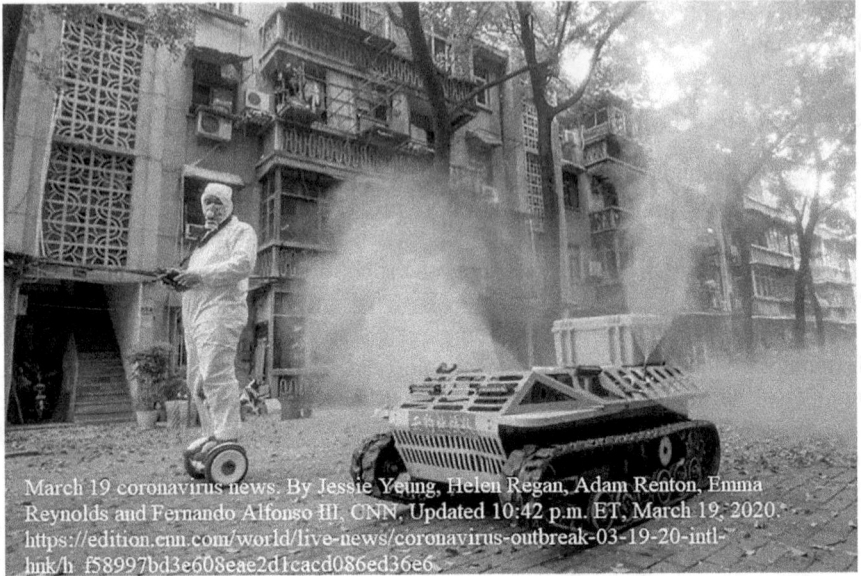

March 19 coronavirus news. By Jessie Yeung, Helen Regan, Adam Renton, Emma Reynolds and Fernando Alfonso III. CNN. Updated 10:42 p.m. ET, March 19, 2020. https://edition.cnn.com/world/live-news/coronavirus-outbreak-03-19-20-intl-hnk/h_f58997bd3e608eae2d1cacd086ed36e6.

FIGURE 4.4 The presence of robotic medical assistants. Figure 4.4 displays a volunteer operates a remote controlled disinfection robot to disinfect a residential area amid the coronavirus outbreak in Wuhan in China's central Hubei province on March 16. Stringer/AFP/Getty Images.

Source: March 19 coronavirus news. By Jessie Yeung, Helen Regan, Adam Renton, Emma Reynolds and Fernando Alfonso III. CNN. Updated 10:42 p.m. ET, March 19, 2020.

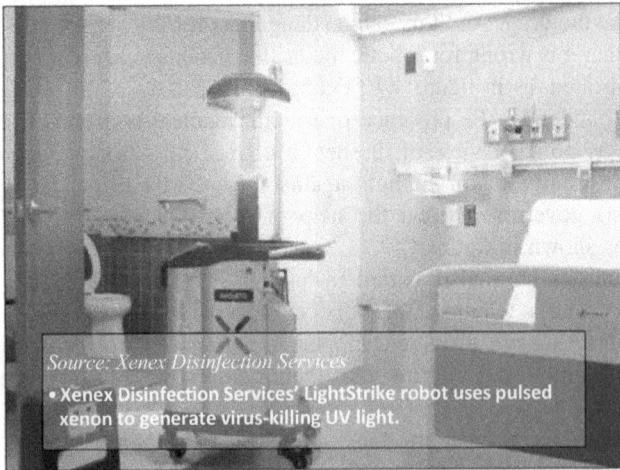

Source: Xenex Disinfection Services
• Xenex Disinfection Services' LightStrike robot uses pulsed xenon to generate virus-killing UV light.

FIGURE 4.5 The presence of robotic medical assistants.

Source: Xenex Disinfection Services and Big data in healthcare (Sabyasachi Dash et al., 2019).

In addition to robots, many technologies are currently being used in healthcare. These technologies work in parallel with robots. Examples of such technologies are: augmented reality, virtual reality, computer vision, deep learning, machine learning, etc.

4.5   TECHNOLOGIES IN HEALTHCARE

Rapid technological development has also had an impact on the healthcare sector. The integration of (smart) technologies in healthcare has taken this sector several levels forward.

In fact, many technological possibilities are used in healthcare. And these technological capabilities interact with each other to enable the proper management of the health sector. "Technologies in healthcare" topic has two parts:

1. Technologies
2. Applications

We can consider the following items.

4.5.1   TECHNOLOGIES

The technologies we will cover in Part 1 are as follows in figure 4.6.

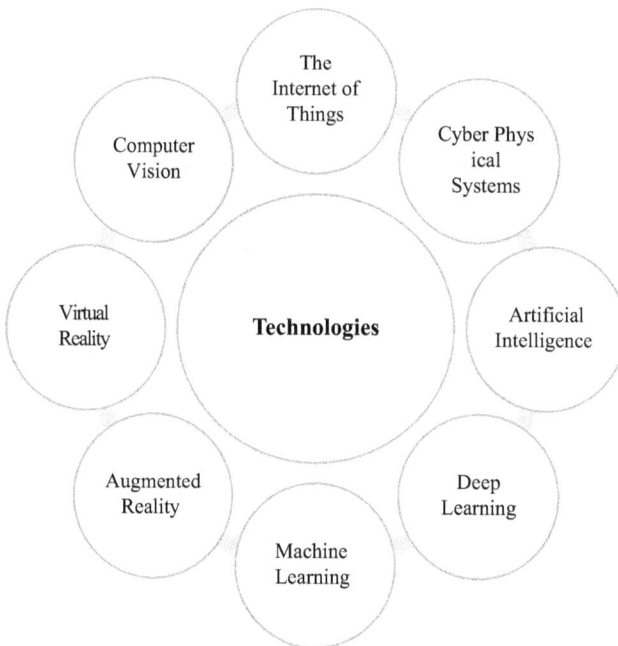

FIGURE 4.6   Technologies in the healthcare. Figure 4.6 presents the technologies applied in healthcare.

Source: Author's owner.

4.5.1.1   Internet of Medical Things

The Internet of Things (IoT) ecosystem, in which information is exchanged through the interaction of smart devices with each other, forms the basis of many other technologies today. Also, the Internet of Things technology applied in many fields has become a part of our daily life (Rani et al., 2021).

One of the main areas where Internet of Things technology is used is the healthcare sector (Khang et al., 2023a). The integration of this technology into the health sector has created a new concept. This concept has been adopted as the Internet of Medical Things (IoMT).

The main function of IoT technology in healthcare is based on the same logic. Thus, the main logic of the Internet of Things technology is the interaction of smart devices with each other (reducing the participation of the human factor in this direction) and data exchange with each other (Khang et al., 2023b).

This will form the basis of proper management at the next stage. Proper data exchange is an indispensable tool for any sector. The correct and especially timely exchange of information is even more important for the health sector (Mathad & Khang, 2023).

In healthcare, many smart devices collect data through sensors, analyze it by sending it to the cyber environment, and send it back to the physical environment. In fact, this is done with the help of the joint use of relatively few technologies. So, the above-mentioned event – AI, CPS, and big data – happens when they work together (Khang et al., 2023e).

Through the Internet of Things technology, remote monitoring of the patient can be carried out, which is called telemedicine.

One of the most well-known applications of Internet of Medical Things technology is "smart medicine containers". These medicine containers perform one of the functions of medical assistant robots. Reminds the patient of the time to take the medicine.

In addition, there are also the following applications:

1. AdhereTech: Medication boxes with wireless network connectivity send a message or alert to the patient when the patient forgets to take medication.
2. Stanley Healthcare: Visualization of the location and status of all staff, equipment, and patients to better understand hospital workflow processes.
3. HealthPatch: A sensor used to monitor acute and chronic diseases. It sends changes in patients' biometric and vital signs to doctors via Bluetooth.
4. Continuous glucose monitor (CGM): A device that helps diabetics monitor their blood sugar levels continuously over several days by taking regular measurements. The first CGM system was approved by the U.S. Food and Drug Administration (FDA) in 1999, and a number of smart CGMs have been released in recent years.
5. Proteus Digital Health: Pills that dissolve in the stomach and produce a small signal that is picked up by this sensor attached to the body. The data is then transferred to a smartphone app and checked to see if the patient is using the medication as directed.
6. Measuring depression with the Apple Watch monitor: Designed to track and assess patients with major depressive disorder in 2017.

7. Coagulation system with Bluetooth: This device is the first of its kind for anticoagulated patients and has been demonstrated by self-testing to help patients stay within therapeutic range and reduce the risk of heart attack or bleeding.
8. ADAMM: A device for monitoring patients with asthma.

The Internet of Medical Things technology has the following positive aspects:

1. Patients are provided with better healthcare devices, medicines, etc. at affordable prices. This reduces overall costs for patients.
2. It offers better treatment results.
3. Provides more confidence to doctors. This is due to the fact that IoMT technologies increase the capabilities of doctors and researchers.
4. Errors are reduced to a greater extent.
5. Medication intake can be monitored and controlled.
6. It is easy to ensure the use of medical devices in such an IoMT network.
7. Diseases are better controlled.

4.5.1.2 Medical Cyber Physical Systems

Cyber physical systems are systems of interaction between the cyber environment and the physical environment. In this interaction, data from the physical environment is collected through sensors and sent to the cyber environment. This data is then analyzed and, if necessary, sent back to the physical environment, which happens in case of user queries, etc.

- The Cyber Physical Systems – Internet of Things – Big data trinity acquires, analyzes, and feeds back patient data to both the patient and the physician.
- CPS here basically represents the "bridge" created. The Internet of Things receives information from the physical environment, CPS sends this information through a "bridge" to the cyber environment. Big data analytics begins its work and analyzes the data. Ready information is available (Khang et al., 2022a).

The following are the advantages of CPS applied in healthcare:

1. Availability of the network – the possibility of correct data exchange is realized through the network created with the help of CPS.
2. Human interaction – since the main purpose of CPS is to connect the physical and cyber environment, with its help, human-machine interaction happens more easily (Khang et al., 2023c).
3. Better system execution (performance) – Interconnection of sensors and network infrastructure enables CPS to have higher performance.
4. Scalability – CPS can use other technological capabilities to expand the system as needed. For example, it can use the features of cloud computing.
5. Faster response time – CPS can respond to user requests faster by using other technological capabilities in parallel, etc.

Applications of cyber physical systems in healthcare include electronic medical records, virtual reality, and smart checklist, etc. We will consider these applications separately (Babasaheb et al., 2023).

4.5.1.3 Artificial Intelligence

Artificial intelligence includes many other concepts. In general, almost all technologies are based on the concept of artificial intelligence, Internet of Things, CPS, etc. However, since these two concepts exist relatively separately, we mentioned their possibilities separately.

The technologies that we will mention from now on are only technologies with artificial intelligence–based progress, machine learning, deep learning, augmented and virtual reality, and computer vision technology.

With the application of these artificial intelligence–based technologies in healthcare, new opportunities have been achieved.

4.5.1.3.1 *Machine Learning*

Machine learning, a subsystem of artificial intelligence, is a technological field that mimics human learning by considering how data and algorithms are used. Through simulation, many models are used to develop the project before it is fully created. In this way, a forecast is given in advance for the project to be created. Machine learning is mainly closely related to neural networks and deep learning.

Thus, deep learning is considered a subsystem of neural networks, and neural networks are considered a subsystem of machine learning.

Machine learning is primarily a data-driven concept. Any next step in machine learning is based on data. In this regard, personnel in any field will learn how to properly work with data, as well as, accordingly, indirectly learn how much machine learning works.

Machine learning is an important component of the growing field of data science. Using statistical methods, algorithms are trained to make classifications or predictions and uncover key concepts in data mining projects. These insights then drive decision-making within applications and businesses and ideally impact key growth metrics.

Machine learning is used in fields such as medicine, construction, gaming, banking, as well as in applications such as speech recognition, computer vision, etc.

In the healthcare sector, machine learning is used for a variety of purposes, such as managing patient data and electronic records, predicting and treating disease, providing medical diagnostics, and discovering and developing new drugs.

In addition, another application of machine learning is telemedicine. The most common application of traditional machine learning in healthcare is precision medicine – it is possible to predict which treatment protocols will be successful in a patient based on various patient attributes and treatment context.

Neural networks, a subsystem of machine learning, are applied in the proper management of data in healthcare. Neural networks with a layered feature filter the received information to get a more accurate output.

The presence of hidden layers in the layers in neural networks allows for additional data acquisition. The use of such networks is mainly applied in analyzes

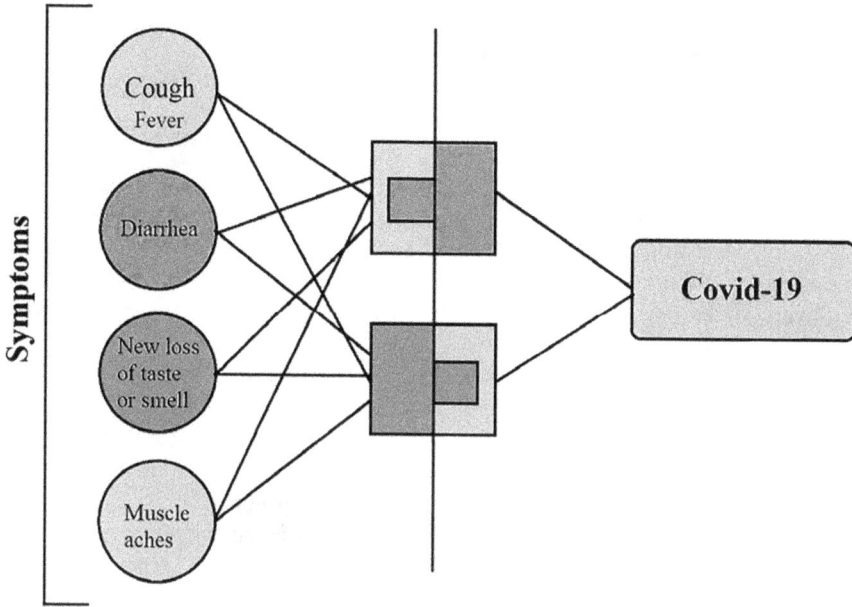

FIGURE 4.7   Diagnostics with neural networks. Figure 4.7. presents the diagnosis of the patient's disease with neural networks.

Source: Author's owner.

related to oncological diseases. In particular, machine learning, neural networks, deep learning, and big data are the most important technologies used in cancer treatment and data analytics.

In the simplest case, based on the input data, the diagnosis of the disease can be made as follows. For example, based on the entered data, it can be understood that the patient has COVID-19 or flu, as follows in figure 4.7.

For example, if it is known that there is more loss of taste and smell, then it will be known that the disease is not the usual flu, but COVID-19. However, the symptoms of flu and COVID-19 are very similar.

4.5.1.3.2   Deep Learning

Deep learning, also known as hierarchical learning or deep structured learning, is a subsystem of neural networks. It also carries features such as machine learning using a layered architecture.

This multi-level strategy allows deep learning models to perform classification tasks such as identifying subtle abnormalities in medical images, grouping patients with similar characteristics into risk-based groups, or highlighting relationships between symptoms and outcomes within large amounts of unstructured data.

Unlike other types of machine learning, deep learning has the added advantage of being able to make decisions with significantly less input from human trainers.

In contrast, machine learning is a relatively human-based activity.

Deep learning is also used for various purposes, such as in image analysis, research, and discovery of new drugs.

In general, both machine learning and deep learning are key enablers in making accurate clinical decisions.

4.5.1.3.3 Augmented Reality (AR) and Virtual Reality (VR)

At its simplest, augmented reality is a technology that transfers the virtual world into the physical world. That is, pictures and videos in the virtual world are reflected in the real world. In other words, it is an imitation technology. The VR technology that everyone knows today is a technology that is used by the younger generation, especially during games.

The main goal of these technologies is to enhance the human experience. With augmented reality, it is possible to get closer to augmented humanity.

Today, these technologies are used not only in the gaming sector, but also in many vital areas. For example, in some areas, it is safer to try imitation for the first time. Military and medical fields can be cited as examples of such fields. In addition, these two technologies are widely used in some other areas: the construction sector, the education sector, as well as the gaming sector, which we mentioned above.

With AR, an augmented version of the real world is offered (presented). With virtual reality, users continue to interact with the virtual world. Virtual has 75% virtuality and AR has 25% virtuality. In AR, users interact with the real world.

With VR, it is possible to create a completely fictional-fantasy world, and with this technology, it is possible to come into contact with this world.

VR, AR, and MR technologies are among the technologies that are in demand in healthcare, as shown in figure 4.8.

4.5.1.3.4 Computer Vision

Computer vision (or machine vision) is a branch of artificial intelligence that includes algorithms for visual object detection, tracking, classification, image depth estimation,

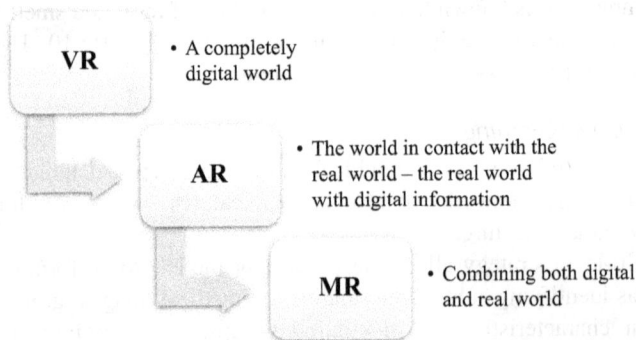

FIGURE 4.8   VR, AR, and MR. Figure 4.8 presents the definitions of VR, AR, and MR technologies.

Source: Author's owner.

pattern and semantic segmentation, etc. Computer vision (CV) attempts to model the mechanism of visual information reception and processing in the human brain.

At its simplest, computer vision uses an object recognition algorithm. So, the sector that uses this technology must have a certain database for it. For example, to recognize any object, a description of that object is entered. Then, objects with similar properties are selected. Then other details are considered and that object is separated from the selected objects.

It is used for diagnostics in healthcare without computer vision. So, from the entered description, it can be known to which category the disease belongs. Of course, for this, there should be a database with the characteristics of diseases.

The following features relate to the positive aspects of computer vision for use in healthcare:

1. Greater security (Khang et al., 2022b)
2. Better service
3. Empowers people's opportunities more
4. Faster execution of routine tasks
5. Autonomy (Hajimahmud et al., 2022)

4.6 APPLICATIONS

Technologies used in healthcare have some applications. Thus, several technologies are generally used in these applications.

These applications include telemedicine, biomedicine, electronic medical records, etc. We will review these three applications. By joint use, for example, in tele-medicine, technologies such as the Internet of Things, big data, and machine learning are used together.

4.6.1 BIOMEDICINE

Biomedicine is a field of medicine that deals with the application of the principles of biology and biochemistry to medical research or practice. Biomedicine, also re-ferred to as Western medicine or traditional medicine, is a branch of medical sci-ence that applies biological and physiological principles to clinical practice.

Traditional medicine, biomedicine, also makes extensive use of the possibilities of technology. In this field, some of the above-mentioned technologies are widely used: Internet of Things, machine learning, deep learning, cloud computing, and big data.

Internet of Things devices are applied in biomedicine in patient monitoring and treatment.

The IoT is being used by hospitals to provide remote care as well as in biomedical applications to improve the performance of athletes. Assessment of sleep patterns can be a key parameter for athletes' performance and motivation (Khang et al., 2022c).

The Internet of Things and big data interact. Information in big data is collected through Internet of Things devices. In particular, data got through sensors is stored in databases and used in conjunction with data analysis packages. Currently, the

Internet of Things is of great importance in big data and cloud computing for data storage and analysis.

Machine learning and deep learning perform far better than a human worker in terms of accuracy. Thus, ML and DL can reveal "hidden" information that can escape the eyes of a human worker. Machine learning is applied to modeling in biomedicine.

Common classes of machine learning methods include:

1. Supervised learning in which groups of information are associated with a specific outcome; categorical data (e.g., disease versus normal) are based on classification methods, whereas continuous values (e.g., strength of response to therapy) are used in regression methods,
2. Unsupervised or semi-supervised methods for grouping data into discrete groups.
3. Machine learning, where the results of multiple computational models are combined to create a final prediction, can lead to more accurate predictions by allowing models to better generalize to new data.
4. Deep learning using artificial neural networks, modeled formalization in the human brain, is useful for recognizing patterns or associations in data, especially when dealing with unstructured data such as images, speech and text, and Bayesian learning, where prior knowledge is encoded into the learning process, is particularly useful in data-poor situations.

In general, it is also used for the following purposes:

- Imaging and prognosis: Biomedical imaging and cardiovascular studies.
- Big data and machine learning: From big data sets to improved patient care.

4.6.2 TELEMEDICINE

Telemedicine is the transmission of medical services and information using electronic, information, and telecommunication technologies. Telemedicine is also considered as long-distance medicine.

With this technology, which also allows long-distance communication, patients who cannot come to the hospital can receive treatment. In addition, it is possible to constantly monitor patients.

Remote delivery of medical care is accomplished using electronic information and technology such as computers, cameras, videoconferencing, satellites, wireless communications, and the Internet. This is also called telehealth.

Telemedicine is based on Internet of Things devices.

With IoT devices, patients can use wearables and other medical devices to check their blood pressure, temperature, and heart rate at home, and transmit the results for analysis by their doctors.

Patients can use wearables and other medical devices to check their blood pressure, temperature, and heart rate at home and transmit the results for analysis by their doctors (Robots and Telemedicine, 2023).

IoT technology enables unprecedented levels of patient-generated data to be delivered to healthcare, making PGD an increasingly critical component of decision-making and delivery, and has significant potential to improve outcomes, reduce costs, increase service accessibility, and improve patient experience (Robots and Telemedicine, 2023)

4.6.3 ELECTRONIC MEDICAL RECORDS

In healthcare, the concepts of EHR and EMR exist. Although some professionals use the terms *EHR* and *EMR* interchangeably, the services they offer vary. An EMR (electronic medical record) is a digital version of a chart with patient information stored on a computer, and an EHR (electronic health record) is a digital record of health information (Jennifer Bresnick, 2023).

An electronic (digital) collection of medical information about a person stored on a computer. An electronic medical record contains information about a patient's health history, such as diagnoses, medications, tests, allergies, vaccinations, and treatment plans (Jennifer Bresnick, 2023).

An EHR is an important part of health IT and can contain a patient's medical history, diagnoses, medications, treatment plans, immunization dates, allergies, radiology images, and lab and test results and allows access to evidence-based tools that providers can use to make decisions about patient care.

The system includes IoT readers and tags. An RFID tag is attached to each item with a unique number recorded in the inventory software. The hospital has IoT readers that receive RFID signals and transmit the data to the interface part of the system.

The doctor's smartphone or computer receives information on which floor and in which office the required device is located. This "search engine" is useful when staff need to take inventory or urgently need to find an oxygen mask for a newly admitted critical patient (HER, 2021).

In EMR and clinical management software, IoT will enrich old platforms with new functionality. It will enable remote treatment of patients and help the administration control multiple processes, from drug quality control to inventory management (HER, 2021).

Electronic health records themselves also bear similarities to big data and with deep learning technology, grouping can be done from electronic medical records.

4.7 DATA EXCHANGE

The present age is the age of information. With digitization, there has been an extreme increase in information. Information is the most important factor in good management, whether in healthcare or any other sector.

Data exchange plays an important role in the treatment of diseases in healthcare. Timely collection, processing, and transmission of data is necessary for proper exchange of information. A database is important for data storage.

Currently, there are many technological possibilities for working with data. The most important of them are big data (analytics) and cloud technology.

As we mentioned,

Proper data management – (helps) → to make the right decision → Improve the enterprise.

In the development of the healthcare sector, as well as in the treatment of diseases, there is a need for proper management of information – data exchange. The progress achieved during the treatment of previous patients is stored in the databases, analyzed, and the treatment of the disease of those patients is found and developed. This is closely related to data analysis.

4.7.1   BIG DATA (ANALYTICS), CLOUD COMPUTING

4.7.1.1   Big Data Technology

The use and management of big data affects many areas of our society. One of the application fields of big data is the field of healthcare. Traditionally, the healthcare industry has lagged behind other industries in its use of big data. This is because part of the healthcare problem stems from resistance to change, because they are used to making decisions independently using their own clinical judgment rather than relying on treatment decisions.

The following applications of big data in healthcare exist.

4.7.1.1.1   Electronic Health Records (EHRs)

It is the most widespread application of big data in medicine. Each patient has their own digital records, including demographics, medical history, allergies, lab test results, and more.

While EHRs are a great idea, many countries are still struggling to fully implement them. According to HITECH research, the United States has made a big leap with 94% of hospitals adopting EHRs, but the EU still lags behind.

4.7.1.1.2   Using Health Data for Informed Strategic Planning

The use of big data in healthcare enables strategic planning through better understanding of people's motivations. With this, they can analyze screening results between people and determine what factors prevent people from starting treatment.

4.7.1.1.3   Big Data Can Help Treatment of Cancer

Another interesting example of the use of big data in healthcare is the Cancer Moonshot program.

Medical researchers can use vast amounts of data on treatment plans and cancer cure rates to find trends and treatments with the highest success rates in the real world.

For example, researchers can examine tumor samples linked to patient treatment records in biobanks. Using this data, researchers can see things like how certain mutations and cancer proteins interact with different treatments and find trends that lead to better patient outcomes.

However, patient databases from disparate institutions such as hospitals, universities, and non-profit organizations need to be linked to make such insights more accessible.

One potential big data use case in healthcare would be to genetically sequence cancer tissue samples from clinical research patients and submit this information to a larger cancer database.

4.7.1.1.4 Smart Staffing and Personal Management

Without a collaborative and engaged workforce, patient care will decline, service rates will decline, and errors will occur. However, with big data in the healthcare field, it is possible to facilitate workforce management activities in many areas. By working with the right HR analytics, time-stretched healthcare facilities can optimize staffing while predicting operating room demands, ultimately streamlining patient care.

4.7.1.1.5 Advanced Risk and Disease Management

The type of medication, symptoms, and frequency of medical visits, among many others, enable healthcare facilities to provide accurate preventive care and ultimately reduce hospital admissions.

This level of risk assessment will not only result in reduced costs of home care, but will also ensure that space and resources are available for those most in need. This is a clear example of how healthcare analytics can improve and save lives.

4.7.1.2 Cloud Computing Technology

In addition to big data technology, cloud computing technology is also applied in healthcare. Cloud computing is as important as big data analytics for risk management.

Healthcare institutions use all three types of cloud technology (public, private, and hybrid). Healthcare institutions can share and use common health data using public cloud infrastructure (Bhambri et al., 2022). (Patient information is not included here.)

In addition, they also use private cloud infrastructure to securely transfer and share electronic health and medical records. Such information includes patient medical records, physician inquiries, etc.

Hybrid cloud infrastructure can retain all the main and positive features of private and public cloud infrastructure. Healthcare institutions can use the hybrid cloud when collaborating. At this time, they can share shared information as a feature of the public cloud, and they can keep their private patients' information in a confidential form, as a feature of the private cloud (Rani et al., 2023).

4.8 THE FUTURE OF HEALTHCARE

When it comes to the future of healthcare, many different ideas come to mind. The future of healthcare is not limited to the slogan "a healthy world". Rather, a completely sane future thinking is full of uncertainties. However, the right management of health care can bring us closer to this motto.

The correct use of technology makes it possible to analyze diseases in the correct form and make a correct diagnosis. In this respect, future healthcare may be ahead of current healthcare. The main condition is the correct management of technological capabilities. Data exchange is the foundation of these opportunities.

Big data, cloud computing – respectively Internet of Things, machine learning, deep learning, reinforced learning, artificial intelligence – are all areas that need proper data management.

In fact, the basic purpose and field of use of all technologies are directed towards the same point.

Diagnosis. Storing data collected through Internet of Things devices in a database. Then the operations performed on this data. With proper data management, the machine can give correct diagnosis. The basis of this is based on previous experiences and the information got from these experiences.

From the foundation to the final development of any healthcare institution (completion of development is a vague concept because development must continue. Shortly after the development stops, the stage of bankruptcy occurs), the stages of development can be ranked as follows:

1. Provision of the basic design of the healthcare facility
2. Complete design and project planning
3. Implementation of the plan

This standard is intended for the external and internal image project of the enterprise. And the main stages in internal management

1. Equipping the enterprise with latest model technologies
2. Establishing management infrastructure
3. Staff training
4. Continuous and continuous exchange
5. Conducting analytics and assessing existing risks

Implementation of joint work between technology and live staff (this is especially important, because steps are taken to justify new technological trends in human-based systems).

4.9 CONCLUSION

With the slogan "Healthy World", not only should people be promised a life in which they are physically healthy, but also spiritually healthy. In modern times, our health is entrusted not only to humans, but also to smart machines (Rana et al., 2021).

However, it should also be taken into account that today is a period when human communication begins to weaken. It's true that robotic medical assistants are one of the most loyal assistants for doctors (as well as patients). Nevertheless, is this any kind of machine that sick people would like to see next to them (around them) in their spiritual and physical "battles", or are they living beings that can understand their thoughts (Khanh & Khang, 2021).

In this era when people become robots and robots become human, there is a greater need for human "touch" and "breath" in any field, in any sector. There are ongoing studies on this topic today; CPSSs are one of the main examples of this.

Placing the person in the center of the system, as it was in the "past" time, is an important factor (Rani et al., 2022).

We should not see robots as anything more than assistants. It is, of course, appropriate to use robots – auxiliary machines in areas that are difficult for people, in areas where there is a lack of human personnel (Khang et al., 2022e).

However, a world in which only robots work instead of humans will be a world of robots, not humans, which, even if it sounds "funny", will create danger for the human "race" (Khang et al., 2022a).

In general, the following results are from the topic:

1. Today, the development of healthcare, the service provided by healthcare institutions is closely related to its design and location. Most of all, people will choose their home as the place where they feel most comfortable. In this regard, creating a "home" environment for patients receiving hospital treatment is the greatest moral service.
2. Modern healthcare is a sector that needs to use technological capabilities at a high level. And now a wide range of technologies are applied in healthcare. Big data, Internet of Things, machine learning, deep learning, etc. (Khang et al., 2023c).
3. One of the most important factors in the healthcare sector is data exchange and proper data management (Khang et al., 2023d).

REFERENCES

Babasaheb J., Sphurti B., Khang A., "Industry Revolution 4.0: Workforce competency models and designs," *Designing Workforce Management Systems for Industry 4.0: Data-Centric and AI-Enabled Approaches*, (1st ed.), (2023), pp. 14–31. CRC Press. 10.1201/9781003357070-2

Bhambri P., Rani S., Gupta G., Khang A., "Cloud and fog computing platforms for internet of things," ISBN: 978-1-032-101507, (2022). CRC Press. 10.1201/9781003213888

Bresnick J., "What is deep learning and how will it change healthcare?" (2023) Retrieved from https://healthitanalytics.com/features/what-is-deep-learning-and-how-will-it-change-healthcare

Dash S., Shakyawar S. K., Sharma M., Kaushik S., "Big data in healthcare: management, analysis and future prospects," *Journal of Big Data volume 6, Article number: 54 (2019) Published: 19 June 2019.* https://link.springer.com/article/10.1186/s40537-019-0217-0

Hajimahmud V. A., Khang A., Hahanov V., Litvinova E., Chumachenko S., Alyar A. V., "Autonomous robots for smart city: Closer to augmented humanity," *AI-Centric Smart City Ecosystems: Technologies, Design and Implementation* (1st Ed.), (2022). CRC Press. 10.1201/9781003252542-7

HER, (Electronic Health Record) vs. EMR (Electronic Medical Records)). (2021). Retrieved from https://www.practicefusion.com/blog/ehr-vs-emr/

Khang A., Chowdhury S., Sharma, S. (Eds.), *The Data-Driven Blockchain Ecosystem: Fundamentals, Applications, and Emerging Technologies* (1st ed.), (2022a). CRC Press. 10.1201/9781003269281

Khang A., Gupta S. K., Hajimahmud V. A., Babasaheb J., Morris G., *AI-Centric Modelling and Analytics: Concepts, Designs, Technologies, and Applications* (1st Ed.), (2023a). CRC Press. 10.1201/9781003400110

Khang A., Gupta S. K., Rani S., Karras D. A., (Eds.), *Smart Cities: IoT Technologies, Big Data Solutions, Cloud Platforms, and Cybersecurity Techniques* (1st Ed.), (2023b). CRC Press. 10.1201/9781003376064

Khang A., Gupta S. K., Shah V., Misra A., (Eds.), *AI-Aided IoT Technologies and Applications in the Smart Business and Production* (1st Ed.), (2023c). CRC Press. 10.1201/9781003392224

Khang A., Hahanov V., Abbas G. L., Hajimahmud V. A., "Cyber-Physical-Social System and İncident Management," *AI-Centric Smart City Ecosystems: Technologies, Design and Implementation* (1st Ed.), (2022b). CRC Press. 10.1201/9781003252542-2

Khang A., Hahanov V., Litvinova E., Chumachenko S., Hajimahmud V. A., Alyar A. V., "The key assistant of smart city – Sensors and tools," *AI-Centric Smart City Ecosystems: Technologies, Design and Implementation* (1st ed.), (2022c). CRC Press. 10.1201/9781 003252542-17

Khang A., Ragimova N. A., Hajimahmud V. A., Alyar A. V., "Advanced technologies and data management in the smart healthcare system," *AI-Centric Smart City Ecosystems: Technologies, Design and Implementation* (1st Ed.), (2022d). CRC Press. 10.1201/9781003252542-16

Khang A., Rana G., Tailor R. K., Hajimahmud V. A., (Eds.), *Data-Centric AI Solutions and Emerging Technologies in the Healthcare Ecosystem* (1st Ed.), (2023d). CRC Press. 10.1201/9781003356189

Khang A., Rani S., Gujrati R., Uygun H., Gupta S. K., (Eds.), *Designing Workforce Management Systems for Industry 4.0: Data-Centric and AI-Enabled Approaches* (1st Ed.), (2023e). CRC Press. 10.1201/99781003357070

Khang A., Rani S., Sivaraman A. K., *AI-Centric Smart City Ecosystems: Technologies, Design and Implementation* (1st Ed.), (2022e). CRC Press. 10.1201/9781003252542

Khanh H. H., Khang A., "The role of artificial intelligence in blockchain applications," *Reinventing Manufacturing and Business Processes through Artificial Intelligence*, pp. 20–40, (2021). CRC Press. 10.1201/9781003145011-2

Mathad K., Khang A., "Hospital 4.0: Capitalization of health and healthcare in Industry 4.0 economy," *Data-Centric AI Solutions and Emerging Technologies in the Healthcare Ecosystem.* (1st ed.), (2023), P (4). CRC Press. 10.1201/9781003356189-19

Ragimova N. A., Abdullayev V. H., Mikayilzada L. A., "The role of big data in the healthcare: Its applications, benefits, affects and future", *The 17th International Conference on "Technical and Physical Problems of Engineering"*, 18–19 October 2021, Istanbul Rumeli University, Istanbul, Turkey. http://www.iotpe.com/IJTPE/IJTPE-2021/IJTPE-Issue47-Vol13-No2-Jun2021/16-IJTPE-Issue47-Vol13-No2-Jun2021-pp98-106.pdf

Rana G., Khang A., Sharma R., Goel A. K., Dubey A. K., "Reinventing manufacturing and business processes through artificial intelligence", (Eds.). (2021). CRC Press. 10.1201/9781003145011

Rani S., Bhambri P., Kataria A., Khang A., "Smart city ecosystem: Concept, sustainability, design principles and technologies," *AI-Centric Smart City Ecosystems: Technologies, Design and Implementation* (1st Ed.), (2022). CRC Press. 10.1201/9781003252542-1

Rani S., Bhambri P., Kataria A., Khang A., Sivaraman A. K. (Eds.), *Big Data, Cloud Computing and IoT: Tools and Applications* (1st Ed.), (2023). Chapman and Hall/CRC. 10.1201/9781003298335

Rani S., Chauhan M., Kataria A., Khang A., "IoT equipped intelligent distributed framework for smart healthcare systems," *Networking and Internet Architecture*, (Eds.), (2021). CRC Press. 10.48550/arXiv.2110.04997

Robots and Telemedicine, *What America can learn from China's use of robots and telemedicine to combat the coronavirus?* (2023) Retrieved from https://www.cnbc.com/2020/03/18/how-china-is-using-robots-and-telemedicine-to-combat-the-coronavirus.html

Vrushank S., Vidhi T., Khang, A., 2023. "Electronic health records security and privacy enhancement using blockchain technology," *Data-Centric AI Solutions and Emerging
Technologies in the Healthcare Ecosystem.* (1st ed.), (2023), P (1). CRC Press. 10.1201/
9781003356189-1

Yeung J., Regan H., Renton A., Reynolds E., Alfonso F. III, CNN. Updated 10:42 p.m. ET,
*Wuhan will need 14 days without new cases to consider lifting restrictions, official says.
March 19 coronavirus news.* (March 19, 2020) https://edition.cnn.com/world/live-news/
coronavirus-outbreak-03-19-20-intl-hnk/h_f58997bd3e608eae2d1cacd086ed36e6

5 Deep Transfer-Learning Model for COVID-19 Diagnosis with Feature Extraction-Based SVM and KNN Classifiers

Rahul Gowtham Poola, Siva Sankar Y., and Uday Sankar V.

CONTENTS

5.1 INTRODUCTION

Global health is in distress due to the unique COVID-19 pandemic, which is still a major concern. One of the first lines of defense against this pandemic is preliminary infection diagnosis, which aims to stop the spread of illnesses. The contemporary yardstick for COVID-19 diagnosis is RT-PCR (Khang et al., 2022a).

However, a considerable hurdle has been created by the sudden spread of COVID-19 and the lack of laboratory kits. As a result, during the COVID-19 pandemic, radiological exams have gained more appeal as a means of diagnosing infections. It is unrealistic to rely entirely on chest CT scans coupled with the fact that they have been proved to be more trustworthy because of the growing number of patients and the resulting rise in radiological testing (Tailor et al., 2022).

Due to the significant burden that a heavy reliance on CT scans will place on radiology professionals, X-ray chest radiographs are a more feasible option for COVID-19 diagnosis. The development of lung anomalies should be monitored throughout time, even though CXRs are thought to be less sensitive in the early stages of pulmonary involvement in COVID-19.

Numerous radiographic symptoms of COVID-19, including consolidation, reticular interstitial thickening, ground-glass opacities, lung nodules, and pleural effusion, have been detected and characterized in other research.

The classification of medical images has been significantly aided by the use of ML and DL, two branches of AI. For research, modeling, and pattern detection, the use of ML and DL has taken center stage (Khanh & Khang, 2021).

The expansion of medical image and radiography databases, along with recent advancements in these fields, open up new possibilities for enhancing medical decision-making systems. Deep learning model-based medical-imaging can be utilized with COVID-19 to examine X-ray chest radiographs. Deep learning algorithms perform better than conventional machine learning models, according to research literature (Khang et al., 2023c).

In the diagnosis of pharmaceutical targets, the feed-forward network outperformed SVM and random forest models, according to Mayr (2018). Similar results were discovered that deep learning models beat random forest and SVM in determining the vulnerability of landslides. Deep neural networks outperformed SVM in a variety of drug discovery tasks, according to Korotcov, (2017).

Although each of the aforementioned experiments has a different focus, they have all demonstrated that DL models surpass conventional ML models. Deep learning has additional advantages over conventional machine learning models, including the ability to learn multiple tasks at once and the ability to automatically extract complicated characteristics. This demonstrates how deep learning may be quite helpful for the key issue of COVID-19 identification (Rana et al., 2021).

Three cutting-edge models, NASNet-Large, InceptionNet-ResNet-V2, and InceptionNet-V3 have been used in the past to classify data without the use of supplementary classifiers with minimal data (Rani et al., 2021). The accuracy of the final result and the overall accuracy of the model are both improved by InceptionNet V3.

Working with scaled images is made easier by InceptionNet V3's inclusion of features from V1 and V2. The InceptionNet-ResNet-V2 has been applied to classify breast cancer tissue images, and it has shown enhanced performance when employing data augmentation. Studies have shown that trained image-net algorithms perform better. ResNet has been applied to the task of detecting COVID-19 in chest X-ray images.

The outcome revealed a sensitivity of 96.0% and an AUC of 0.952. DL models are fine-tuned with the aid of transfer learning. Data augmentation can be used to manage a small dataset (Bhambri et al., 2022).

A deep learning image classification issue can benefit from data augmentation in terms of training efficiency. The diagnoses of prevalent thoracic disorders and the distinction between bacterial and viral pneumonia using deep learning have both been demonstrated to be highly effective (Rani et al., 2022).

The issue also lies in creating an algorithm that can recognize a patient with COVID-19. Even so, COVID-19 can exhibit radiographic characteristics that are comparable to those of other kinds of pneumonia, making this work problematic. When the training dataset solely contained cases of bacterial pneumonia, MobileNet performed poorly at differentiating COVID-19 cases from other cases, according to the authors.

The COVID-19 against non-COVID classification presents a considerable gap regarding the amount of COVID-19 against non-COVID-19 samples.

5.2 OVERVIEW OF DEEP TRANSFER-LEARNING IN MEDICAL IMAGING

Several ML and DL research have been carried out for the monitoring of chest disorders generally rather than being done specifically for the diagnosis of COVID-19. For the purpose of identifying disorders that affect the chest, Arimura (2002) used a template-matching technique.

In order to locate hernias, Lehmann (2003) made use of the conventional K-nearest neighbor method. To classify chest radiographs, Kao (2006) used two feature-based systems that can take advantage of body symmetry and backdrop information. Computed CT performed by Jian-Xin Yang accurately identified lung atelectasis consolidations in 81 patients.

Pietka (1992) proposed a method to distinguish radiographs for the detection of chest illness. It used a neural network approach utilizing the properties of the projection profiles to classify the radiographs. Similar to this, Kao et al.'s (2006) technique for establishing a view-invariant mechanism for diagnosing chest infections was presented.

To diagnose pneumonia, Luo (2020) used Bayes' decision theory. In addition to the aggregate intensity of the ROI, the criteria they employed included the presence and form of the anatomical components. Using Vgg-16 and ResNet-101 in deep learning, it categorized lung images into ten categories with 90% accuracy and estimated tuberculosis levels using a 3D block residual network and CT lung images.

An analysis highlighted the benefits of CNN for COVID-19 diagnosis using X-rays. To address tiny dataset issues, transfer learning was applied. The COVID-19 dataset includes 224 sample X-ray chest radiographs.

In order to attain the highest results, transfer learning was combined with a DeTraC architecture by Abbas (2020). His model had a 95.12% accuracy rate and a 97.91% sensitivity rate, respectively. The segmentation model based on UNet++ was used by Chen to predict whether patients were COVID-19 infected or not.

COVID-19 diagnostic has demonstrated the effectiveness of using DL algorithms to manipulate the extracted characteristics. The detection of COVID-19 based on X-rays is accomplished by Wang using a deep CNN model.

The model had a 98.9% accuracy rate. In order to automatically identify people with coronavirus infections using chest X-ray radiographs, Hemdan (2020) developed a COVIDX-Net.

With regard to COVID cases, COVIDX-classification Net's accuracy was 91%. For the categorization of COVID-19 from chest X-ray chest radiographs, Narin et al. (2003) proposed distinct CNN algorithms, including InceptionNet-ResNet-V2, ResNet-50, and InceptionV3. In comparison to the other models, ResNet50 had a classification accuracy of 98%.

Sethy and Behera (2020) employed the pre-trained transfer learning model ResNet-50 to extract the image attributes from the patients infected. The developed model's classification accuracy was 95.3%. For the pre-trained ResNet-50 architecture, Farooq and Hafeez (2020) presented fine-tuned multistage technique. The created model is known as COVIDResNet.

COVIDResNet reported 96.23% accuracy. For the diagnosis of COVID-19, Asnaoui (2020) performed an evaluation of multiple transfer learning approaches. Classification accuracy of 96% was offered by MobileNet-V2 and Inception-V3. Decompose, Transfer, and Compose (DeTraC) is a deep CNN that Abbas (2020) described for differentiating COVID symptoms using chest radiographs; 95.12% accuracy and 97.91% sensitivity were attained with the DeTraC model.

The detection of coronavirus infection on chest radiographs was proposed by Chowdhury (2020) using a transfer-learning model based on image augmentation. Four popular pre-trained methods—ResNet-18, DenseNet-201, SqueezeNet and AlexNet—are utilized for classification. For the purpose of early COVID-19 symptom detection in patients, Alqudah et al. (2021) employed ML techniques, based on random forest and SVM. They extracted features using the CNN model.

To diagnose COVID-19 through a chest radiograph, Ghoshal and Tucker (2020) applied Bayesian-based CNN. BCNN's classification accuracy was 90%. A trained CNN model was used by Salman (2020) to detect coronavirus infection on X-ray chest radiographs.

The model yielded 100% accuracy in terms of sensitivity and specificity. A deep CNN model called COVID-Xpert was developed by Li and Zhu (2020) to capture image attributes from X-ray chest radiographs. In order to automatically identify COVID-19 symptoms, Karim (2020) developed a Deep COVID Explainer model that employed an ensemble method that included image processing and transfer learning strategies.

In order to identify coronavirus patterns from the patient's X-rays, it engaged a transfer learning approach. Using chest X-ray scans, Ozturk (2020) created a DarkNet Model for categorizing binary and multiclass tasks of COVID X-rays. It achieved classification accuracy ratings of 98.08% for binary and 87.02% for multi-class.

Using X-ray chest radiographs, Deep CNN was employed to identify and classify coronavirus infection. Asif and Wenhui (2020) suggested a COVID-19 intelligent detection approach using X-ray chest radiographs. Inception-V3 with transfer learning was employed to find the infection in the X-ray chest radiographs.

For the purpose of detecting COVID-19 in chest X-rays, Ozturk T (2020) built a GAN-based deep learning technique including ResNet-18, GoogleNet, and AlexNet.

In a study of seven alternative deep learning architectures for identifying COVID-19 symptoms in X-ray chest radiographs, (Asnaoui, Chawki, & Idri, 2020) conducted a comparative analysis.

5.3   PROPOSED METHODOLOGY

The methodology is intended to assess the efficiency and precision of several deep transfer learning models. Seven key stages make up the suggested methodology. The initial stage is data collection, followed by data pre-processing that gets the chest X-ray chest radiographs ready for feature extraction, where a number of edge features of X-ray chest radiographs are extracted (Rani et al., 2023).

VGG-19, Inception-V3, SqueeezeNet, VGG-16, ResNet-50, and AlexNet are among the deep transfer-learning models that are trained using the retrieved features in the fourth stage. The deep transfer-learning models' training accuracy and loss function are assessed.

The COVID and non-COVID X-ray chest radiographs are classified using SVM and KNN classifiers using the deep transfer-learning model, which has a high degree of accuracy and a low loss function (Khang et al., 2022b). As a reference for classification, the classifiers employ the feature label established during the training phase based on the features extracted as in figure 5.1.

5.3.1   DATASET COLLECTION STAGE

The dataset includes the COVID and non-COVID classes. The proposed methodology employs 30% of the dataset for validation and 70% of the dataset for training. The dataset includes 10192 non-COVID and 3616 COVID X-ray chest radiographs. All of the images have a resolution of either $1024 \times 1024 \times 3$ pixels or $229 \times 229 \times 3$ pixels and are stored in the .PNG file format.

To standardize the dataset for smooth execution, the photos were reduced to $229 \times 229 \times 1$ pixel before being fed into a pre-trained model for feature extraction.

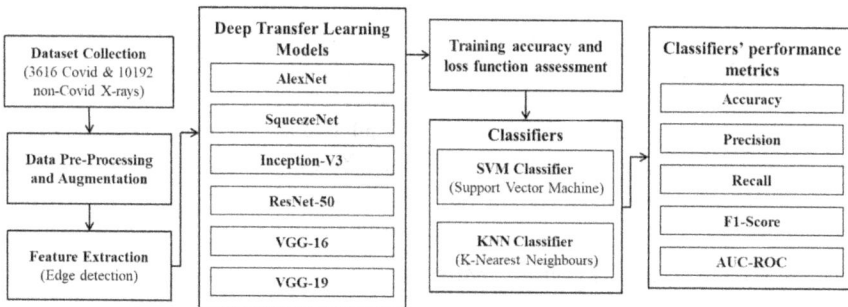

FIGURE 5.1 Proposed methodology.

Source: Author's owner.

5.3.2   Data Pre-processing and Augmentation Stage

Lowering the computational complexity is the main objective of adopting deep transfer learning models in most image classification tasks. To decrease the computational load and speed up processing, the original images were downsized from $1024 \times 1024 \times 3$ to $224 \times 224 \times 1$ pixel.

For eliminating unwanted noise from the given image, pre-processing techniques can be significant. Hidden information that is present in the low range of the gray level image is revealed by adjusting the pixel intensity.

Image rotation, scaling, flipping, and translation are forms of data augmentation techniques. Stretching, rotating, reflecting, scaling, and shearing existing photographs are all examples of data augmentation strategies.

5.3.3   Feature Extraction Stage

The method of extracting numerical features from unfiltered raw data while retaining the data from the source image is known as feature extraction. Compared to directly applying machine learning to the raw data, it produces better outcomes.

In order to extract features from images, feature extraction employs specialized algorithms. The important areas of an image are represented as a small feature vector by a feature extraction algorithm. Computer vision applications such as classification, object identification, image registration, and content-based image retrieval call for an efficient representation of image features.

Erosion, dilation, border clearing, boundary tracing, and feature extraction as a string value are all tasks carried out during the feature extraction stage. To remove unwanted objects, the ROI's bounds are eroded. The ROI borders are then dilated to incorporate the final ROI boundary objects. After that, "imclearborder" and "bwareopen" are used to clear the borders of any remaining minor edge fragments.

By using "bwboundary," which traces the boundaries, the feature extraction result is transformed into a mathematical string value. The number of edges found in the input image is represented by the mathematical string value.

The number of edges found in the input image is represented by the mathematical string value. The number of edges constitutes the features of the images extracted to classify COVID and non-COVID X-ray chest radiographs.

A feature label set is created based on the feature extraction decision condition. The number of edges that were retrieved from the input photos is listed in the feature label set. With feature extraction values in the range below 100 are classified as COVID classes, while images with a value range beyond 100 are classified as non-COVID classes. The feature label is used to classify chest X-ray radiographs into COVID and non-COVID categories using classifiers.

5.3.4   Deep Transfer-Learning Models

Transfer learning in machine learning is the use of a model that has already been trained on an unfamiliar task. In transfer learning, the algorithm actionable intelligence acquired from a previous assignment enhances prediction about a new task.

The initial layer of neural networks used in computer vision aims to detect images, the intermediate layer handles image processing, and the latter layers collect task-specific features. Reduced training time and enhanced neural network performance are the two most significant benefits of transfer learning.

A pre-trained model is trained by deep transfer-learning and reused for different tasks based on the features extracted from the images. Transfer learning usually makes it faster and simpler to make minor adjustments to a previously trained network than to start from zero and train a network with randomly initialized weights.

Image input, convolution, max pooling, ReLu activation, fully connected, softmax, batch normalization, concatenation, dropout, global average pooling, depth concatenation, and output classification layers are the layers that make up deep transfer-learning models. Deep transfer-learning models like VGG-19, Inception-V3, SqueeezeNet, VGG-16, ResNet-50, and AlexNet are optimized to classify COVID X-ray chest radiographs based on feature extraction-based model training.

5.3.4.1 Layer Description of Deep Transfer-Learning Models

Convolutional layer, sometimes called the base layer of CNN, is in charge of identifying patterns in input images. The CNN is assisted in extracting low-level and high-level features by a filter made up of feature maps and kernels that are applied to images from the training dataset.

A 3×3 or 5×5 matrix that is part of the filter layer's kernel transforms with the input image matrix. The stride parameter controls how many steps will be tweaked to shift over the input matrix. After gathering similar data in the area around the region of interest, the pooling layer, sometimes referred to as a down-sampling layer, outputs the dominating response in the image.

The activation function's job is to modify the weighted sum input of one node for a layer and use it to activate the node for the specific input. The fully connected layer, which is employed for classification at the conclusion of the deep CNN network, is the most important layer of CNN. The features that were collected from the network at various levels are used as the input for this stage, and the outputs from all the layers before it are compared.

The batch normalization layer enables the network's layers to undergo learning more independently. The output of the earlier layers is normalized, which aids in tackling issues caused by the internal covariance shift.

By randomly skipping some units or connections within the deep CNN network with a particular probability, dropout is utilized to add regularization and demonstrate generalization. Several flattened network architectures are produced as a result of the elimination of some random links or components. Inputs are concatenated along a specific dimension using a concatenation layer.

Except for the concatenation dimension, all of the inputs need to be the same size. In traditional CNNs, fully connected layers are to be replaced with a pooling technique called global average pooling. For each category that corresponds to the classification problem, a feature map is intended to be provided in the final convolution layer.

Instead of constructing fully connected layers on top of the feature maps, the average feature map is computed, and the vector result is directed to the softmax layer. The neural network's final layer, the classification output layer, is where the

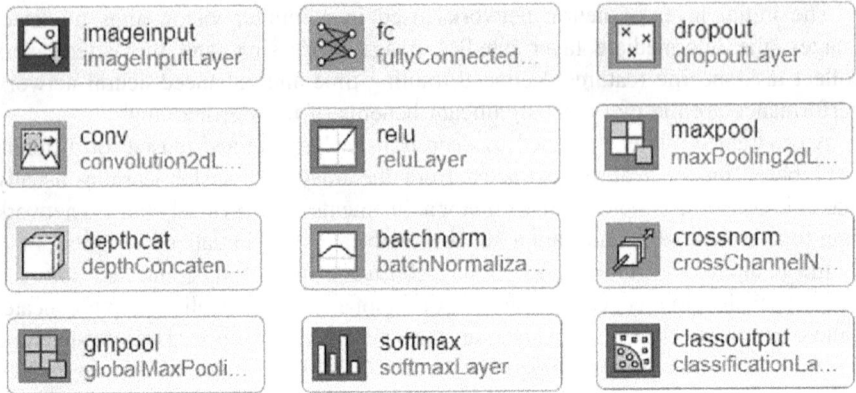

FIGURE 5.2 Layer description of deep transfer-learning models.

Source: Author's owner.

intended predictions are made. A neural network has a single output layer that generates the desired outcome, as in figure 5.2.

5.3.4.2 AlexNet

The winner of ILSVRC 2012 was the AlexNet architecture, which greatly outperformed the hand-crafted features. With 24 connections between each layer, the AlexNet model has a depth of 25 layers. The input image layer size is optimized to 229 × 229 × 1 dimensions in the AlexNet architecture.

Following each convolution layer, there are max pooling layers for sampling and ReLU activation layers. The resulting architecture for classifying the images consists of 5 convolution, 3 fully connected, 7 nonlinear activation (ReLu), 3 max pooling, 2 dropout, 1 softmax, 1 cross channel normalization, and an output layer for classification. The following figure 5.3 illustrates an optimized AlexNet architecture.

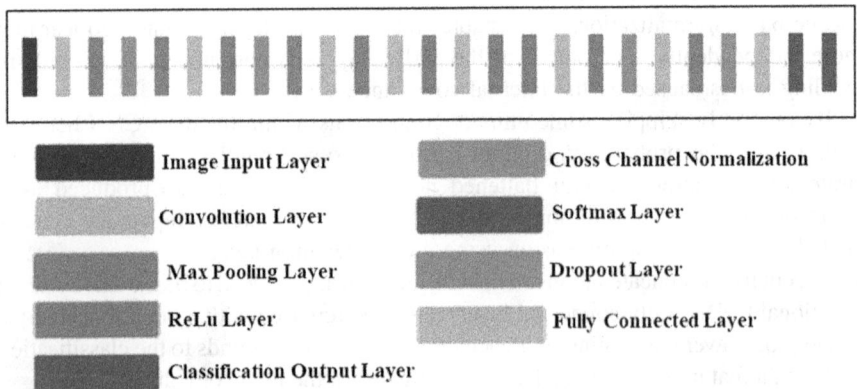

FIGURE 5.3 AlexNet architecture.

Source: Author's owner.

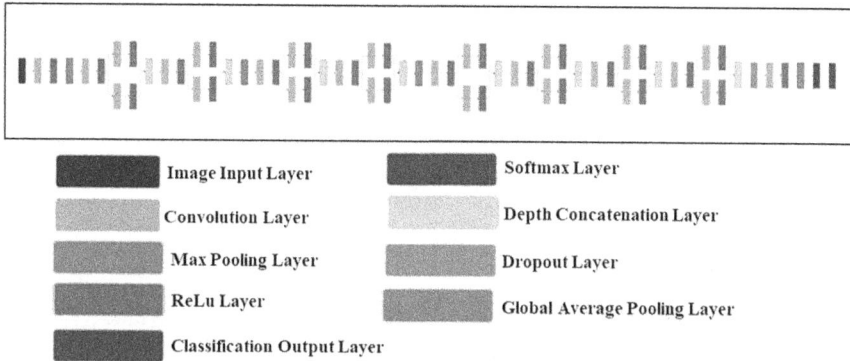

FIGURE 5.4   SqueezeNet architecture.

Source: Author's owner.

5.3.4.3   SqueezeNet

A compact architecture termed *SqueezeNet* employs the fire module concept. With 75 connections between each layer, the SqueezeNet model has a depth of 68 layers. The input image layer size is optimized to $229 \times 229 \times 1$ dimensions in the SqueezeNet architecture.

The resulting architecture for classifying the pictures consists of 26 convolution layers, 26 ReLu nonlinear activation, 3 max pooling, 1 dropout, 1 softmax, 8 depth concatenation, 1 global average pooling, and a classification output layer.

SqueezeNet employ filters of (3×3) with a stride of 1 in the convolution layers and filters of 2×2 with a stride of 2 in the max pooling layers, as shown in figure 5.4.

5.3.4.4   Inception-V3

Label smoothing and an auxiliary classifier are used by Inception-V3 to convey label information down the network, along with batch normalization for side head layers. It has smaller convolutions for faster training and a smaller grid to get over the limitations of computing expenses.

The approaches include dimension reduction, regularization, factorized convolutions, and parallel calculations. With 349 connections between each layer, the Inception-V3 model has a depth of 315 layers.

The input image layer size is optimized to $229 \times 229 \times 1$ dimensions in the Inception-V3 architecture. The resulting architecture for classifying the images consists of 94 convolution layers, 1 fully connected layer, 93 ReLu nonlinear activation layers, 5 max pooling layers, 10 average pooling layers, 1 softmax layer, 94 batch normalization layers, 15 depth concatenation layers, and a classification output layer to classify the images.

In the max pooling layers, Inception-V3 employs filters of (3×3) with a stride of 1 and 5×5 with a stride of 1 in the convolution layers and filters of (2×2) with a stride of 2 in the ReLu activation and max pooling layers. The following figure 5.5 illustrates optimized Inception-V3 architecture.

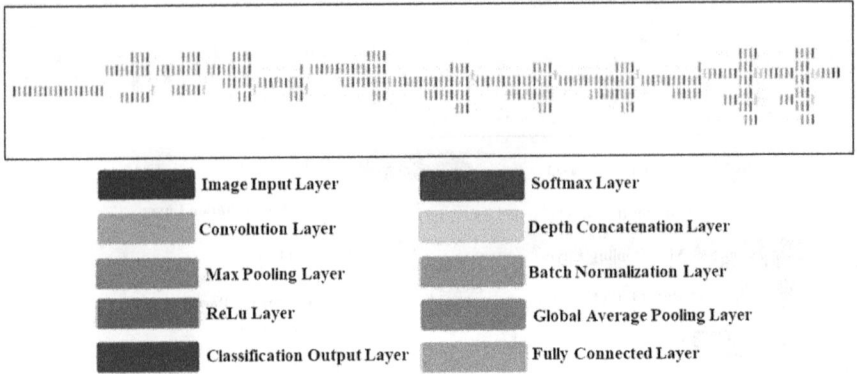

FIGURE 5.5   Inception-V3 architecture.

Source: Author's owner.

5.3.4.5   ResNet-50

"Residual network" is referred to as ResNet. Compared to other systems, this architecture is intended to be far more robust. With 192 connections between each layer, the ResNet-50 model has a depth of 177 layers. The input image layer size is optimized to 229 × 229 × 1 dimensions in the ResNet-50 architecture.

The resulting architecture for classifying the images consists of 53 convolution, 1 fully connected, 49 ReLu nonlinear activation, 1 max pooling, 1 global pooling, and 53 batch normalization, 1 softmax, and an output layer for classification. ResNet-50 employs filters of (3 × 3) with a stride of 2 in convolution layers and (3 × 3) with a stride of 2 in the max pooling layers.

It has the capacity to classify images into many classes. The following figure 5.6 illustrates optimized ResNet-50 architecture.

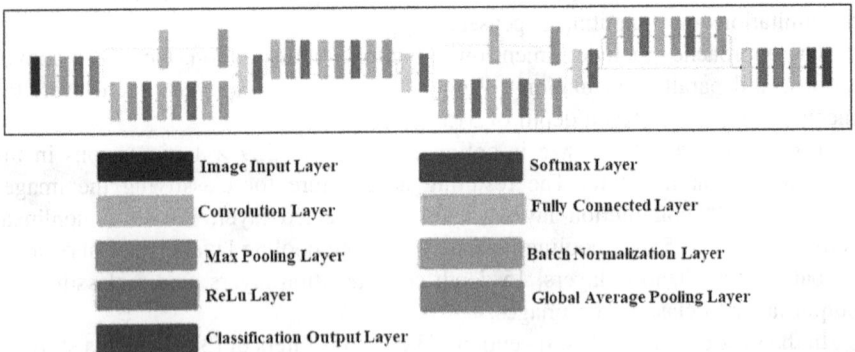

FIGURE 5.6   ResNet-50 architecture.

Source: Author's owner.

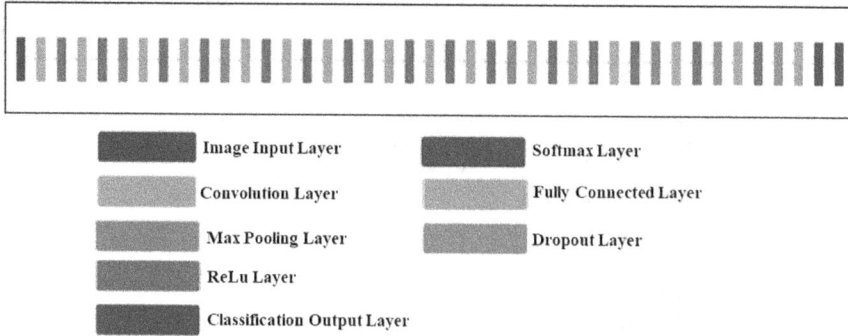

FIGURE 5.7   VGG-16 architecture.

Source: Author's owner.

5.3.4.6   VGG-16

VGG stands for the visual geometry group. The main idea behind VGG architectures is to create a deep network while maintaining a moderate and consistent convolution size. The number "16" in the VGG-16 architecture stands for a total of 3 fully connected layers and 13 convolution layers.

With 40 connections between each layer, the VGG-16 model has a depth of 41 layers. The input image layer size is optimized to $229 \times 229 \times 1$ dimensions in the VGG16 architecture. The resulting architecture for classifying the images consists of 13 convolution, 3 fully connected, 15 ReLu nonlinear activation, 5 max pooling, 2 dropout, 1 softmax, and an output layer for classification.

VGG-16 employs filters of 3×3 with a stride of 1 in the convolution layer, filters of (2×2) with a stride of 2 in the ReLu activation layer and max pooling layers as shown in figure 5.7.

5.3.4.7   VGG-19

In the VGG-19 design, the number "19" stands for a total of 16 convolutions and 3 fully connected layers. With 46 connections between each layer, the VGG-19 model has a depth of 47 layers. The input image layer size is optimized to $229 \times 229 \times 1$ dimensions in the VGG-19 architecture.

The resulting architecture for classifying the images consists of 16 convolution, 3 fully connected, 18 ReLu nonlinear activation, 5 max pooling, 2 dropout, 1 softmax, and an output layer for classification. VGG-19 employs a filter of (3×3) with a stride of 1 in the convolution layer, a filter of (3×3) with a stride of 1 in the convolution layer, filter of (2×2) with a stride of 2 in the ReLu activation, and max pooling layers as figure 5.8.

5.4   RESULTS AND DISCUSSION

To classify COVID and non-COVID X-ray chest radiographs, deep transfer-learning models including VGG-19, Inception-V3, SqueeezeNet, VGG-16, ResNet-50, and AlexNet are trained by employing the features retrieved from edge detection.

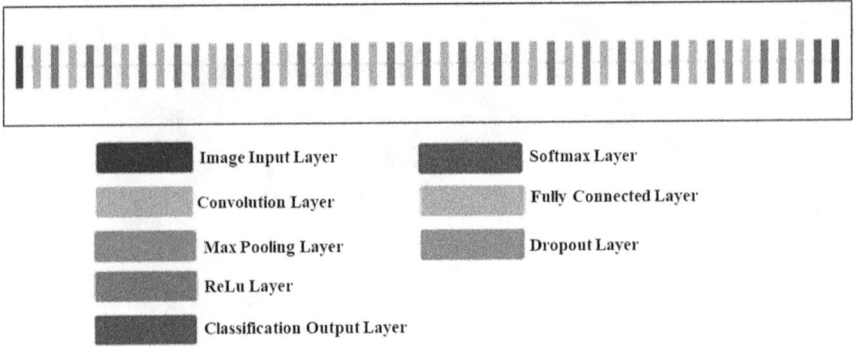

FIGURE 5.8 VGG-19 architecture.

Source: Author's owner.

Monitoring the training process is frequently helpful when a network is trained for a deep learning application. The training progress is examined by plotting different metrics throughout the training.

Deep transfer-learning model training performance evaluation criteria include accuracy and loss function. On each individual mini-batch, training accuracy defines classification accuracy. On the full validation set, validation accuracy defines classification accuracy. Losses on each mini-batch and losses on the validation set are defined, respectively, by training loss and validation loss.

The methodology includes evaluating the deep transfer-learning models' accuracy and loss function. For 30 successive epochs, the accuracy and loss-function metrics were recorded. The learning rate was established at 0.01 (SGDM solver). The optimized VGG-19, Inception-V3, SqueeezeNet, VGG-16, ResNet-50, and AlexNet models' accuracy and loss function curves are illustrated in figure 5.9.

The feature label created during the training phase based on the features retrieved is used as a reference for classification by the classifiers.

The x-axes in this graph represent the number of iterations per epoch, and the y-axes represent accuracy and loss function measurements. The following table 5.1 tabulates the accuracy and loss function of optimized deep transfer learning models.

Based on the findings, the optimized Inception-V3-based deep transfer-learning model achieves the best accuracy and least loss function.

5.4.1 Optimized Inception-V3-Based Classifiers' Quality Metrics

Different forms of SVM and KNN classifiers were used to assess the quality metrics for the optimized Inception-V3. Confusion matrix, accuracy, recall, precision, F1 score, and area under the receiver operating characteristic curve are among the quality metrics for classifiers. Frequently, a confusion matrix is used to measure the effectiveness of a model on a test dataset with established actual values.

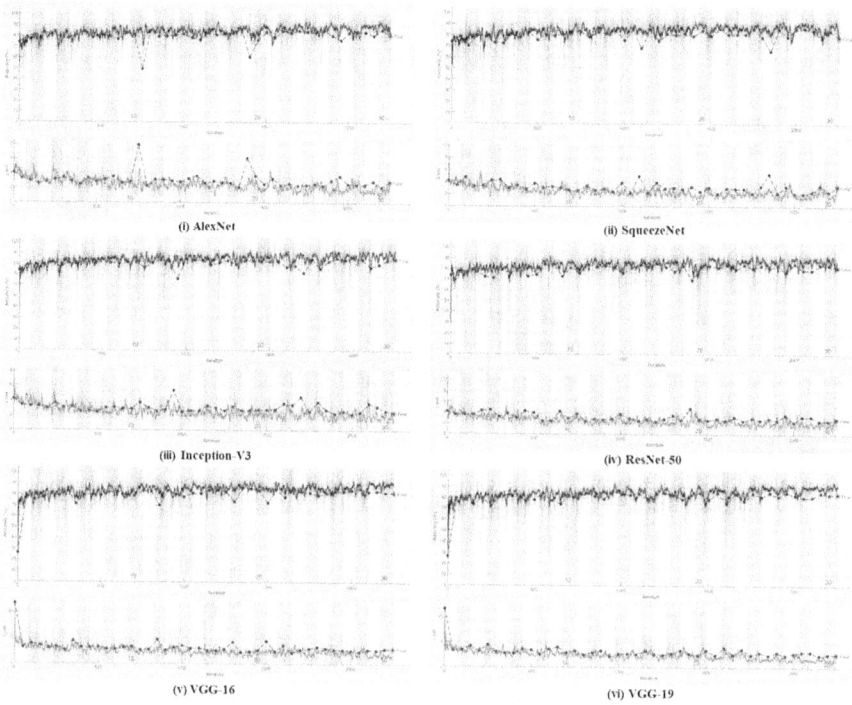

(i) AlexNet

(ii) SqueezeNet

(iii) Inception-V3

(iv) ResNet-50

(v) VGG-16

(vi) VGG-19

FIGURE 5.9 VGG-19 architecture.

Source: Author's owner.

TABLE 5.1

Accuracy and Loss-Function of Optimized Deep Transfer Learning Models

Model	Accuracy	Loss Function
AlexNet	81.73%	3.1%
SqueezeNet	78.64%	3.7%
Inception-V3	84.79%	2.4%
Resnet-50	82.02%	2.6%
VGG-16	81.58%	2.8%
VGG-19	83.44%	2.3%

Source: Author's owner.

Metrics for precision and recall show how often model predictions are accurate. False positives are taken into account by the Precision metric while false negatives are addressed by the Recall metric.

The Harmonic mean of the Precision and Recall measures is represented by the F1 score. The amount of accurate predictions out of all data samples is given by

Accuracy, which evaluates the performance of the approach as a whole. A graph displaying the effectiveness of a classification model at each classification threshold is known as a ROC curve.

The entire two-dimensional region that sits underneath the actual ROC curve is calculated by the AUC. Regardless of the categorization threshold that is used, it evaluates the accuracy of the model's predictions.

5.4.2   SVM (Support Vector Machine) Classifier

The SVM classification system is prioritized for problems involving classifications and regression under supervision. Data classification issues frequently employ it. SVM uses a technique similar to that of the kernel function to construct a linear hyper-plane among classes. SVM is superior to other classifiers for its efficiency, productivity, and reliability.

For the classification of huge datasets, it is also hailed as the best method. When there are precisely two classes in a dataset, SVM is employed. SVM classifiers work well in big dimensional domains and when the dimensionality is greater than the amount of samples. The characteristic of SVM Classifiers is customizable. If there are more features than samples, SVM has an over-fitting issue.

SVM classifiers can be classified as linear or non-linear. For data with linear separability, linear SVM is employed. For data that is not linearly separable, non-linear SVM is employed. Among the non-linear SVMs are the Cubic, Quadratic, Coarse, and Medium Gaussian classifiers. In order to categorize data, a fundamental linear SVM classifier draws a linear boundary between two groups.

All of the data points along one side of the partition will represent one category, while the data points on either side of the line will represent distinct classes. Linear SVM is easy to interpret and less flexible. Quadratic SVM is hard to interpret and moderately flexible. When dealing with the problem of limited memory, the cubic SVM classifier is effective. In multidimensional space, SVM identifies a hyper-plane that best divides the classes.

Cubic SVM is hard to interpret and moderately flexible. When learning from nonlinear datasets, Gaussian SVM is used. It is typically used to create the traditional SVM for nonlinear applications. Fine Gaussian (Hard Interpretability and High Flexibility), Medium Gaussian (Hard Interpretability and Medium Flexibility), and Coarse Gaussian (Hard Interpretability and Low flexibility) are three variants of Gaussian SVMs, as shown in figure 5.10.

The SVM classifiers whose quality metrics are reported in the corresponding table 5.2 are linear, quadratic, cubic, medium, and coarse Gaussian SVM.

The confusion matrix for every SVM classifier, both linear and nonlinear, are shown in figure 5.11.

5.4.3   KNN (K-Nearest Neighbor) Classifier

One of the nonparametric learning algorithms used for classification is KNN. Additionally, it is one of the most widely used machine learning algorithms, with several applications in areas like pattern recognition research.

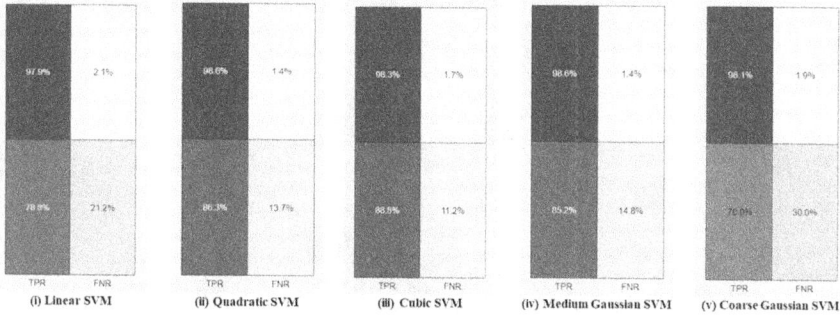

97.9% 2.1%	98.6% 1.4%	98.3% 1.7%	98.6% 1.4%	98.1% 1.9%
78.8% 21.2%	86.3% 13.7%	88.8% 11.2%	85.2% 14.8%	70.0% 30.0%
TPR FNR	TPR FNR	TPR FNR	TPR FNR	TPR FNR
(i) Linear SVM	(ii) Quadratic SVM	(iii) Cubic SVM	(iv) Medium Gaussian SVM	(v) Coarse Gaussian SVM

FIGURE 5.10 Confusion matrix of SVM classifiers.

Source: Author's owner.

TABLE 5.2
Quality Metrics of SVM Classifiers

SVM Types	Accuracy	Precision	Recall	F1 Score	AUC
Linear	92.9%	0.979	0.8219	0.89	0.97
Quadratic	95.4%	0.986	0.878	0.928	0.98
Cubic	95.8%	0.983	0.8977	0.9384	0.99
Medium Gaussian	95.1%	0.986	0.869	0.953	0.98
Coarse Gaussian	90.8%	0.981	0.765	0.859	0.95

Source: Author's owner.

KNN needs a training data set, a metric to gauge neighbor closeness, and an integer k to represent the total number of neighbors utilized for classification. The sample class is defined by the closest neighbors when k is equal to 1.

The KNN algorithm relies on the assumption that new data and existing data are similar, and it places the new example in the category that best matches the categories already in existence. A new set of data is classified using the KNN algorithm, depending on how similar the existing data is and recorded.

The KNN algorithm uses a lazy learner. Due to its laziness, the algorithm can generate models without using any training data. The testing phase is slowed down and training is accelerated as a result.

Different KNN classifiers include Fine KNN, Medium KNN, Cosine KNN, Coarse KNN, Weighted KNN, and Cosine KNN. An exceptionally accurate categorization of classes is produced by the Fine KNN classifier when the count of neighbors is set to 1.

In comparison to a Fine KNN, the Medium KNN classifier produces limited classifications when the configured count of neighbors is set to 10. The coarse KNN classifier provides crude classifications between classes when the count of neighbors is configured to 100.

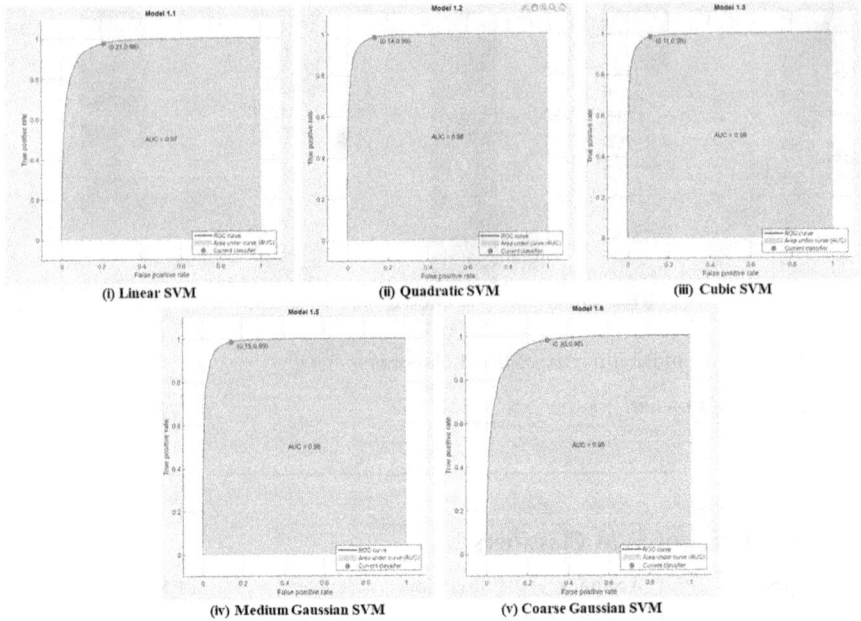

FIGURE 5.11   AUC-ROC graphs of the SVM classifiers.

Source: Author's owner.

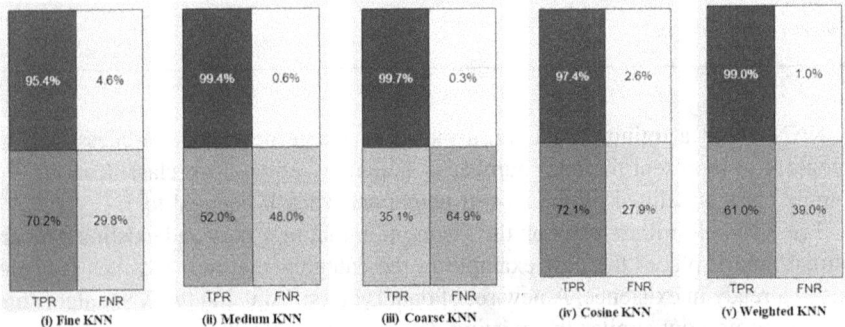

FIGURE 5.12   Confusion matrix of KNN classifiers.

Source: Author's owner.

Cosine and cubic distance measures are used by the Cosine KNN classifier and the Cubic KNN classifier, respectively. Distance weighting is a classification method used by a weighted KNN classifier as in figure 5.12 (table 5.3).

The confusion matrix for all KNN classifiers is shown in figure 5.12. The AUC-ROC graphs of the KNN classifiers employed for optimized Inception-V3-based classification are illustrated in figure 5.13.

TABLE 5.3

Quality Metrics of KNN Classifiers

KNN types	Accuracy	Precision	Recall	F1 score	AUC
Fine	88.8%	0.954	0.761	0.847	0.83
Medium	86.9%	0.994	0.674	0.803	0.94
Coarse	82.7%	0.997	0.605	0.753	0.94
Cosine	90.8%	0.974	0.777	0.864	0.95
Weighted	89.0%	0.99	0.717	0.831	0.94

Source: Author's owner.

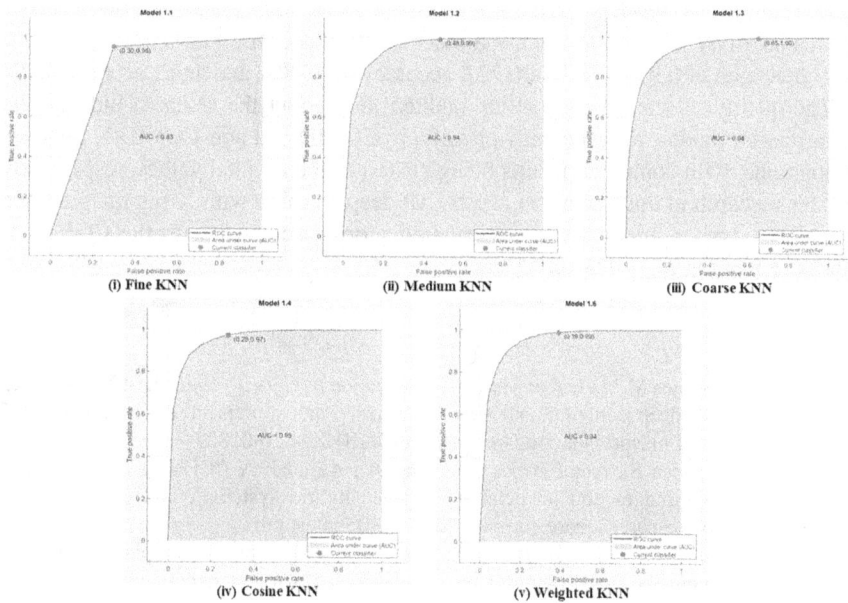

FIGURE 5.13 AUC-ROC graphs of the KNN classifiers.

Source: Author's owner.

5.5 CONCLUSION

A widespread epidemic of COVID-19 has taken effect. To prevent, diagnose, and monitor the spread, it is essential to accurately and promptly detect the presence of COVID-19 in suspected patients (Vrushank, Vidhi & Khang, 2023).

Six deep transfer-learning models, namely VGG-19, Inception-V3, SqueeezeNet, VGG-16, ResNet-50, and AlexNet, are optimized in this study to classify COVID and non-COVID X-ray chest radiographs.

The training accuracy and loss-function of the deep transfer-learning models were evaluated. The Inception-V3 dominates the six deep transfer-learning models, according to the assessment results, with a training accuracy of 84.79% and a loss function of 2.4%. Using a dataset of 3000 COVID X-ray chest radiographs and 13000 normal radiographs, the deep transfer-learning models are optimized to get a more precise diagnosis.

During training, the classification of X-ray chest radiographs based on the feature extraction stage outcome is transformed into a feature label set containing the reclassified image data, with a feature string value reflecting the number of edges detected following edge detection. Edge detection is used to extract the image features (Khang et al., 2023b).

To audit the quality metrics of the enhanced Inception-V3 deep transfer-learning model, the feature label set is further examined using SVM and KNN classifiers. The performance of Cubic SVM was superior to that of the other SVM classifiers, with an AUC score of 0.99, precision of 0.983, recall of 0.8977, accuracy of 95.8%, and F1 score of 0.9384.

Cosine KNN fared better than the other KNN classifiers with an AUC score of 0.95, precision of 0.974, recall of 0.777, accuracy of 90.8%, and an F1 score of 0.864.

The quality metric scores that are audited throughout the research indicate that the proposed model was efficiently classifying COVID and non-COVID X-ray chest radiographs, with computed results being closest to the optimal values, respectively.

This research in this chapter suggests that deep learning with X-ray imaging may be able to extract important biological indicators associated with the COVID-19 illness (Khang et al., 2023d).

REFERENCES

Abbas A., Abdelsamea M.M., Gaber M.M. "Classification of COVID-19 in chest X-ray images using detrac deep convolutional neural network". arXiv preprint. arXiv: 2003.13815, 2020. https://link.springer.com/article/10.1007/s10489-020-01829-7

Alqudah A.M., Qazan S., Alquran H., Qasmieh I.A., Alqudah A. "COVID-2019 detection using X-ray images and artificial intelligence hybrid systems", 2021. 4(3): 18–25. https://www.researchsquare.com/article/rs-24305/latest.pdf

Arimura H., Katsuragawa S., Li Q., Ishida T., Doi K. "Development of a computerized method for identifying the poster anterior and lateral views of chest radiographs by use of a template matching technique". Med Phys 2002, 29(7): 1556–1561. https://aapm.onlinelibrary.wiley.com/doi/abs/10.1118/1.1487426

Asif S., Wenhui Y. "Automatic detection of COVID-19 using X-ray images with deep convolutional neural networks and machine learning". medRxiv, 2020. https://onlinelibrary.wiley.com/doi/abs/10.1111/exsy.13099

Asnaoui K.E., Chawki Y., Idri A. "Automated methods for detection and classification pneumonia based on X-ray images using deep learning". arXiv preprint. arXiv: 2003.14363, 2020. https://link.springer.com/chapter/10.1007/978-3-030-74575-2_14

Bhambri P., Rani S., Gupta G., Khang A. "Cloud and fog computing platforms for Internet of Things". ISBN: 978-1-032-101507, 2022, CRC Press. 10.1201/9781003213888

Chowdhury M.E., Rahman T., Khandakar A., Mazhar R., Kadir M.A., Mahbub Z.B., et al. "Can AI help in screening viral and COVID-19 pneumonia? arXiv preprint". arXiv: 2003.13145, 2020. https://ieeexplore.ieee.org/abstract/document/9144185/

Farooq M., Hafeez A. "COVID-ResNet: A deep learning framework for screening of COVID19 from radiographs". arXiv preprint. arXiv: 2003.14395, 2020. https://arxiv.org/abs/2003.14395

Ghoshal B., Tucker A. "Estimating uncertainty and interpretability in deep learning for coronavirus (COVID-19) detection". arXiv preprint. arXiv: 2003.10769, 2020. https://arxiv.org/abs/2003.10769

Hemdan EE-D, Shouman M.A., Karar M.E. "COVIDX-Net: A framework of deep learning classifiers to diagnose COVID-19 in X-ray images". arXiv preprint. arXiv: 2003.11055, 2020. https://arxiv.org/abs/2003.11055

Kao E.F., Lee C., Jaw T.S., Hsu J.S., Liu G.C. "Projection profile analysis for identifying different views of chest radiographs". *Acad Radiol* 2006; 13(4): 518–525. https://www.sciencedirect.com/science/article/pii/S1076633206000171

Karim M., Döhmen T., Rebholz-Schuhmann D., Decker S., Cochez M., Beyan O., et al. 2020. https://www.scirp.org/journal/paperinformation.aspx?paperid=118603

Khang A., Gupta S.K., Shah V., Misra A., (Eds.) *AI-Aided IoT Technologies and Applications in the Smart Business and Production* (1st Ed.), 2023a. CRC Press. 10.1201/97810033 92224

Khang A., Hahanov V., Abbas G.L., Hajimahmud V.A. "Cyber-physical-social system and incident management". *AI-Centric Smart City Ecosystems: Technologies, Design and Implementation* (1st Ed.), 2022a. CRC Press. 10.1201/9781003252542-2

Khang A., Hahanov V., Litvinova E., Chumachenko S., Hajimahmud V.A., Alyar A.V. "The Key Assistant of smart city – Sensors and tools". *AI-Centric Smart City Ecosystems: Technologies, Design and Implementation* (1st ed.), 2022b. CRC Press. 10.1201/9781 003252542-17

Khang A., Hahanov V., Litvinova E., Chumachenko S., Triwiyanto, Hajimahmud V.A., Ali R.N., Alyar A.V., Anh P.T.N., "The analytics of hospitality of hospitals in healthcare ecosystem". *Data-Centric AI Solutions and Emerging Technologies in the Healthcare Ecosystem.* (1st ed.), p. 4, 2023b.CRC Press. 10.1201/9781003356189-4

Khang A., Hahanov V., Litvinova E., Chumachenko S., Triwiyanto, Kadarningsih A., Avromovic Z., Ali R.N., Hajimahmud A.V., "Cloud platform and data storage systems in healthcare ecosystem". *Data-Centric AI Solutions and Emerging Technologies in the Healthcare Ecosystem.* (1st ed.), p. 4, 2023c. CRC Press. 10.1201/9781003356189-21

Khang A., Rana G., Tailor R.K., Hajimahmud V.A., (Eds.) *Data-Centric AI Solutions and Emerging Technologies in the Healthcare Ecosystem* (1st Ed.), 2023d. CRC Press. 10.1201/9781003356189

Khanh H.H., Khang A. "The role of artificial intelligence in blockchain applications". *Reinventing Manufacturing and Business Processes through Artificial Intelligence*, pp. 20–40, 2021, CRC Press. 10.1201/9781003145011-2

Korotcov A., Tkachenko V., Russo D.P., Ekins S. "Comparison of deep learning with multiple machine learning methods and metrics using diverse drug discovery data sets". *Mol Pharm* 2017; 14(12): 4462–4475. https://pubs.acs.org/doi/abs/10.1021/acs.molpharmaceut.7b00578

Lehmann T.M., Güld O., Keysers D., Schubert H., Kohnen M., Wein B.B. "Determining the view of chest radiographs". *J Digit Imaging* 2003; 16(3): 280–291. https://link.springer.com/article/10.1007/s10278-003-1655-x

Li X., Zhu D. "COVID-Xpert: An AI powered population screening of COVID-19 cases using chest radiography images". arXiv preprint. arXiv: 2004.03042, 2020. https://europepmc.org/article/ppr/ppr346252

Luo L., Yu L., Chen H. et al. "Deep mining external imperfect data for chest X-ray disease screening". *IEEE Transactions on Medical Imaging* 2020; 39(11): 3583–3594. https://ieeexplore.ieee.org/abstract/document/9110911/

Mayr A., Klambauer G., Unterthiner T., et al. "Large-scale comparison of machine learning methods for drug target prediction on ChEMBL". *Chem Sci (Camb)* 2018; 9(24): 5441–5451. 10.1039/C8SC00148K PMID: 30155234

Morris G., Babasaheb J., Khang A., Gupta S.K., Hajimahmud V.A., *AI-Centric Modelling and Analytics: Concepts, Designs, Technologies, and Applications* (1st Ed.), 2023. CRC Press. 10.1201/9781003400110

Narin A., Kaya C., Pamuk Z. "Automatic detection of coronavirus disease (covid-19) using x-ray images and deep convolutional neural networks". arXiv preprint 2003. https://link.springer.com/article/10.1007/s10044-021-00984-y

Ozturk T., Talo M., Yildirim E.A., Baloglu U.B., Yildirim O., Acharya U.R. "Automated detection of COVID-19 cases using deep neural networks with X-ray images". *Comput Biol Med* 2020: 103792. https://www.sciencedirect.com/science/article/pii/S0010482520301621

Pietka E., Huang H.K. "Orientation correction for chest images". *J Digit Imaging* 1992; 5(3): 185–189. https://link.springer.com/article/10.1007/BF03167768

Rana G., Khang A., Sharma R., Goel A.K., Dubey A.K. "Reinventing manufacturing and business processes through artificial intelligence", (Eds.), 2021. CRC Press. 10.1201/9781003145011

Rani S., Bhambri P., Kataria A., Khang A. "Smart city ecosystem: Concept, sustainability, design principles and technologies". *AI-Centric Smart City Ecosystems: Technologies, Design and Implementation* (1st Ed.), 2022. CRC Press. 1 (20). 10.1201/9781003252542-1

Rani S., Bhambri P., Kataria A., Khang A., Sivaraman A.K. (Eds.) *Big Data, Cloud Computing and IoT: Tools and Applications* (1st Ed.), 2023. Chapman and Hall/CRC. 10.1201/9781003298335

Rani S., Chauhan M., Kataria A., Khang A. "IoT equipped intelligent distributed framework for smart healthcare systems". *Networking and Internet Architecture*, (Eds.), 2021. CRC Press. 2 (30). 10.48550/arXiv.2110.04997

Salman F.M., Abu-Naser S.S., Alajrami E., Abu-Nasser B.S., Alashqar B.A. "COVID-19 detection using artificial intelligence". *Int J Acad Eng Res* 2020; 4 (3): 18–25. http://dstore.alazhar.edu.ps/xmlui/handle/123456789/587

Sethy P.K., Behera S.K. "Detection of coronavirus disease (COVID-19) based on deep features". Preprints 2020:2020030300. *Phys. Rev.*2020; 47: 777–780. https://pdfs.semanticscholar.org/9da0/35f1d7372cfe52167ff301bc12d5f415caf1.pdf

Tailor R.K., Pareek R., Khang A., (Eds.) "Robot process automation in blockchain". In Khang A., Chowdhury, S., & Sharma S. (Eds.) *The Data-Driven Blockchain Ecosystem: Fundamentals, Applications, and Emerging Technologies* (1st ed.), pp. 149–164, 2022. CRC Press. 10.1201/9781003269281-8

Vrushank S., Vidhi T., Khang, A., "Electronic health records security and privacy enhancement using blockchain technology". In Khang A., Rana G., Tailor R.K., Hajimahmud V.A. (Eds.) *Data-Centric AI Solutions and Emerging Technologies in the Healthcare Ecosystem.* (1st ed.), p. 1, 2023. CRC Press. 10.1201/9781003356189-1

6 Heart Disease Prediction Using Logistic Regression and Random Forest Classifier

Praveen Kumar Misra, Narendra Kumar, Anuradha Misra, and Alex Khang

CONTENTS

DOI: 10.1201/9781003356189-6

6.1   INTRODUCTION

Machine Learning (ML) is a way of manipulating and extraction of implicit, previously unknown/known, and potential useful information about data (Rani et al., 2023). Machine learning is a very vast and diverse field and its scope and implementation is increasing day by day.

Machine learning incorporates various classifiers of supervised, unsupervised, and ensemble learning, which are used to predict and find the accuracy of the given dataset (Rana et al., 2021).

We can use that knowledge in our work of HDPS as it will help a lot of people. Cardiovascular diseases are very common these days; they describe a range of conditions that could affect your heart. The World Health Organization estimates that 17.9 million global deaths are from (cardiovascular diseases) CVDs (Dangare & Apte, 2012).

It is the primary reason of deaths in adults. Our work can help predict the people who are likely to be diagnosed with a heart disease by help of their medical history (Shinde et al., 2015). It recognizes who all are having any symptoms of heart disease such as chest pain or high blood pressure and can help in diagnosing disease with less medical tests and effective treatments, so that they can be cured accordingly.

This work focuses on mainly three data mining techniques, namely

- Logistic regression
- Random forest classifier

The accuracy of our work is 92% for which is better than the previous system where only one data mining technique is used. So, using more data mining techniques increased the HDPS accuracy and efficiency (Bashir, Qamar & Javed, 2014). Logistic regression falls under the category of supervised learning. Only discrete values are used in logistic regression.

The objective of this work is to check whether the patient is likely to be diagnosed with any cardiovascular heart diseases based on their medical attributes such as gender, age, chest pain, fasting sugar level, etc. A dataset is selected from the UCI repository with patient's medical history and attributes.

By using this dataset, we predict whether the patient can have a heart disease or not. To predict this, we use 14 medical attributes of a patient and classify him if the patient is likely to have a heart disease. These medical attributes are trained under three algorithms (Ordonez, 2006).

Most efficient of these algorithms is logistic regression, which gives us the accuracy of 92% and finally we classify patients that are at risk of getting heart disease or not and also this method is totally cost efficient.

6.1.1 KEY FACTS

1. Cardiovascular diseases (CVDs) are the leading cause of death globally (World Health Organization).
2. An estimated 17.9 million people died from CVDs in 2019, representing 32% of all global deaths. Of these deaths, 85% were due to heart attack and stroke.
3. Over three-quarters of CVD deaths take place in low- and middle-income countries.
4. Out of the 17 million premature deaths (under the age of 70) due to non-communicable diseases in 2019, 38% were caused by CVDs.
5. Most cardiovascular diseases can be prevented by addressing behavioral risk factors such as tobacco use, unhealthy diet and obesity, physical inactivity, and harmful use of alcohol.
6. It is important to detect cardiovascular disease as early as possible so that management with counselling and medicines can begin.

6.1.2 PROBLEM STATEMENT

The major challenge in heart disease is its detection. There are instruments available that can predict heart disease but either they are expensive or are not efficient to calculate the chance of heart disease in humans. Early detection of cardiac diseases can decrease the mortality rate and overall complications.

However, it is not possible to monitor patients every day in all cases accurately and consultation of a patient for 24 hours by a doctor is not available since it requires more patience, time, and expertise.

Since we have a good amount of data in today's world, we can use various machine learning algorithms to analyze the data for hidden patterns. The hidden patterns can be used for health diagnosis in medicinal data (Khanh & Khang, 2021).

6.2 RELATED WORK

Numerous work has been done related to disease prediction systems using different data mining techniques and machine learning algorithms in medical centers (Kumar et al., 2023).

Polaraju and Prasad (2017) proposed prediction of heart disease using a multiple regression model and proves that multiple linear regression is appropriate for predicting heart disease chances. The work is performed using training data set that consists of 3000 instances with 13 different attributes, which was mentioned earlier.

The data set is divided into two parts: 70% of the data are used for training and 30% used for testing. Based on the results, it is clear that the classification accuracy of regression algorithm is better compared to other algorithms.

Sultana and Haider al. (2017) developed heart disease prediction using KStar, j48, SMO, and Bayes Net and Multilayer perception using WEKA software. Based on performance from different factors, SMO and Bayes Net achieve optimum performance than KStar, multilayer perception, and J48 techniques using k-fold cross validation.

The accuracy performances achieved by those algorithms are still not satisfactory. Therefore, the accuracy's performance is improved more to give a better decision to diagnosis of disease.

Shedole and Deepika (2016) focuses on techniques that can predict chronic disease by mining the data contained in historical health records using Naïve Bayes, decision tree, support vector machine (SVM), and artificial neural network (ANN).

A comparative study is performed on classifiers to measure the better performance on an accurate rate. From this experiment, SVM gives the highest accuracy rate, whereas for diabetes, Naïve Bayes gives the highest accuracy (Vrushank, Vidhi & Khang, 2023).

Dwivedi (2016) recommended different algorithms like Naive Bayes, classification tree, KNN, logistic regression, SVM, and ANN. The logistic regression gives better accuracy compared to other algorithms.

Shahi and Gurm (2017) suggested a heart disease prediction system using data mining techniques. WEKA software was used for automatic diagnosis of disease and to give qualities of services in healthcare centers.

The chapter used various algorithms like SVM, Naïve Bayes, association rule, KNN, ANN, and decision tree. The chapter recommended SVM as effective and provides more accuracy compared with other data mining algorithms (Vrushank & Khang, 2023).

Chala Beyene et al. (2018) recommended prediction and analysis of the occurrence of heart disease using data mining techniques. The main objective is to predict the occurrence of heart disease for early automatic diagnosis of the disease within result in short time (Hajimahmud et al., 2022).

The proposed methodology is also critical in healthcare organizations with experts that have no more knowledge and skill. It uses different medical attributes such as blood sugar and heart rate, age, sex are some of the attributes are included to identify if the person has heart disease or not. Analyses of dataset are computed using WEKA software (Khang et al., 2022a).

Sharmila and Chellammal (2018) proposed to use a nonlinear classification algorithm for heart disease prediction. It proposed to use big data tools such as Hadoop Distributed File System (HDFS) and MapReduce along with SVM for prediction of heart disease with optimized attribute set.

This work made an investigation on the use of different data mining techniques for predicting heart diseases. It suggests to use HDFS for storing large data in different nodes and executing the prediction algorithm using SVM in more than one node simultaneously using SVM. SVM is used in a parallel fashion, which yielded better computation time than sequential SVM (Vrushank & Khang, 2023).

Patel et al. (2017) suggested heart disease prediction using data mining and machine learning algorithm. The goal of this study is to extract hidden patterns by applying data mining techniques. The best algorithm J48 based on UCI data has the highest accuracy rate compared to LMT.

Purushottam et al. (2016) proposed an efficient heart disease prediction system using data mining. This system helps medical practitioner to make effective decision making based on the certain parameter. By the testing and training phase of a certain parameter, it provides 86.3% accuracy in testing phase and 87.3% in training phase.

6.2.1 LOGISTIC REGRESSION ALGORITHM

Logistic regression is one of the most popular machine learning algorithms, which comes under the supervised learning technique. It is used for predicting the categorical dependent variable using a given set of independent variables (Morris et al., 2023).

Logistic regression predicts the output of a categorical dependent variable. Therefore, the outcome must be a categorical or discrete value. It can be either yes or no, 0 or 1, true or false, etc. but instead of giving the exact value as 0 and 1, it gives the probabilistic values that lie between 0 and 1.

6.2.2 RANDOM FOREST ALGORITHM

Random forest is a supervised learning algorithm. It is an extension of machine learning classifiers that include the bagging to improve the performance of decision trees. It combines tree predictors, and trees are dependent on a random vector that is independently sampled.

The distribution of all trees is the same. Random forests split nodes using the best among a predictor subset that are randomly chosen from the node itself, instead of splitting nodes based on the variables.

The time complexity of the worst case of learning with random forests is O (M (dnlogn)), where M is the number of growing trees, n is the number of instances, and d is the data dimension. It can be used both for classification and regression. It is also the most flexible and easy-to-use algorithm. A forest consists of trees. It is said that the more trees it has, the more robust a forest is.

The greater number of trees in the forest leads to higher accuracy and prevents the problem of overfitting.

6.2.3 ASSUMPTIONS

Since the random forest combines multiple trees to predict the class of the dataset, it is possible that some decision trees may predict the correct output, while others may not. But together, all the trees predict the correct output. Therefore, below are two assumptions for a better random forest classifier:

- There should be some actual values in the feature variable of the dataset so that the classifier can predict accurate results rather than a guessed result.
- The predictions from each tree must have very low correlations.

6.2.4 MACHINE LEARNING

Machine learning is a subset of artificial intelligence. Machine learning is the study of computer algorithms that improve automatically through experience and by the use of data (Tailor et al., 2022).

Machine learning algorithms build a model based on sample data, known as "training data", machine learning is a science of designing and applying algorithms that are able to learn things from past cases. If some behavior exists in past, then you may predict if or it can happen again. This means if there are no past cases, then there is no prediction (Khang et al., 2022b).

Machine learning uses complex algorithms that constantly iterate over large datasets, analyzing the patterns in data facilitating machines to respond different situations for which they have not been explicitly programmed.

6.2.5 DATA SOURCE

An organized dataset of individuals had been selected, keeping in mind their history of heart problems and in accordance with other medical conditions. Heart disease is the diverse condition by which the heart is affected. According to the World Health Organization (WHO), the greatest number of deaths in middle-aged people are due to cardiovascular diseases.

We take a data source that is comprised of the medical history of 304 different patients of different age groups. This dataset gives us the much-needed information i.e. the medical attributes such as age, resting blood pressure, fasting sugar level, etc. of the patient that helps us in detecting the patient that is diagnosed with any heart disease or not.

This dataset contains 13 medical attributes of 304 patients that helps us detecting if the patient is at risk of getting a heart disease or not and it helps us classify patients that are at risk of having a heart disease and that who are not at risk. This heart disease dataset is taken from the UCI repository.

6.3 DATA DESCRIPTION

According to this dataset, the pattern which leads to the detection of patient prone to getting a heart disease is extracted. These records are split into two parts: training and testing. This dataset contains 303 rows and 14 columns, where each row corresponds to a single record, as shown in table 6.1.

6.4 DATA ANALYSIS

6.4.1 ANALYSIS

Data analysis is the process of systematically applying statistical and/or logical techniques to describe and illustrate, condense and recap, and evaluate data.

TABLE 6.1
Variable Description Table

Variable Name	Description
Age	Patient age (in years)
Sex	Gender of patients (0 = male, 1 = female)
Cp	Chest pain type (4 values; 0,1,2,3)
Trestbps	Resting blood pressure (in mm Hg)
Fbs	Fasting blood sugar >120 mg/dl (1 = true; 0 = false)
Restecg	electrocardiographic results (values 0,1,2)
Thalach	Maximum heart rate achieved
Exang	Exercise induced angina
Oldpeak	ST depression induced by exercise relative to rest
Slope	The slope of the peak exercise ST segment(values 0,1,2)
Ca	Number of major vessels (0–4) colored by flourosopy
Thal	(3 = normal; 6 = fixed defect; 7 = reversable defect)
Chol	Serum cholestoal (in mg/dl)
Target	Target column (1 = yes; 0 = No)

Source: Author's owner.

6.4.2 SUMMARY OF DATASET

The function df.describe () shows the basic statistical information about our dataset such that mean, standard deviation, quartiles, minimum, and maximum values as figure 6.1.1, 6.1.2, and 6.2.

	age	sex	cp	trestbps	chol
count	303.000000	303.000000	303.000000	303.000000	303.000000
mean	54.366337	0.683168	0.966997	131.623762	246.264026
std	9.082101	0.466011	1.032052	17.538143	51.830751
min	29.000000	0.000000	0.000000	94.000000	126.000000
25%	47.500000	0.000000	0.000000	120.000000	211.000000
50%	55.000000	1.000000	1.000000	130.000000	240.000000
75%	61.000000	1.000000	2.000000	140.000000	274.500000
max	77.000000	1.000000	3.000000	200.000000	564.000000

FIGURE 6.1.1   Dataset summary.

Source: Author's owner.

fbs	restecg	thalach	exang	oldpeak
303.000000	303.000000	303.000000	303.000000	303.000000
0.148515	0.528053	149.646865	0.326733	1.039604
0.356198	0.525860	22.905161	0.469794	1.161075
0.000000	0.000000	71.000000	0.000000	0.000000
0.000000	0.000000	133.500000	0.000000	0.000000
0.000000	1.000000	153.000000	0.000000	0.800000
0.000000	1.000000	166.000000	1.000000	1.600000
1.000000	2.000000	202.000000	1.000000	6.200000

FIGURE 6.1.2 Dataset summary.

Source: Author's owner.

slope	ca	thal	target
303.000000	303.000000	303.000000	303.000000
1.399340	0.729373	2.313531	0.544554
0.616226	1.022606	0.612277	0.498835
0.000000	0.000000	0.000000	0.000000
1.000000	0.000000	2.000000	0.000000
1.000000	0.000000	2.000000	1.000000
2.000000	1.000000	3.000000	1.000000
2.000000	4.000000	3.000000	1.000000

FIGURE 6.2 Dataset summary.

Source: Author's owner.

6.4.3 DATA VISUALIZATION

Histogram of all the attributes: df.hist (figsize = (12, 12), layout = (5, 3)); as figure 6.3.

From the sex histogram we can conclude that there are approximately 95 female patients and 205 male patients. The histogram of target attribute shows that there

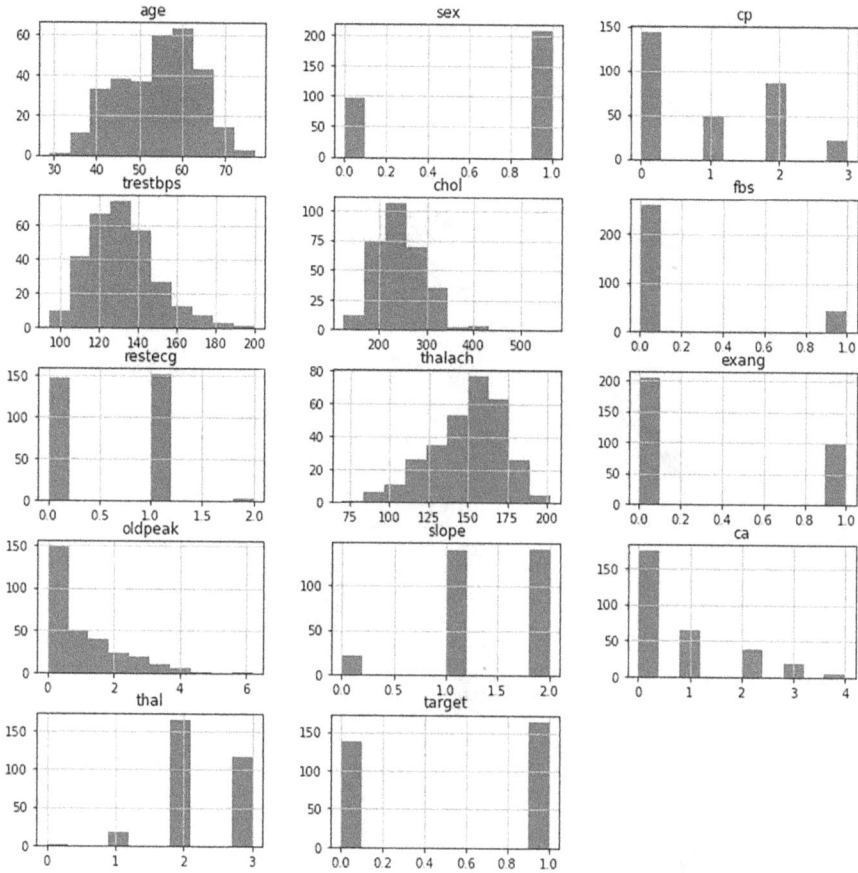

FIGURE 6.3 We can see the histogram of all the attributes in the above.

Source: Author's owner.

are approximately 140 female patients and 160 male patients who has found heart disease. Correlation among the attributes:

```
plt.figure (figsize = (20, 10))
sns.heatmap (df.corr (), annot = True, cmap = 'terrain')
```

The correlation matrix in machine learning is used for feature selection. It represents dependency between various attributes (figure 6.4).

- The magnitude 1 indicating strongly correlation and negative values indicating no correlations.
- The darker the color the stronger will be the relational, whereas fader the color will be loosely the relation will be
- Age is strongly related with the blood pressure and cholesterol, whereas it is not having any relation with maximum heart rate achieved.

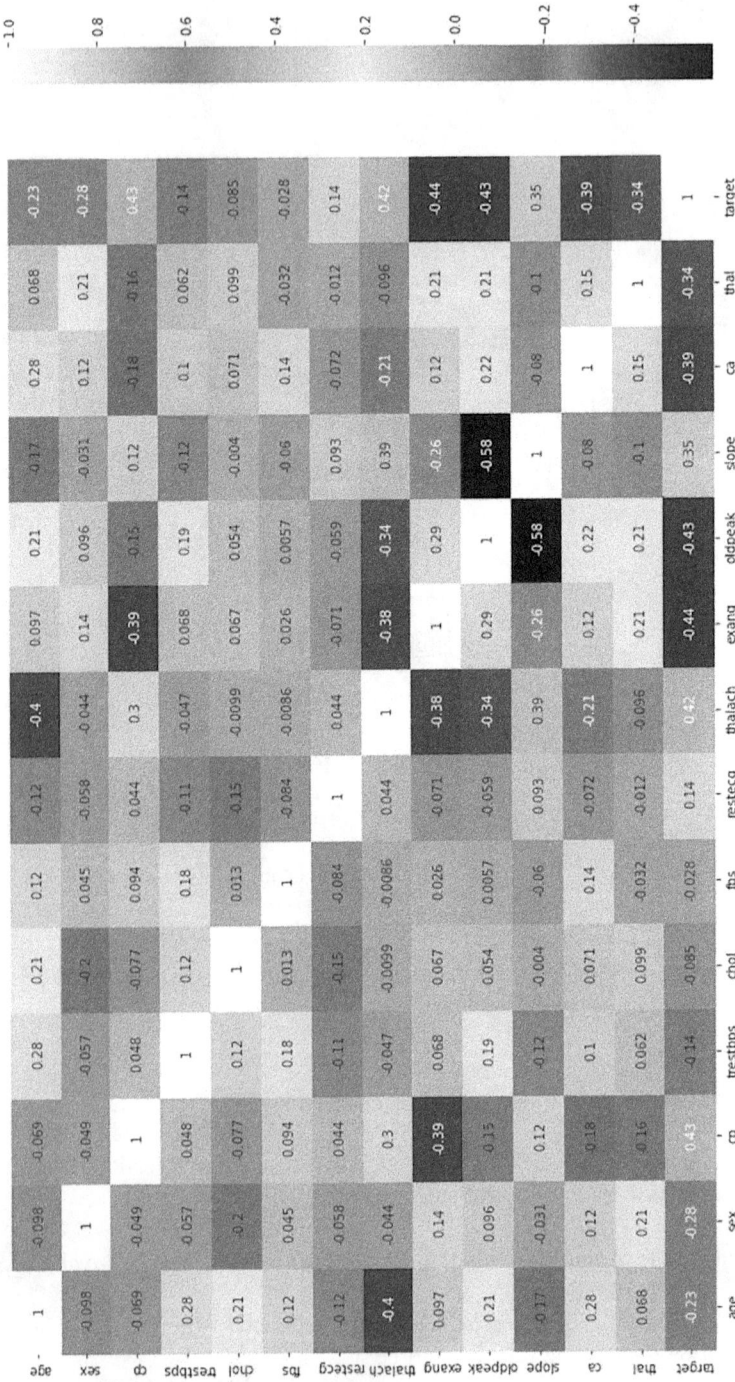

FIGURE 6.4 Co-relation matrix.

Source: Author's owner.

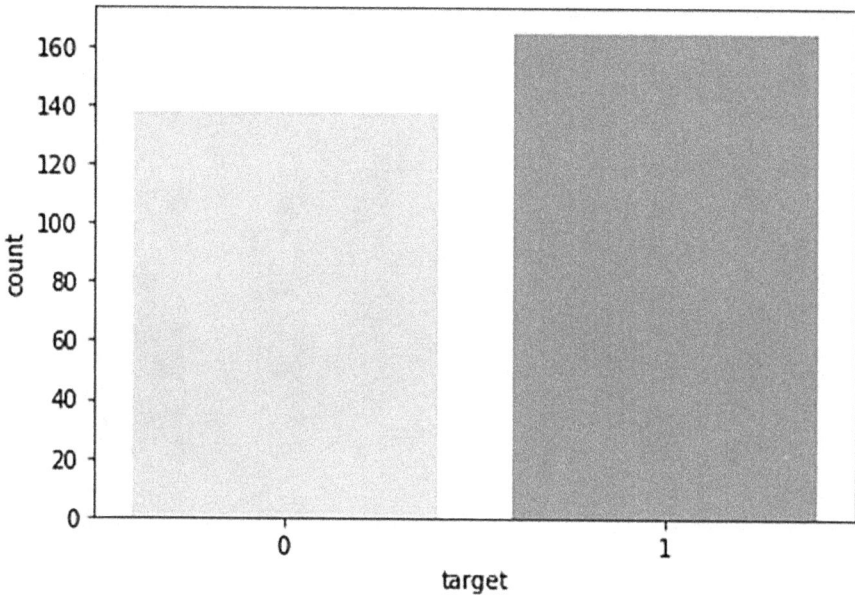

FIGURE 6.5   Count plot.

Source: Author's owner.

- Similarly, resting BP is also related with the cholesterol level and old peak. Maximum heart rate does not have any link with old peak (figure 6.5).

```
Countplot (target) sns.countplot
(x='target',palette='BuGn', data=df)
```

6.4.4   GRAPHICAL REPRESENTATION OF DIFFERENT ATTRIBUTE SEX (GENDER) DISTRIBUTION

Code for graphical representation of different attribute sex (gender) distribution (figure 6.6).

```
# --- Setting Colors, Labels, Order ---
    Colors = color_mix [2:4]
    Labels= ['Female', 'Male']
    Order = df ['sex'].value_counts ().index
# --- Size for Both Figures ---
    plt.figure (figsize = (16, 8))
    plt.suptitle ('Sex (Gender) Distribution', fontweight =
    'heavy', fontsize = '16', fontfamily = 'sans-serif',
    color = black_grad
    [0])
```

Sex (Gender) Distribution

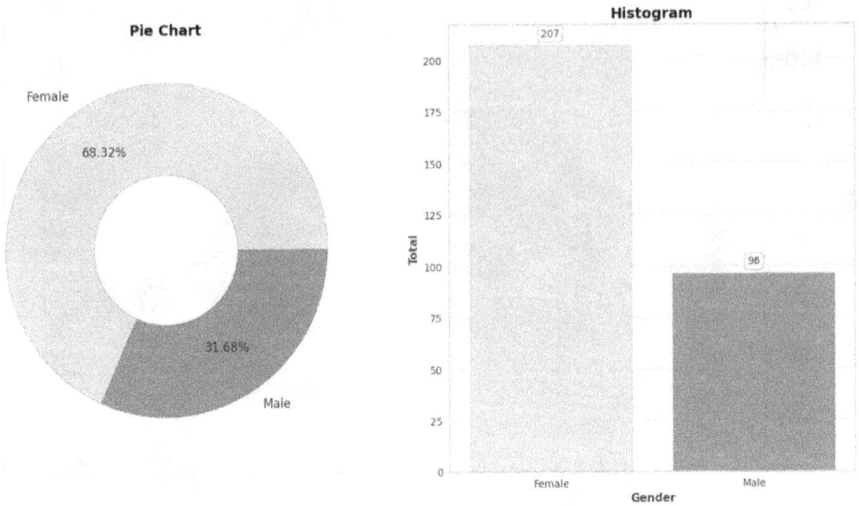

FIGURE 6.6　Graphical representation of different attribute sex (gender) distribution.

Source: Author's owner.

6.4.4.1　Chest Pain (cp) Type Distribution

Code for chest pain (cp) type distribution (figure 6.7).

```
# --- Pie Chart ---

    plt.subplot (1, 2, 1)

    plt.title ('Pie Chart', fontweight = 'bold', fontsize = 14,
    fontfamily = 'sans-serif', color = black_grad [0])

    plt.pie (df ['cp'].value_counts (), labels = labels, colors =
    colors, pctdistance = 0.7, autopct = '%.2f%%', textprops =
    {'fontsize':12}, wedgeprops = dict (alpha=0.8, edgecolor =
    black_grad [1]))

    centre = plt.Circle ((0, 0), 0.45, fc='white', edgecolor =
    black_grad [1])

    plt.gcf ().gca ().add_artist (centre)

# --- Histogram ---

    countplt = plt.subplot (1, 2, 2)

    plt.title ('Histogram', fontweight='bold', fontsize=14,
    fontfamily = 'sans-serif', color=black_grad [0])

    ax = sns.countplot (x='cp', data=df, palette=colors,
    order=order, edgecolor=black_grad[2], alpha=0.85)
```

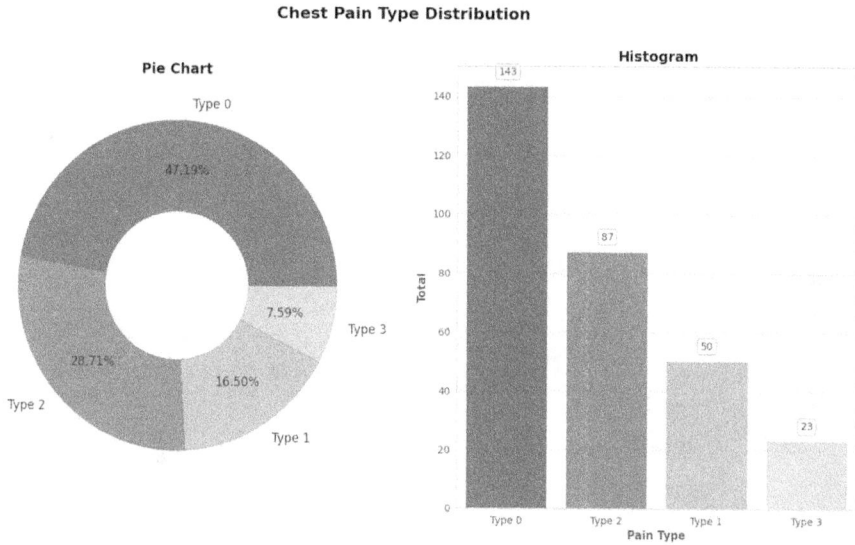

FIGURE 6.7 Chest pain (cp) type distribution.

Source: Author's owner.

```
for rect in ax.patches: ax.text (rect.get_x () +
rect.get_width ()/2, rect.get_height () + 4.25,
rect.get_height (), horizontalalignment = 'center',
fontsize= 10, bbox=dict (facecolor = 'none', edgecolor =
black_grad [0], linewidth = 0.25, boxstyle = 'round'))

    plt.xlabel ('Pain Type', fontweight='bold',
    fontsize=11, fontfamily = 'sans-serif',
    color=black_grad [1])

    plt.ylabel ('Total', fontweight='bold', fontsize=11,
    fontfamily = 'sans-serif', color=black_grad [1])

    plt.xticks ([0, 1, 2, 3], labels)

    plt.grid (axis='y', alpha=0.4)

countplt
```

6.4.4.2 Exercise-Induced Angina (exang) Distribution

Code for exercise-induced angina (exang) distribution (figure 6.8).

```
# --- Count Categorical Labels w/out Dropping Null Walues ---
    Print ('*' * 35)
    print ('\033[1m'+'.: Exercise Induced Angina Total:.' +
    '\033[0m')

    print ('*' * 35)
```

Exercise Induced Angina Distribution

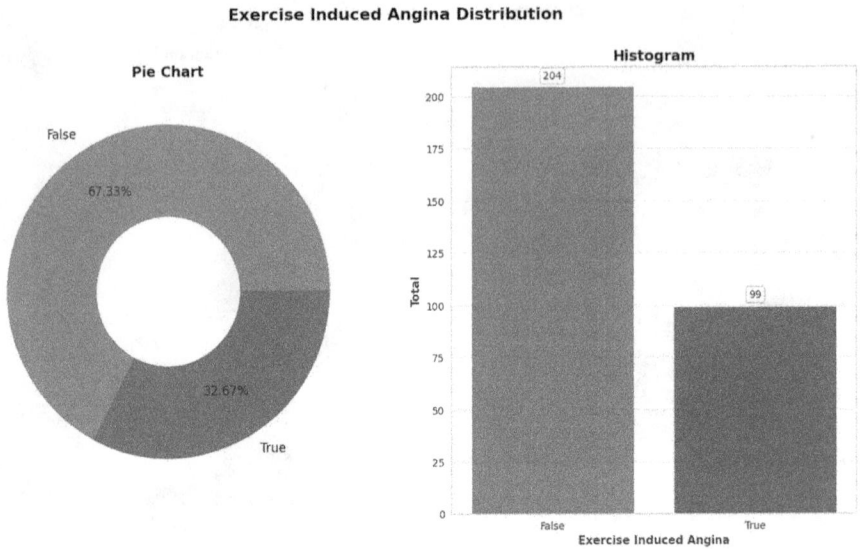

FIGURE 6.8 Exercise-induced angina (exang) distribution.

Source: Author's owner.

6.4.4.3 Slope of the Peak Exercise (Slope) Distribution

Code for slope of the peak exercise (slope) distribution (figure 6.9).

```
# --- Count Categorical Labels w/out Dropping Null Walues ---
    print('*' * 20)
    print('\033[1m'+'.: Slope Total:.'+'\033[0m')
    print('*' * 20)
    df.slope.value_counts (dropna=False)
```

6.4.4.4 Fasting Blood Sugar Distribution

Graphical representation of fasting blood sugar distribution (figure 6.10).

6.4.4.5 Resting Electrocardiographic (restecg) Distribution

Graphical representation of resting electrocardiographic (restecg) distribution (Figure 6.11).

6.4.4.6 Thal Distribution

Graphical representation of Thal distribution (figure 6.12).

6.4.4.7 Number of Major Vessels (ca) Distribution

Graphical representation of number of major vessels (ca) distribution (figure 6.13).

Slope of the Peak Exercise Distribution

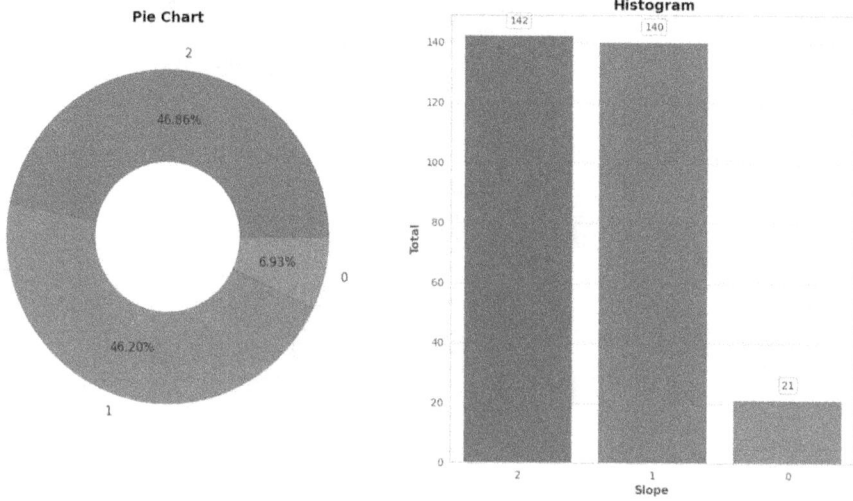

FIGURE 6.9 Slope of the peak exercise (slope) distribution.

Source: Author's owner.

Fasting Blood Sugar Distribution

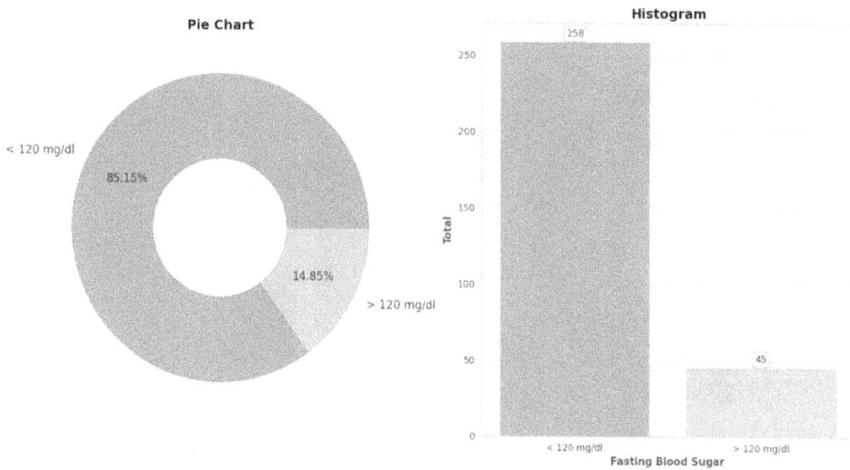

FIGURE 6.10 Fasting blood sugar distribution.

Source: Author's owner.

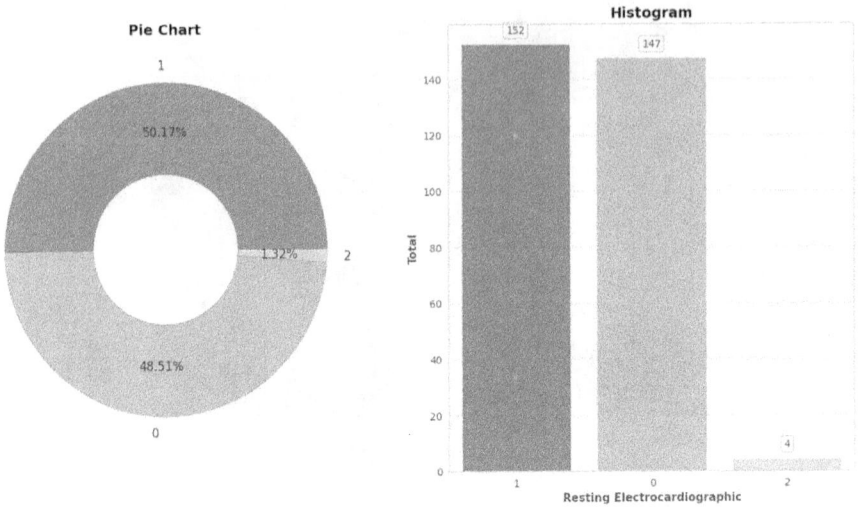

FIGURE 6.11   Resting electrocardiographic (restecg) distribution.

Source: Author's owner.

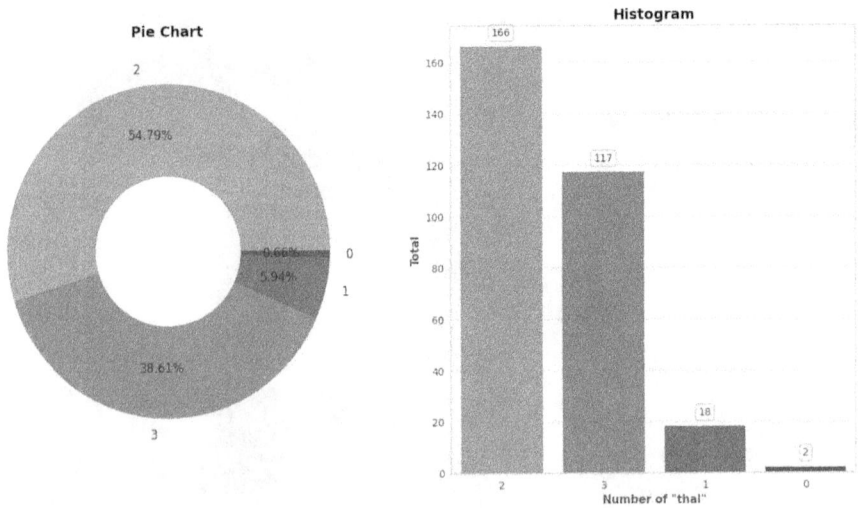

FIGURE 6.12   Graphical representation of thal distribution.

Source: Author's owner.

Number of Major Vessels Distribution

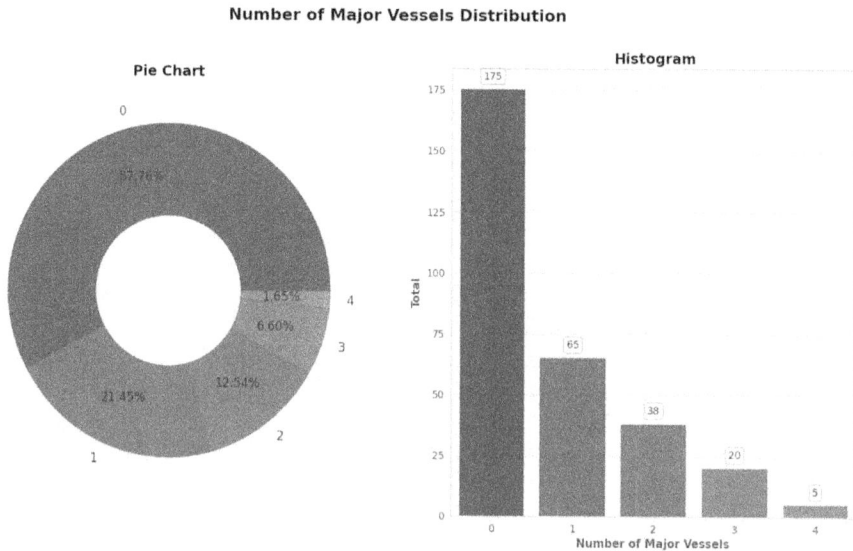

FIGURE 6.13   Graphical representation of number of major vessels (ca) distribution.

Source: Author's owner.

6.4.4.8   Age Column

Graphical representation of age column distribution (figure 6.14).

In this column, the kurtosis value is −0.5, which indicates that the column is platikurtic. From the Q-Q plot, the data values tend to closely follow the 45 degree, which means the data is likely normally distributed (Rani et al., 2021).

6.4.4.9   Serum Cholestoral Column

Code for serum cholestoral column distribution (figure 6.15).

```
# --- Box Plot ---
    ax_3=fig.add_subplot (1, 2, 1)
    plt.title ('Box Plot', fontweight='bold', fontsize=14,
    fontfamily='sans-serif', color=black_grad[1])
    sns.boxplot (data=df, y=var, color=color, boxprops = dict
    (alpha=0.8), linewidth=1.5)
    plt.ylabel ('Serum Cholestoral', fontweight='regular',
    fontsize=11, fontfamily='sans-serif', color = black_grad[1])
    plt.show()
```

There are some outliers detected at the upper part of the boxplot. At the upper part of the Q-Q plot, there is a gap at the upper part of the Q-Q plot with 45-degree line, which means the data is likely highly right skewed. In this column, the kurtosis value is 4.5, which indicates that the column is leptokurtic (Bhambri et al., 2022).

Age Column Distribution

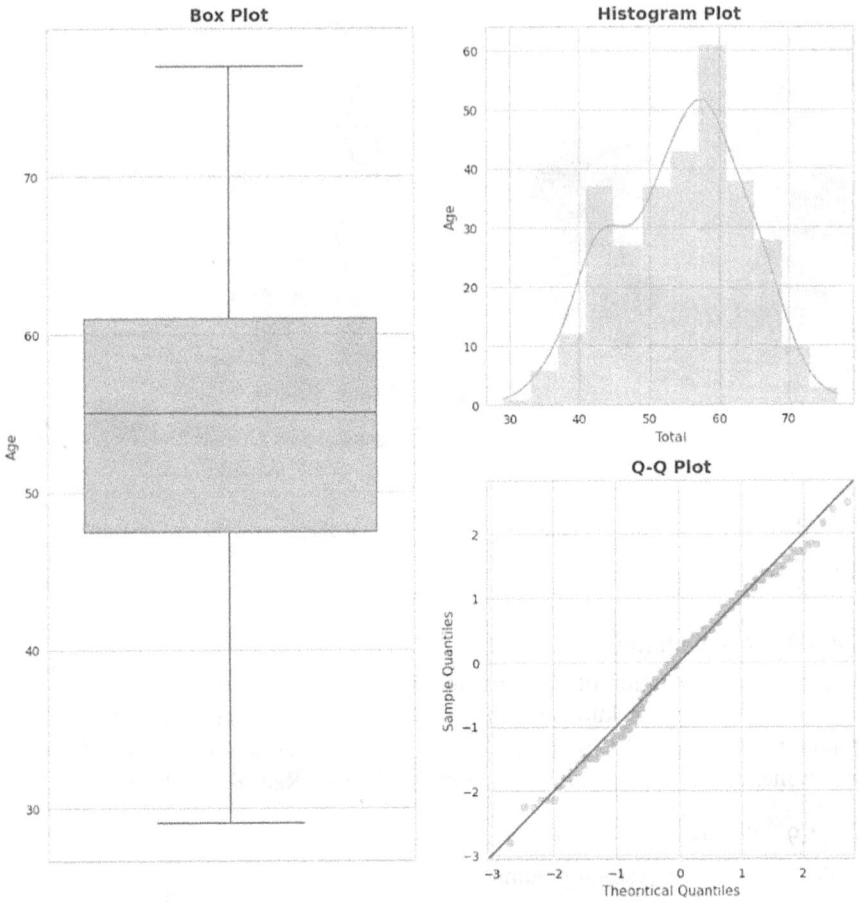

FIGURE 6.14   Graphical representation of age column distribution.

Source: Author's owner.

6.4.4.10   "thalach" (Maximum Heart Rate)

Box plot, Q-Q plot, and histogram representation for "thalach" (maximum heart rate) (figure 6.16).

There is an outlier detected at the bottom of boxplot. At the upper part of the Q-Q plot, there is a gap at the bottom part of the Q-Q plot with the 45-degree line, which means the data is likely moderately left skewed. The kurtosis value is –0.06, which indicates that the column is platikurtic.

6.4.4.11   "oldpeak" Column Skewness and Kurtosis

Skewness and kurtosis measurement (figure 6.17).

Serum Cholestoral Column Distribution

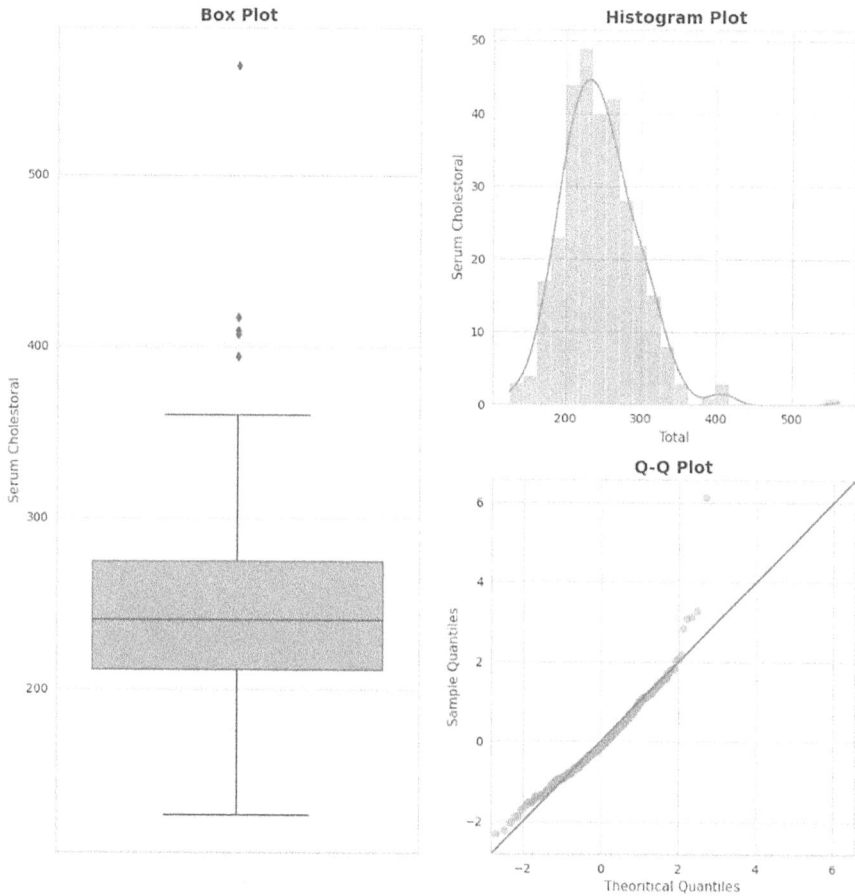

FIGURE 6.15 Graphical representation serum cholestoral column distribution.

Source: Author's owner.

There are some outliers detected at the upper part of the boxplot. At the upper part of the Q-Q plot, there is a gap at the bottom part of the Q-Q plot with the 45-degree line, which means the data is likely highly right skewed. The kurtosis value is 1.57, which indicates that the column is platikurtic.

6.4.4.12 Heart Disease Prediction (target)

Code for heart disease prediction (target) model (figure 6.18).

```
# --- Setting Colors, Labels, Order ---
    Colors = color_mix[3:5] labels=['True', 'False']
    Order = df['target'].value_counts().index
```

Maximum Heart Rate Column Distribution

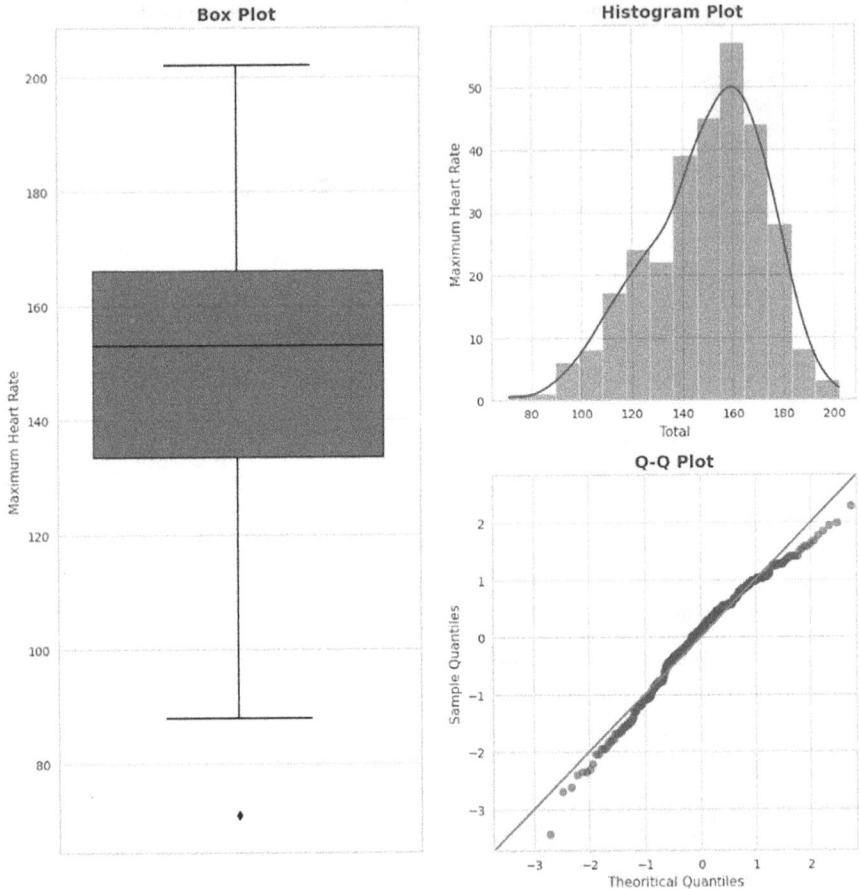

FIGURE 6.16 Box plot, Q-Q plot, and histogram representation for "thalach" (maximum heart rate).

Source: Author's owner.

```
# --- Size for Both Figures ---
    plt.figure (figsize = (16,8)) plt.suptitle ('Heart Diseases
    Distribution', fontweight='heavy', fontsize=16,
    fontfamily='sans-serif', color=black_grad [0])
# --- Pie Chart ---
    plt.subplot(1, 2, 1)
    plt.title ('Pie Chart', fontweight='bold', fontsize=14,
    fontfamily='sans-serif', color=black_grad [0])
    plt.pie (df['target'].value_counts(), labels = labels,
    colors = colors, wedgeprops = dict (alpha=0.8, edgecolor =
    black_grad [1]), autopct = '%.2f%%', pctdistance = 0.7,
    textprops = {'fontsize':12})
```

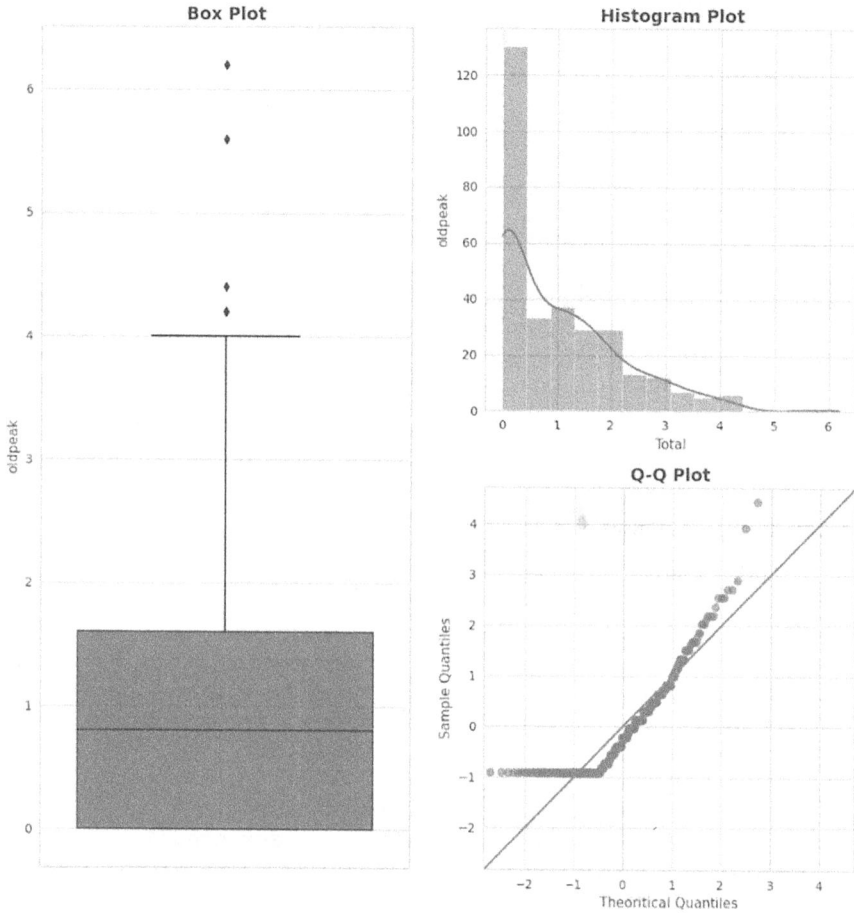

FIGURE 6.17 Skewness and kurtosis measurement.

Source: Author's owner.

```
centre = plt.Circle ((0, 0), 0.45, fc='white', edgecolor =
black_grad [1])
plt.gcf ().gca ().add_artist (centre)
# --- Histogram ---
countplt = plt.subplot (1, 2, 2)
plt.title ('Histogram', fontweight='bold', fontsize=14,
fontfamily='sans-serif', color=black_grad[0])
ax = sns.countplot (x='target', data=df, palette=colors,
order=order, edgecolor=black_grad[2], alpha=0.85)
for rect in ax.patches:
    ax.text (rect.get_x () + rect.get_width()/2,
    rect.get_height () + 4.25, rect.get_height (),
```

Heart Diseases Distribution

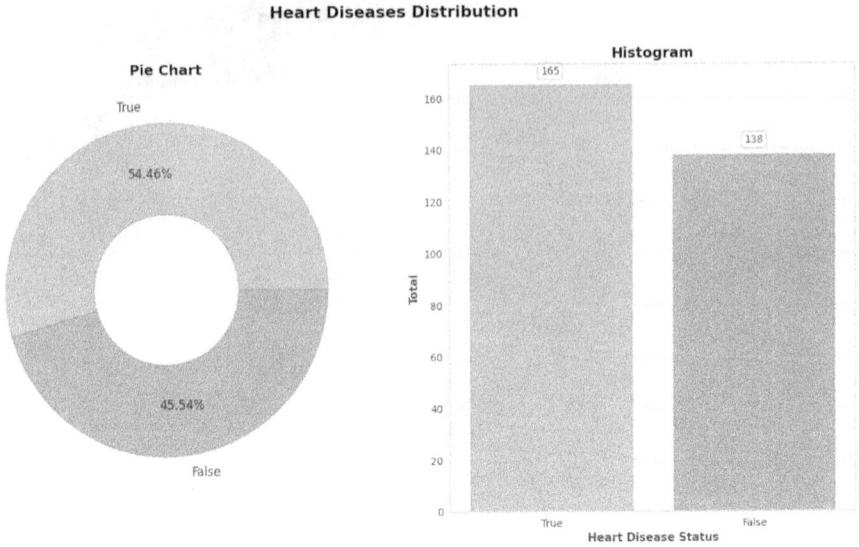

FIGURE 6.18   Heart diseases distribution.

Source: Author's owner.

```
        horizontalalignment='center',fontsize=10,
        bbox=dict (facecolor='none', edgecolor=black_grad[0],
        linewidth=0.25, boxstyle='round'))
        plt.xlabel('Heart Disease Status', fontweight='bold',
        fontsize=11, fontfamily='sans-serif',
        color=black_grad[1])
        plt.ylabel('Total', fontweight='bold', fontsize=11,
        fontfamily='sans-serif', color=black_grad[1])
        plt.xticks([0, 1], labels)
        plt.grid(axis='y', alpha=0.4)
    countplt
# --- Count Categorical Labels w/out Dropping Null Walues ---
    Print ('*' * 45)
    Print ('\033[1m'+'.: Heart Diseases Status (target)
    Total:.'+'\033[0m')
    Print ('*' * 45)
    df.target.value_counts (dropna=False)
```

6.4.4.13   Heart Disease Distribution Based on Gender

Graphical representation of heart disease distribution based on gender (figure 6.19).

There are a total of 96 male patients and 207 female patients and those who have found heart disease are 72 males and 93 females.

6.4.4.14   Heart Disease Scatter Plot Based on Age

Graphical representation of heart disease scatter plot based on age (figure 6.20).

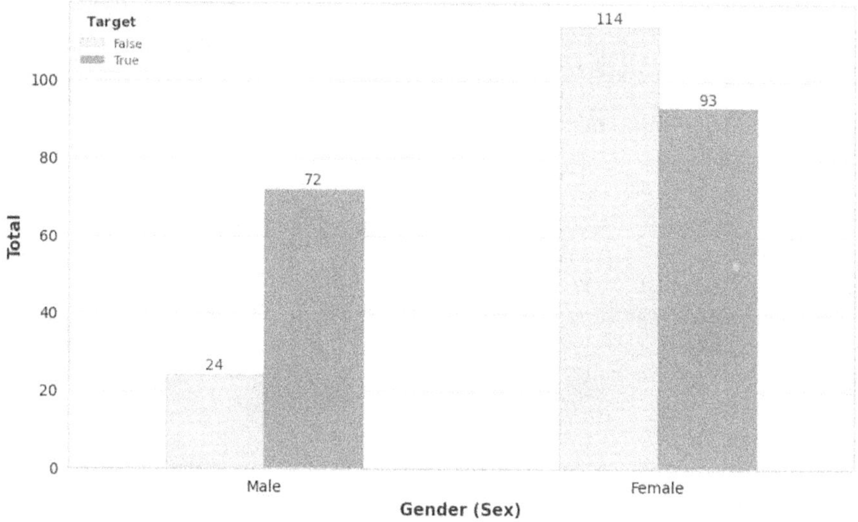

sant_ pro

FIGURE 6.19 Graphical representation of heart disease distribution based on gender.

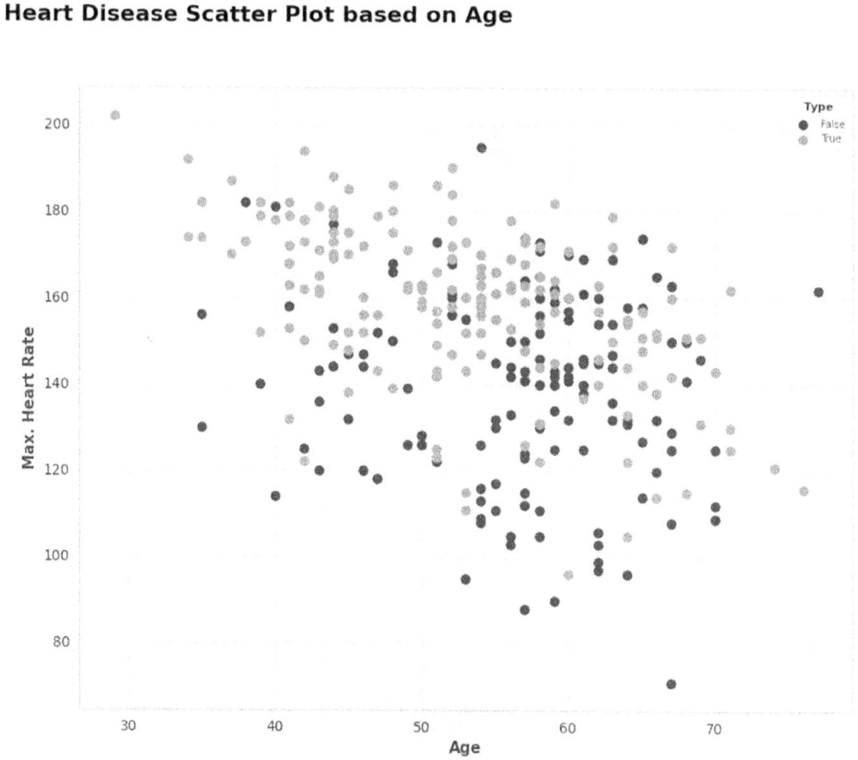

Heart Disease Scatter Plot based on Age

FIGURE 6.20 Graphical representation of heart disease scatter plot based on age.

Source: Author's owner.

6.5 MODEL IMPLEMENTATION

6.5.1 LOGISTIC REGRESSION

6.5.1.1 Model Implementation Using Logistic Regression

Code for model implementation using logistic regression

```
from sklearn.linear_model import LogisticRegression
lr=LogisticRegression()
model1=lr.fit(X_train,y_train)
prediction1=model1.predict(X_test)
from sklearn.metrics import confusion_matrix
cm=confusion_matrix(y_test,prediction1) cm
sns.heatmap(cm, annot=True,cmap='BuPu')
```

Run above code; the result of model implementation using logistic regression is shown in figure 6.21.

6.5.1.2 Accuracy

Code for accuracy of Logistic Regression Model

```
TP=cm[0][0]
TN=cm[1][1]
```

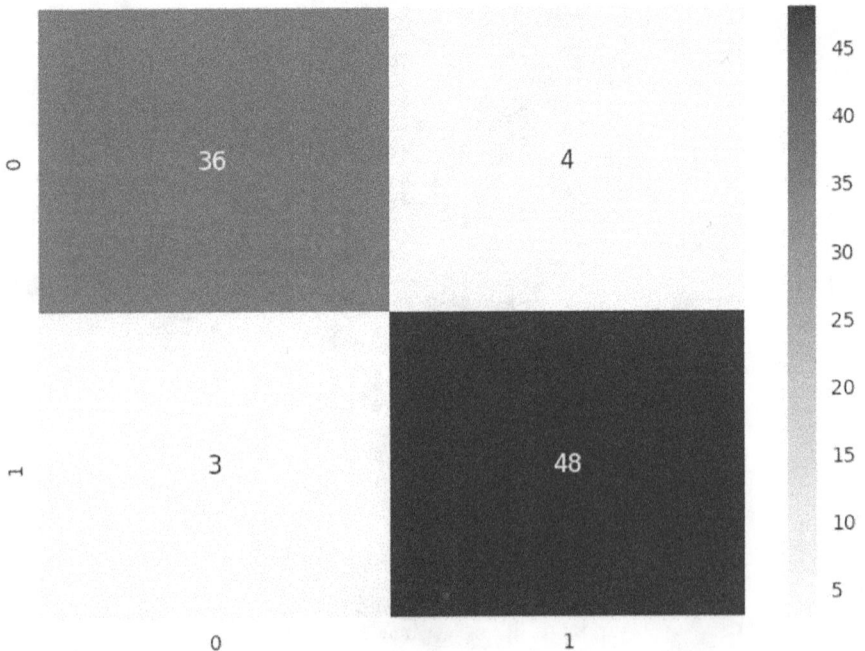

FIGURE 6.21 Model implementation using logistic regression.

Source: Author's owner.

```
FN=cm[1][0] FP=cm[0][1]
print ('Testing Accuracy:', (TP+TN)/(TP+TN+FN+FP))

    0.9230769230769231

from sklearn.metrics import accuracy_score
accuracy_score(y_test,prediction1)

    0.9230769230769231

from sklearn.metrics import classification_report
print (classification_report(y_test, prediction1))
```

Run above code, the data output by using precision and accuracy of logistic regression model is as shown in figure 6.22.

6.5.2 RANDOM FOREST CLASSIFIER

6.5.2.1 Model Implementation Using Random Forest Classifier

Code for implementation of model using random forest classifier (figure 6.23).

```
from sklearn.ensemble import RandomForestClassifier
rfc=RandomForestClassifier() model2 = rfc.fit(X_train,
y_train) prediction2 = model2.predict(X_test)
c_m=confusion_matrix(y_test, prediction2) c_m
```

6.5.2.2 Accuracy

Code for accuracy of random forest classifier model (figure 6.24).

```
accuracy_score (y_test, prediction2)

    0.8791208791208791

print (classification_report(y_test, prediction2))
```

	precision	recall	f1-score	support
0	0.92	0.90	0.91	40
1	0.92	0.94	0.93	51
accuracy			0.92	91
macro avg	0.92	0.92	0.92	91
weighted avg	0.92	0.92	0.92	91

FIGURE 6.22 Precision and accuracy of logistic regression model.

Source: Author's owner.

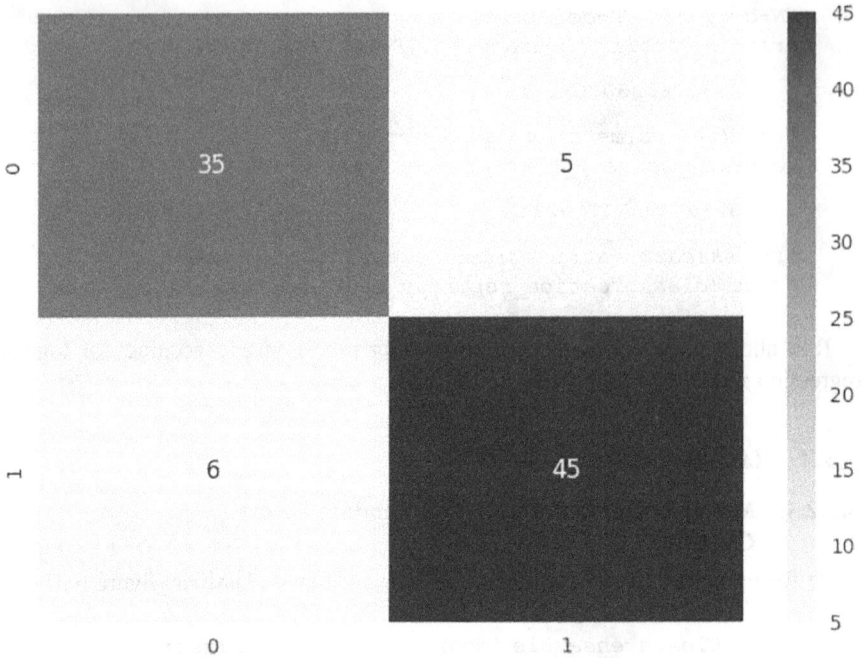

FIGURE 6.23 Model implementation using random forest classifier.

Source: Author's owner.

	precision	recall	f1-score	support
0	0.87	0.85	0.86	40
1	0.88	0.90	0.89	51
accuracy			0.88	91
macro avg	0.88	0.88	0.88	91
weighted avg	0.88	0.88	0.88	91

FIGURE 6.24 Precision and accuracy table of random forest classifier.

Source: Author's owner.

6.6 COMPARISON OF ACCURACY IN BOTH MODELS

Comparison of both the model in terms of precision and accuracy shows that the logistic regression algorithm has better accuracy than the random forest classifier (figure 6.25).

```
logistic regression : 0.9230769230769231
random forest classifier : 0.8791208791208791
```

FIGURE 6.25 Comparison of accuracy in both models.

Source: Author's owner.

```
print ('logistic regression:', accuracy_score(y_test,
prediction1))
print('random forest classifier:', accuracy_score(y_test,
prediction2))
```

6.7 CONCLUSION

This work predicts people with cardiovascular disease by extracting the patient medical history that leads to a fatal heart disease from a dataset that includes patients' medical history such as chest pain, sugar level, blood pressure, etc.

This heart disease detection system assists a patient based on his/her clinical information of them been diagnosed with a previous heart disease. The algorithms used in building the given model are logistic regression and random forest classifier. Logistic regression algorithm has better accuracy.

Use of more training data ensures the higher chances of the model to accurately predicting whether the given person has a heart disease or not. By using these computer-aided techniques, we can predict the patient faster and better and the cost can be reduced very much (Khang et al., 2022b).

There are a number of medical databases that we can work on as these machine learning techniques are better and they can predict better than a human being, which helps the patient as well as the doctors. If all the attributes are taken into consideration, then the efficiency of the model becomes less (Khang et al., 2023a).

To increase efficiency, attribute selection is done. In this the features have to be selected for evaluating the model, which gives more accuracy. The correlation of some features in the dataset is almost equal and so they are removed. If all the attributes present in the dataset are taken into account, then the efficiency decreases considerably (Khang et al., 2023b; Babasaheb et al., 2023).

In this paper, the two different machine learning algorithms used to measure the performance are logistic regression algorithm and random forest classifier applied on the dataset. Hence, the aim is to use various evaluation metrices like confusion matrix, accuracy, precision, recall, and f1-score, which predict the disease efficiently (Kavita & Khang, 2023).

Comparing both classifiers, logistic regression and random forest classifier, logistic regression gives the highest accuracy of 92%.

REFERENCES

According to the World Health Organization (WHO), cardiovascular diseases are the leading cause of death globally (source: https://www.who.int/news-room/factsheets/detail/cardiovascular-diseases-(cvds)

Babasaheb, J., B. Sphurti, Khang A., "Industry Revolution 4.0: Workforce Competency Models and Designs," *Designing Workforce Management Systems for Industry 4.0: Data-Centric and AI-Enabled Approaches*, (1st ed.), (2023), pp 14–31. CRC Press. 10.1201/9781003357070-2

Bashir, S., U. Qamar & M.Y. Javed. "An ensemble-based decision support framework for intelligent heart disease diagnosis," *In International Conference on Information Society* (i-Society 2014), (2014, November), 259–264. IEEE. https://ieeexplore.ieee.org/abstract/document/7009056/

Beyene, Mr. C., Prof. P. Kamat, "Survey on Prediction and Analysis the Occurrence of Heart Disease Using Data Mining Techniques," *International Journal of Pure and Applied Mathematics*, (2018). https://www.researchgate.net/profile/Pooja-Kamat/publication/323277772_Survey_on_prediction_and_analysis_the_occurrence_of_heart_disease_using_data_mining_techniques/links/5fba166e458515b797607125/Survey-on-prediction-and-analysis-the-occurrence-of-heart-disease-using-data-mining-techniques.pdf

Bhambri, P., S. Rani, G. Gupta, Khang A., "Cloud and Fog Computing Platforms for Internet of Things," ISBN: 978-1-032-101507, (2022), CRC Press. 10.1201/9781003213888

Dangare, C.S. & S.S. Apte. "Improved study of heart disease prediction system using data mining classification techniques," *International Journal of Computer Applications*, 47(10), (2012), 44–48. https://citeseerx.ist.psu.edu/document?repid=rep1&type=pdf&doi=546aa1fb27c8428a87da3b54cd2d3e76a7b331f2

Dwivedi, A.K., "Evaluate the performance of different machine learning techniques for prediction of heart disease using ten-fold cross-validation," Springer, (17 September 2016). https://link.springer.com/article/10.1007/s00521-016-2604-1

Hajimahmud, V.A., Khang A., V. Hahanov, E. Litvinova, S. Chumachenko, A.V. Alyar, "Autonomous Robots for Smart City: Closer to Augmented Humanity," *AI-Centric Smart City Ecosystems: Technologies, Design and Implementation* (1st Ed.), (2022). CRC Press. 10.1201/9781003252542-7

Khang, A., S.K. Gupta, V. Shah, A. Misra, (Eds.). *AI-aided IoT Technologies and Applications in the Smart Business and Production* (1st Ed.), (2023a). CRC Press. 10.1201/9781003392224

Khang, A., V. Hahanov, G.L. Abbas, V.A. Hajimahmud, "Cyber-Physical-Social System and Incident Management," *AI-Centric Smart City Ecosystems: Technologies, Design and Implementation* (1st Ed.), (2022a). CRC Press. 10.1201/9781003252542-2

Khang, A., V. Hahanov, E. Litvinova, S. Chumachenko, V.A. Hajimahmud, A.V. Alyar, "The Key Assistant of Smart City - Sensors and Tools," *AI-Centric Smart City Ecosystems: Technologies, Design and Implementation* (1st ed.), (2022b). CRC Press. 10.1201/9781003252542-17

Khang, A., N.A. Ragimova, V.A. Hajimahmud, A.V. Alyar, "Advanced Technologies and Data Management in the Smart Healthcare System," *AI-Centric Smart City Ecosystems: Technologies, Design and Implementation* (1st Ed.), (2022c). CRC Press. 10.1201/9781003252542-16

Khang, A., S. Rani, R. Gujrati, H. Uygun, S.K. Gupta, (Eds.). *Designing Workforce Management Systems for Industry 4.0: Data-Centric and AI-Enabled Approaches* (1st Ed.), (2023b). CRC Press. 10.1201/99781003357070

Khanh, H.H., Khang A., "The Role of Artificial Intelligence in Blockchain Applications," *Reinventing Manufacturing and Business Processes through Artificial Intelligence*, (2021), 20–40, CRC Press. 10.1201/9781003145011-2

Kumar, D.V.S., R. Chaurasia, A. Misra, P.K. Misra, Khang A., "Heart Disease and Liver Disease Prediction using Machine Learning," *Data-Centric AI Solutions and Emerging Technologies in the Healthcare Ecosystem*. (1st ed.), (2023a), P (4). CRC Press. 10.1201/9781003356189-13

Mathad, K., Khang A., "Hospital 4.0: Capitalization of Health and Healthcare in Industry 4.0 Economy," *Data-Centric AI Solutions and Emerging Technologies in the Healthcare Ecosystem.* (1st ed.), (2023), P (4). CRC Press. 10.1201/9781032398570-19

Morris, G., J. Babasaheb, Khang A., S.K. Gupta, V.A. Hajimahmud, *AI-Centric Modelling and Analytics: Concepts, Designs, Technologies, and Applications* (1st Ed.), (2023). CRC Press. 10.1201/9781003400110

Ordonez, C., "Association rule discovery with the train and test approach for heart disease prediction," *IEEE Transactions on Information Technology in Biomedicine*, 10(2), (2006), 334–343. https://ieeexplore.ieee.org/abstract/document/1613959/

Patel, Prof Jayami, Dr. Tejal Upadhay, Samir Patel, "Heart disease Prediction using Machine Learning and Data mining Technique," (March 2017). https://www.ijresm.com/Vol.2_2019/Vol2_Iss2_February19/IJRESM_V2_I2_89.pdf

Polaraju, K., D. Durga Prasad, "Prediction of Heart Disease using Multiple Linear Regression Model," *International Journal of Engineering Development and Research Development*, https://ejmcm.com/article_3785_56dea6128008c7563d95cb35313a0908.pdf. ISSN: 2321-9939, 2017.

Purushottam, Prof. (Dr.) K. Saxena, R. Sharma, "Efficient Heart Disease Prediction System," (2016), pp. 962–969. https://www.sciencedirect.com/science/article/pii/S187705091630638X Ansari

Rana, G., Khang A., R. Sharma, A.K. Goel, A.K. Dubey. "Reinventing Manufacturing and Business Processes through Artificial Intelligence," (Eds.), (2021). CRC Press. 10.1201/9781003145011

Rani, S., M. Chauhan, A. Kataria, Khang A., "IoT Equipped Intelligent Distributed Framework for Smart Healthcare Systems," *Networking and Internet Architecture*, (Eds.), (2021). CRC Press. 10.48550/arXiv.2110.04997

Rani, S., P. Bhambri, A. Kataria, Khang A., A.K. Sivaraman (Eds.). *Big Data, Cloud Computing and IoT: Tools and Applications* (1st Ed.), (2023). Chapman and Hall/CRC. 10.1201/9781003298335

Shahi, M., R. Kaur Gurm, "Heart Disease Prediction System using Data Mining Techniques," *Orient J. Computer Science Technology*, 6, (2017), 457466. http://www.computerscijournal.org/vol6no4/heart-disease-prediction-system-using-data-mining-techniques/

Sharmila, R., S. Chellammal, "A conceptual method to enhance the prediction of heart diseases using the data techniques," *International Journal of Computer Science and Engineering*, (May 2018). https://www.sciencedirect.com/science/article/pii/S2214785320367675

Shedole, S. Seema, K. Deepika, "Predictive analytics to prevent and control chronic disease," (January 2016). https://www.researchgate.net/punlication/316530782

Shinde, R., S. Arjun, P. Patil, J. Waghmare. "An intelligent heart disease prediction system using k-means clustering and Naïve Bayes algorithm," *International Journal of Computer Science and Information Technologies*, 6(1), (2015), 637–639. https://citeseerx.ist.psu.edu/document?repid=rep1&type=pdf&doi=c0dcb61a41a7f9aeb8f5bf85eed7583ea6d2c77d

Sultana, M., A. Haider, "Heart Disease Prediction Using WEKA Tool and 10 Fold Cross-validation," *The Institute of Electrical and Electronics Engineers* (March 2017). https://beei.org/index.php/EEI/article/view/3242

Tailor, R.K., R. Pareek, Khang A., (Eds.). "Robot Process Automation in Blockchain," *The Data-Driven Blockchain Ecosystem: Fundamentals, Applications, and Emerging Technologies* (1st ed.), (2022), 149–164. CRC Press. 10.1201/9781003269281-8

Vrushank, S., Khang A., "Internet of Medical Things (IoMT) Driving the Digital Transformation of the Healthcare Sector," *Data-Centric AI Solutions and Emerging Technologies in the Healthcare Ecosystem.* (1st ed.), (2023), P (1). CRC Press. 10.12 01/9781003356189-2

Vrushank, S., T. Vidhi, Khang A., "Electronic Health Records Security and Privacy Enhancement using Blockchain Technology," *Data-Centric AI Solutions and Emerging Technologies in the Healthcare Ecosystem.* (1st ed.), (2023), P (1). CRC Press. 10.1201/9781032398570-1

7 Convolutional Neural Network–Based Smart Incubator System for Infant Monitoring Using IoT Technology

Veeramani P., Srinivasan K., Radhika V., and Aravindaguru I.

CONTENTS

7.1   INTRODUCTION

In the 21st century, the birthrate of infants in the world was 17.873 births per 1000 people. In this, infant mortality rate was 2.4 million children deaths in the first month of life.

There is approximately 6500 newborn baby deaths every day. These deaths occur due to the inaccessibility, insufficient, and lack of monitoring. It mainly occurs in the developing countries rather than the developed countries. The mortality rate for developing countries is 93 deaths per 1000.

The average mortality rate of infants in India was at about 28.3 deaths per 1000 live births. The leading causes of death for the infant in the developing countries are improper monitoring, carelessness, and loss of consciousness.

This chapter provides the solution for the above-mentioned problem survey by altering the doctors and parents for the great supervision and monitoring. The smart incubator system monitors the infants continuously and sends the data collection to the cloud storage, where the data are stored (Sai Subhash Reddy et al., 2021).

DOI: 10.1201/9781003356189-7

The purpose of this research is to build a smart incubator system prototype that is based on IoT (Internet of Things) connected with the various sensors to detect the data (Rani et al., 2021). These data are sent to the parents and caretakers for altering them through the mail. The data values can be viewed on computers, laptops, and mobile phones (Ibrahim et al., 2019).

The main aim is to monitor and safeguard the infant by ensuring proper monitoring, using advanced technology, and reducing the workload of the caretaker and parents. It is an IoT-based system that uses the convolutional neural network (CNN) and MATLAB. It overcomes the disadvantages such as signal interfaces, hacking, and false sense of security (Khang et al., 2022a).

By using the CNN technique along with the IR sensor, we can predict the infants' current position (Isthlaq et al., 2021). The data can be viewed in the mail, which is sent to the doctors and parents through mail. So the caretakers can view the data while away from the infants and it also reduces the workload of them (Bhambri et al., 2022).

They can prevent the infant effects from the problem, which is sent in the mail. By these procedures, we can reduce the mortality rate of the babies and improve in the monitoring (Vrushank et al., 2023).

7.2   SYSTEM ARCHITECTURE

In the perspective of the structure, the lightweight architecture is divided into three components – health monitoring, vital check, and IoT-based mail notification (Kiruthika et al., 2021). The smart incubator is a prototype used to monitor the infants and maintain the environmental conditions. This incubator is a smart system that monitors the three internal organs mainly – heart, lungs, and brain. And also, it monitors the motion of the infants and environmental conditions such as temperature and humidity (Zakaria et al., 2018).

It detects the sound of the baby for crying monitoring (Plangsangmas et al., 2021). In the heart, it monitors the heart beat and electrical activity of the heart using chest leads. In the brain, it monitors the electrical activity of the brain using an EEG sensor (Khang et al., 2022b).

In the lungs, it monitors the respiration by using the breathing sensor (Rani et al., 2023). These processes were taken by using the specific sensors for the conditions applied. In our smart incubator system, the data that are detected by the sensor are transferred and stored to the cloud storage (Mittal et al., 2015).

The medical data can be viewed on the computer and mobile phone, which the data results are sent to through the mail by using the IoT (Kiruthika et al., 2021). It is a Wi-Fi-based technology and it acts as a quick manner. When the variations are occurred to the baby, it will send the altering mail to the doctors (hospital management) and parents (Veeramani et al., 2020).

This chapter is a bio-medical application-related project that monitors the infants to improve the stability by using the sensor data, CNN, and IoT-based system, so that the doctors can view the status of the babies and prevent them from problems (Khanh & Khang, 2021).

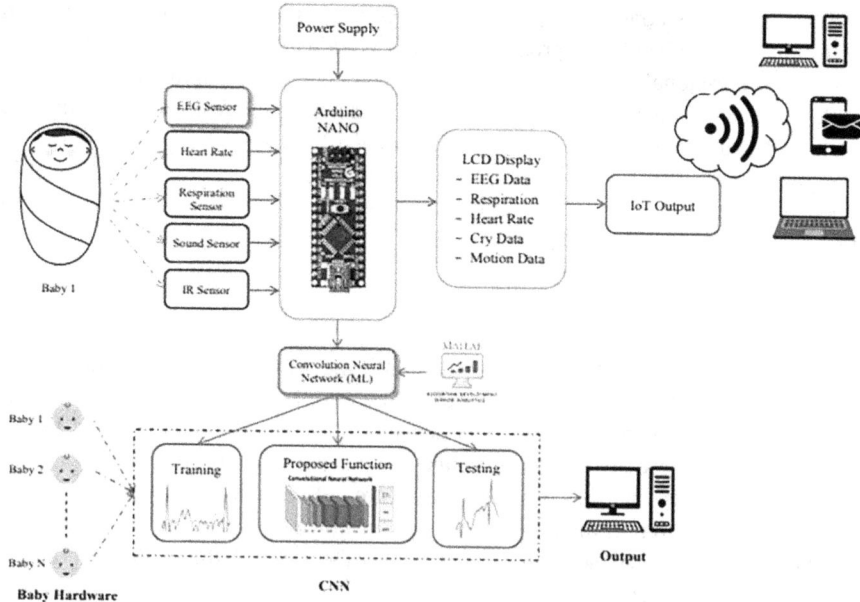

FIGURE 7.1 Block diagram of proposed system.

Source: Author's owner and (P. Sakthi et al., 2021).

The schematic block diagram of the proposed system is shown in figure 7.1. It consists of the electroencephalogram (EEG), heart rate, respiration sensor, IR, and sound, along with the temperature and humidity sensor. The sensors are implemented with the Arduino NANO.

Here, the liquid-crystal display (LCD) is used to display the values of the data that are detected by the sensors. Then they will be processed and analyzed using the CNN, which the datasets are predefined as the input. And it also predicts the position of the baby using the predefined model. Then the data are updated to the IoT (Rana et al., 2021).

It is a Wi-Fi network system that will send the medical data to the caretakers and parents through mail. The data can be viewed on computers, mobile phones, and laptops (Sakthi et al., 2021). This monitoring process can be applied to a number of babies for a better and safer environment also for less risk, as shown in figure 7.1.

7.3 RESULTS AND DISCUSSION

7.3.1 SOFTWARE SIMULATION

The software required for implementing the smart incubator system is Arduino IDE and MATLAB. These are the software used for the implementing the proposed system. In this project, this software is important for implementing the proposed system. The Arduino IDE is software used for adding the library files to the Arduino.

The library files contain the programming code for running the output. It is used for running the embedded C programs for the working of the microcontroller. The Proteus 8 professional is software used for drawing the circuit diagram for the project implementation. The MATLAB is a numeric computing platform that includes the machine learning, deep learning, etc. (Sakthi et al., 2021).

In our project, the convolution neural network is included with the MATLAB in which the input datasets are predefined. The MATLAB is used for the GUI and algorithm development analytics.

7.3.2 HARDWARE SIMULATION

The hardware components for implementing the smart incubator system are Microcontroller – Arduino NANO, temperature sensor, humidity sensor, EEG sensor, respiration sensor, heart rate sensor, IR sensor, sound sensor, LCD display, power supply, and PC. These are the components used for the implementing the apparatus, which are connected and the respected results are delivered as shown in figure 7.2.

The hardware setup of the proposed system is shown in figure 7.2. In the project, the above-mentioned sensors are connected to the pins of the Arduino NANO, which is a crystal oscillator with the frequency of 16 MHz.

The humidity sensor is used to measure the humidity level inside the incubator. The temperature sensor is used for maintaining the temperature inside the incubator. The IR sensor is used for checking the motion of the baby.

The sound sensor is for checking the crying baby. The breathing/respiration sensor is used for the respiration level monitoring. The EEG sensor is to check the

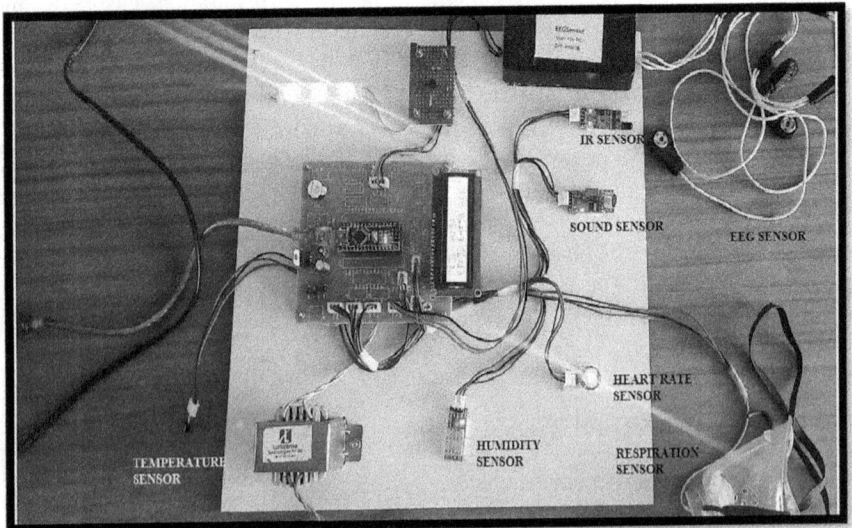

FIGURE 7.2 Hardware setup.

Source: Author's owner.

electrical activity of the brain. The heart rate sensor is used to measure the heart rate of infants.

The Arduino NANO is connected to the power supply that supplies the power to it. The LCD display is connected to the Arduino NANO, which is used for displaying the medical data. Then the data are sent through the IoT-based system to the mentioned persons (Khang et al., 2023).

7.3.3 OUTPUT

The results of the proposed system are mentioned below. The result shows the output of the project, overall kit display, and the software requirements. The sensor detects which is connected with the Arduino. It is connected with the LCD display to display the medical values.

Then the results are sent to the caretakers and parents to alert. The overall kit display of the prototype is shown in figure 7.3.

In the notifications part, enter the email ID and message sending process are taken. Here, the sample mail ID is published to check the output of the project prototype. The software simulation of the MATLAB is shown in figure 7.4.

This is the output of the project, which describes the sensor data, serial port connection, and notification's part. In the sensor data part, the values of the infants are detected by the sensor.

The predefined datasets are applied as the input, which if the data detected by the sensor are above the predefined datasets, will alert the message through the mail based on the IoT system (Khang et al., 2023a). In the serial port connection, the start and stop of the prototype working is controlled.

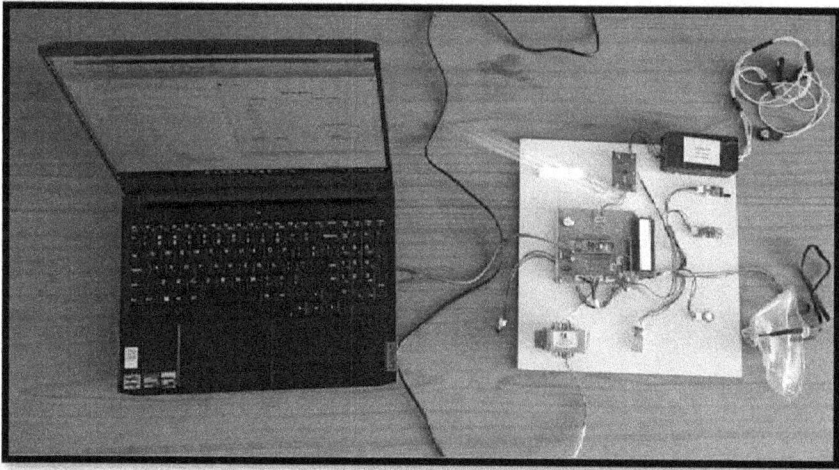

FIGURE 7.3 Figure 7.3 presents the overall kit display of the prototype.

Source: Author's Owner.

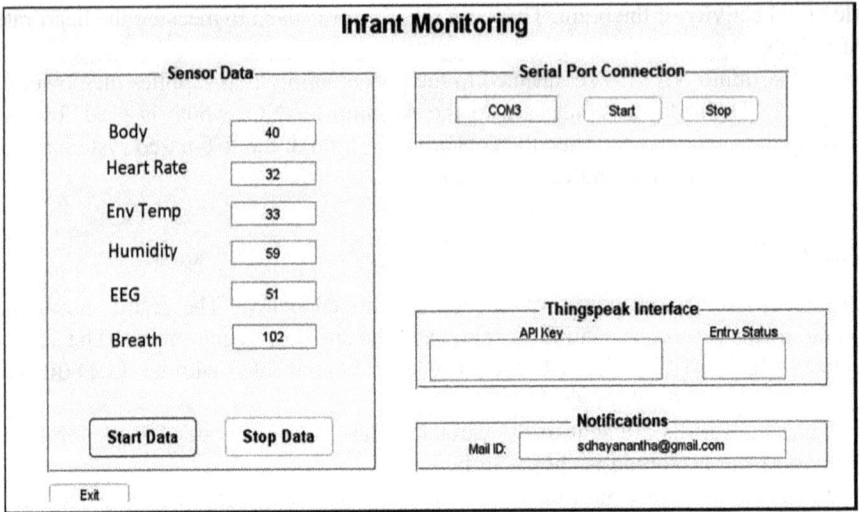

FIGURE 7.4 MATLAB simulation.

Source: Author's owner.

7.4 CONCLUSION

This chapter provides that the baby can be monitored safely with the specific sensors and software using the advanced technology of IoT and CNN (Khang et al., 2022c).

- The sensor detects the values that are connected with the Arduino works on the power supply.
- The LCD will display the output values of the data.
- The data values are sent to the caretakers through the mail which is based on the IoT system. The values are checked for regularly.

The data values are so accurate and it is an economical system will be used for developing countries. It has the great scope in the future to implement the prototype in a real-time monitoring application system (Khang et al., 2022b).

REFERENCES

Bhambri, P., S. Rani, G. Gupta, Khang, A. "Cloud and Fog Computing Platforms for Internet of Things", ISBN: 978-1-032-101507, 2022, CRC Press. 10.1201/9781003213888

Ibrahim, D. M., M. A. A. Hammoudeh, M. Ambreen, "Raspberry Pi-based smart infant monitoring system", *International Journal of Engineering Research and Technology*, 2019. https://www.ripublication.com/irph/ijert19/ijertv12n10_15.pdf

H. M. Isthlaq Salehin, Q. R. Anjum, F. TuzZuhra, "Development of an IOT based smart baby monitoring system with face recognition", *IEEE World AI IOT congress (AIIOT) Conference*, 2021. https://ieeexplore.ieee.org/abstract/document/9454187/

Khang, A., V. Hahanov, E. Litvinova, S. Chumachenko, V. A. Hajimahmud, A. V. Alyar, "The Key Assistant of Smart City - Sensors and Tools", *AI-Centric Smart City Ecosystems: Technologies, Design and Implementation* (1st ed.), 2022a. CRC Press. 10.1201/9781003252542-17

Khang, A., S. Rani, A. K. Sivaraman, *AI-Centric Smart City Ecosystems: Technologies, Design and Implementation* (1st Ed.), 2022b. CRC Press. 10.1201/9781003252542

Khang, A., V. Hahanov, G. L. Abbas, V. A. Hajimahmud, "Cyber-Physical-Social System and İncident Management", *AI-Centric Smart City Ecosystems: Technologies, Design and Implementation* (1st Ed.), 2022c. CRC Press. 10.1201/9781003252542-2

Khang, A., S. K. Gupta, S. Rani, D. A. Karras, (Eds.). *Smart Cities: IoT Technologies, Big Data Solutions, Cloud Platforms, and Cybersecurity Techniques* (1st Ed.), 2023a. CRC Press. 10.1201/9781003376064

Khang, A., S. K. Gupta, Shah V., Misra A., (Eds.). *AI-aided IoT Technologies and Applications in the Smart Business and Production* (1st Ed.), 2023b. CRC Press. 10.1201/9781003392224

Khanh, H. H., Khang, A. "The Role of Artificial Intelligence in Blockchain Applications", *Reinventing Manufacturing and Business Processes through Artificial Intelligence*, pp. 20–40, 2021, CRC Press. 10.1201/9781003145011-2

Kiruthika, S., P. Sakthi, M. Kaviya, S. Vishnupriya, "Blood Bank Monitoring and Blood Identification System Using IoT Device", *Annals of R.S.C.B.*, Vol. 25, No. 6, 2021, pp. 182–192, 2021. https://www.annalsofrscb.ro/index.php/journal/article/view/5270

Kiruthika, S., P. Sakthi, N. Gokul, G. Praveen Kumar, S. Praveenkumar, R. Prem, "Monitoring Soil Quality and Fertigation System Using IoT", *Turkish Journal of Computer and Mathematics Education (TURCOMAT)*, Vol. 12, No. 9, pp. 2884–2893, 2021. https://www.turcomat.org/index.php/turkbilmat/article/view/4682

Mittal, H., L. Mathew, A. Gupta, "Design and Development of an Infant Incubator for Controlling Multiple Parameter", *International Journal of Emerging trends in Electrical and Electronics*, 2015. https://www.academia.edu/download/52840213/FMSS.pdf

Plangsangmas, V., S. Leeudomwong, P. Kongthaworn, "Sound Pressure level in an infant incubator", *Journal of Meteorology Society of India*, 2012. https://link.springer.com/article/10.1007/s12647-012-0030-0

Rana, G., Khang, A. R. Sharma, A. K. Goel, A. K. Dubey, "Reinventing Manufacturing and Business Processes through Artificial Intelligence", (Eds.), 2021. CRC Press. 10.1201/9781003145011

Rani, S., M. Chauhan, A. Kataria, Khang, A. "IoT Equipped Intelligent Distributed Framework for Smart Healthcare Systems", *Networking and Internet Architecture*, (Eds.), 2021. CRC Press. 10.48550/arXiv.2110.04997

Rani, S., P. Bhambri, A. Kataria, Khang, A. "Smart City Ecosystem: Concept, Sustainability, Design Principles and Technologies", *AI-Centric Smart City Ecosystems: Technologies, Design and Implementation* (1st Ed.), 2022. CRC Press. 10.1201/9781003252542-1

Rani, S., P. Bhambri, A. Kataria, Khang, A. A. K. Sivaraman (Eds.), *Big Data, Cloud Computing and IoT: Tools and Applications* (1st Ed.), 2023. Chapman and Hall/CRC. 10.1201/9781003298335

Sai Subhash Reddy, Y., K. S. V. Vamsi, G. Akhila, "An Automated Baby Monitoring System", *International Journal of Engineering and Advanced Technology (IJEAT)*, 2021. https://www.researchgate.net/profile/Akhila-Golla/publication/354221158_An_Automated_Baby_Monitoring_System/links/617014b7435dab3b758369ae/An-Automated-Baby-Monitoring-System.pdf

Sakthi, P., S. Kiruthika, A. Surya, C. Venkatraj, K. S. Vignesh, S. Gokulakrishnan, "Detection Of Driver Drowsiness Using Face Recognition", *Turkish Journal of Computer and Mathematics Education (TURCOMAT)*, Vol. 12, No. 9, pp. 2894–2900, 2021. https://turcomat.org/index.php/turkbilmat/article/view/4684

Veeramani, P. et al., "Billing of Products using Edge Detection in Matlab", *Bioscience BIoTechnology Research Communications*, Vol. 13, 2020. https://www.researchgate.net/profile/Siddig-Noureldin-2/publication/288820215_Potential_mosquito_vectors_of_arboviral_diseases_in_Jazan_Region_Saudi_Arabia/links/56cea79008ae4d8d649998c1/Potential-mosquito-vectors-of-arboviral-diseases-in-Jazan-Region-Saudi-Arabia.pdf

Vrushank S., T. Vidhi, Khang, A. 2023. "Electronic Health Records Security and Privacy Enhancement using Blockchain Technology", *Data-Centric AI Solutions and Emerging Technologies in the Healthcare Ecosystem* (1st ed.), 2023, P (1) CRC Press. 10.1201/9781003356189

Zakaria, N. A., F. N. B. M. Saleh, M. A. A. Razak, "IoT (internet of things) based infant body temperature monitoring", *International conference on bio signal analysis, processing and systems (ICBAPS). Phys. Rev.* Vol. 47, 777–780, 2018. https://ieeexplore.ieee.org/abstract/document/8527408/

8 A Fuzzy Expert System for Alzheimer's Disease Diagnosis Using 2D Wavelet Texture Biomarkers

M. Ramya and A. R. Kavitha

CONTENTS

8.1 INTRODUCTION

Alzheimer's disease (AD), also referred to simply as Alzheimer's, is a chronic neurodegenerative disease that usually starts slowly and finally the whole brain degeneration occurs over time. It is the cause of 60% to 70% of cases of dementia. AD typically begins in people over the age of 65, and its symptoms are frequently misinterpreted as those of normal aging.

An examination of brain tissue is needed for a definite diagnosis of this disease. Previous studies show that the physical changes in the brain that lead to AD begin long before the symptoms, like memory problems, occur. Therefore, methods to identify these brain changes before the occurrence of symptoms are required (Vrushank, Vidhi, Khang, 2023).

DOI: 10.1201/9781003356189-8

8.2 RELATED WORK

Numerous studies have focused on identifying biomarkers for the diagnosis of Alzheimer's disease at various stages. The review paper (Ramya & Cyriac, 2019) explains the different types of non-invasive biomarkers used for the early diagnosis of AD.

Non-invasive biomarkers were categorised as imaging biomarkers, olfactory dysfunction, and signal biomarkers. Imaging biomarkers can be classified as structural or functional biomarkers.

Magnetic resonance imaging (MRI), diffusion tensor imaging (DTI), functional magnetic resonance imaging (fMRI), magnetic resonance spectroscopy (MRS), and fluorodeoxyglucose-positron emission tomography (FDG-PET) are the different imaging modalities used in finding the biomarkers for the diagnosis of AD. It has been found that classification accuracy is improved by using multimodal biomarkers. Some of the research studies focused on soft computing techniques, which were discussed here.

A medical healthcare system was developed (Ramya & Kavitha, 2020a), which has been used to diagnose AD and mild cognitive impairment in cognitively normal subjects. Pre-processing of the ROI (hippocampus and amygdala of the left hemispherical region of the MRI) using the $\mu \pm 3\sigma$ normalization method has been done, followed by the textural features extraction. This system uses the soft computing technique (Khang et al., 2022).

FIS for the classification by using two extracted textural features: skewness and kurtosis. Tumors in the brain MRI were detected using a back propagation neural network to reduce segmentation time and improve accuracy (Kavitha & Chellamuthu, 2016).

In another system, the diagnosis of MCI, including LMCI and AD, has been done by extracting the 2D wavelet textural features (Max norms and standard deviation of the diagonal detail coefficient) using the db2 wavelet at level 2. These extracted 2D wavelet features have been given as input for the classification using Mamdani FIS (Fuzzy Inference System).

The chapter (Ramya & Kavitha, 2020b, Chapter 10, p. 167) analyzes different soft computing techniques like fuzzy inference system, neural network, and genetic algorithm. By reviewing various research works, optimization algorithms for different stages in medical image analysis have been identified.

The application of a genetic algorithm for optimum feature selection along with the fuzzy inference classifier for brain tumor grading in the system (Kavitha & Thyagharajan, 2018) has been found to be better when compared to the classification using the FIS with all the features.

Apparent diffusion coefficient (ADC), fractional anisotropy (FA), and gray matter (GM) features were extracted from DTI and risk status of the AD has been found by using fuzzy expert system (FES). In this system (Kar & Majumder, 2019), application of neuro fuzzy technique for classification detect AD in the early stage.

Based on the visual features extracted from the hippocampus, AD, MCI, and normal control, classification has been done using fuzzy logic (FL) tool (Mallika et al., 2019).

8.3 PROPOSED METHODOLOGY

In the proposed system, three textural biomarkers were extracted from the 10 brain MRI and used for the classification of AD and cognitively normal (CN) subjects (Rana et al., 2021).

Application of FIS enables the classification of the small cohort with 100% accuracy. In this system, the MATLAB (R2018b) tool has been used for the different stages of medical image analysis. A block diagram of the proposed system is represented in figure 8.1.

Basic Algorithm for the Proposed System:

1. T2-weighted MRI acquisition from the ADNI for the CN and AD groups of subjects //Acquisition
2. Do segmentation for all T2-MRIs. //Segmentation
3. The ROI was obtained by free hand segmenting the hippocampal and amygdala from the left hemisphere.
4. Calculate the mean of the ROI. //feature extraction
5. In the 2D wavelet tool of the wavelet analyzer, the Haar wavelet at level 2 has been used to identify the two wavelet features, max norms, and the standard deviation of the diagonal detail coefficient.
6. end for
7. FIS (three textural biomarkers) function // Classification
8. Defining the membership functions for the input and output variables of the FIS.
9. Determine the parameters and the ranges for all the membership functions (Trapezoidal, Gaussian, Generalized Bell, and Sigmoidal MF).
10. Optimal fuzzy rules have been developed by analyzing the membership functions.
11. FIS has been executed by giving three textural features as the input variables and obtaining the values at the output.

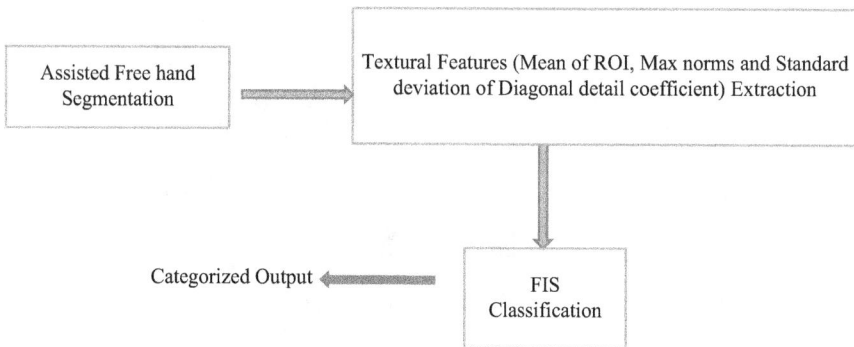

FIGURE 8.1 Block diagram of the proposed system.

Source: Author's owner.

12. Classification has been done based on the values of the output variables that fall in the defined range.
13. for all "subjects,"
14. If (the subject's actual group name ≠ the subject's obtained group name) than
15. Adjust the parameters and the ranges of the MFs of the input variables.
16. Modify the fuzzy rules.
17. Go to step 11.
18. End for
19. Return categorized output
20. End

8.3.1 SUBJECTS AND DATA ACQUISITION

In the proposed system, T2-MRI of the human brain has been acquired for two different research groups (AD and CN) from the ADNI-3 database (ADNI, 2016). From the large number of downloaded images, ten samples of MRI (five MRIs of AD subjects and five MRIs of CN subjects) have been used for this research work (Rani et al., 2021). A few samples of AD subjects' MRIs are shown in figure 8.2. A few samples of CN subjects' MRIs are shown in figure 8.3.

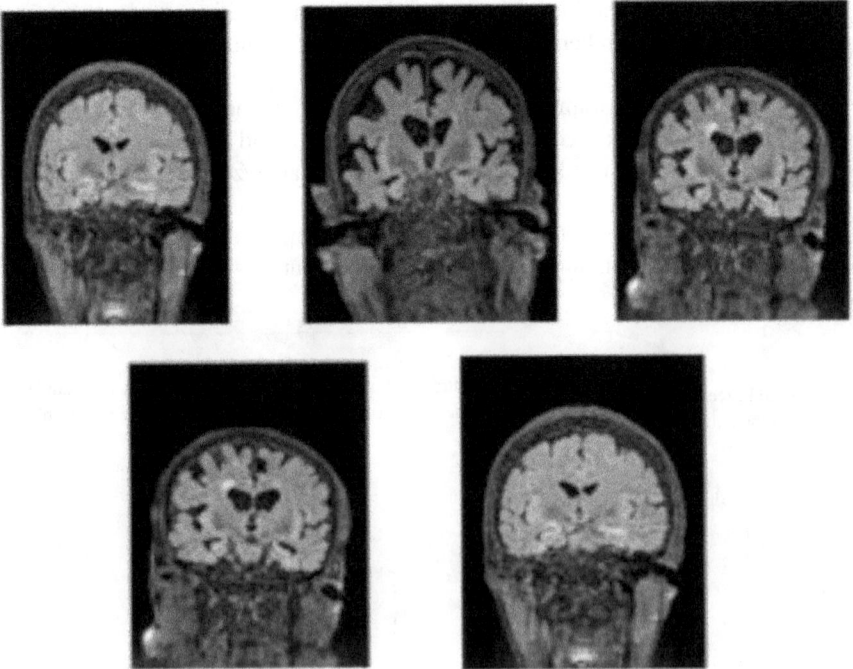

FIGURE 8.2   Samples of acquired AD subjects' MRIs in the coronal view.

Source: Author's owner.

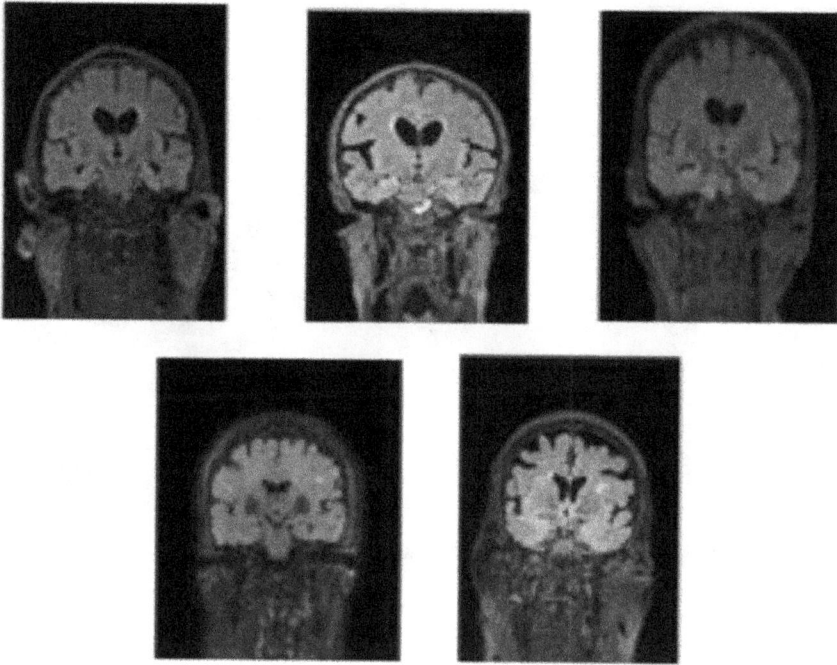

FIGURE 8.3 Samples of acquired CN subjects' MRIs in the coronal view.

Source: Author's owner.

8.3.2 SEGMENTATION

From the acquired MRIs, the hippocampus and amygdala in the left hemispherical region (ROIs) have been segmented with the assisted free hand segmentation technique available in the MATLAB (R2018b) tool.

The snapshot of the Image Segmenter tool is shown in Figure 8.4. In the coronal view of the MRI, the hippocampus looks like that of a seahorse.

8.3.3 FEATURE EXTRACTION

As the hippocampal region has more textural changes prior to its atrophy during the AD progression (Sørensen et al., 2016). Texture may be used as a prognostic biomarker for the early diagnosis of AD.

In this proposed system, the mean of the ROI, max norms, and standard deviation of the diagonal detail coefficient were considered the textural features (Rajaei & Rangarajan, 2011) and extracted using the Haar wavelet at level 2 (In mathematics, the Haar wavelet is a sequence of rescaled "square-shaped" functions that together form a wavelet family or basis). These extracted textural features (max norms and standard deviation) are shown in figure 8.5.

Equations (8.1) and (8.2) show expressions for the ROI mean and the standard deviation of the diagonal detail coefficient.

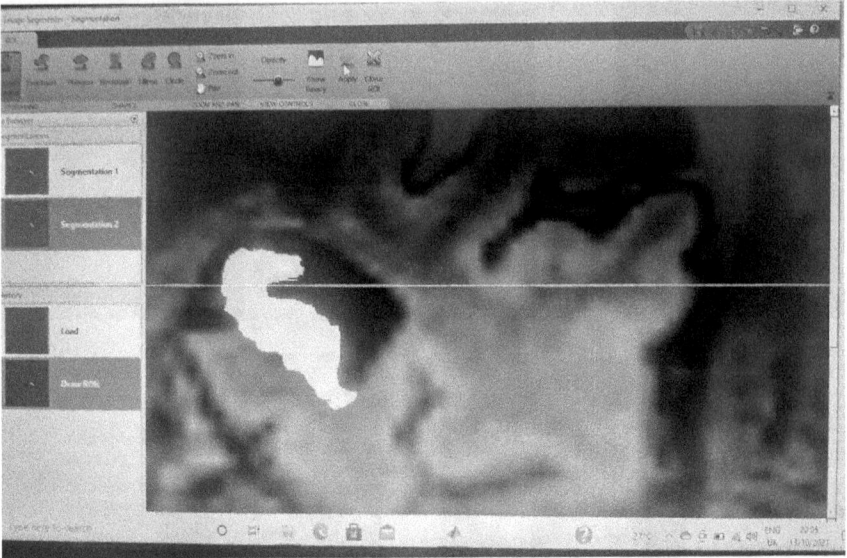

FIGURE 8.4   A snapshot of the image segmenter tool with the segmented ROI.

Source: Author's owner.

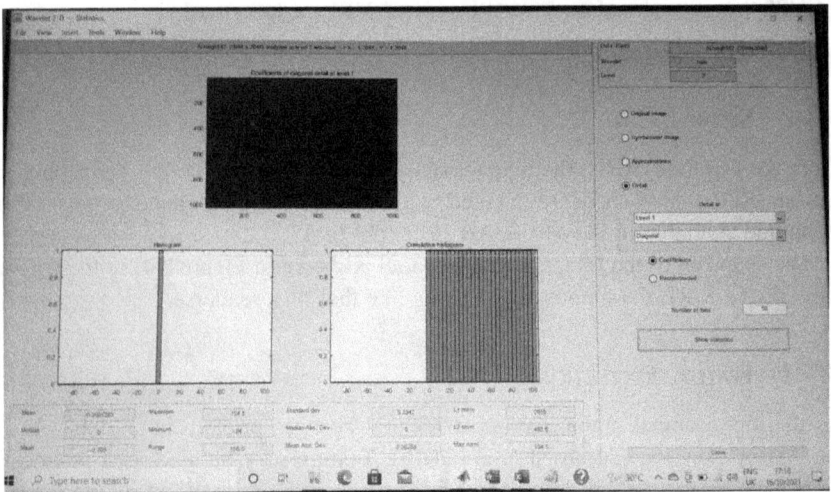

FIGURE 8.5   Textural features.

Source: Author's owner.

$$\text{Mean of ROI } \mu = \frac{\sum_{i=1}^{N} Pi}{N} \qquad (8.1)$$

Pi is the pixel intensity value.

N is the number of pixel elements in the ROI matrix.

$$\text{Standard Deviation of Diagonal Detail coefficient} = \sqrt{\frac{\Sigma_{j=1}^{k} (D_j - M)^2}{K}} \quad (8.2)$$

D_j is a gray value of the pixel element in the diagonal detail coefficient matrix. M is the mean of the pixel elements in the diagonal detail coefficient matrix. K is the number of pixel elements in the diagonal detail coefficient matrix.

8.3.4 CLASSIFICATION

The classification of AD and CN has been done using three extracted textural features as input to the fuzzy classifier. Based on the categorized output from FIS, AD, and CN subjects were classified.

8.4 TEST RESULTS AND DISCUSSION

In this research, T2-MRIs of the AD and CN groups of subjects were acquired from the ADNI-3 database (Bhambri et al., 2022). The image segmenter tool is used for the segmentation of the ROI.

Three textural features are extracted from the ROI (hippocampus and amygdala in the left hemispherical region of the brain MRI). The mean of the ROI has been calculated for all the subjects.

The Two-Dimensional Wavelet 2-D tool from the Wavelet Analyzer has been used to extract the 2D-wavelet textural features (max norm and standard deviation of the diagonal detail coefficient) from the ROI.

2D-wavelet features are extracted using the Haar wavelet at level 2. The mean of the ROI, max norms, and standard deviation of diagonal detail coefficient matrix were stored as the feature vector and given as input to the FIS. The fuzzy logic designer of the proposed system is represented in figure 8.6.

Initially, for classification, membership functions for all the input and output variables have been defined. Parameter values have been assigned for the membership functions (MF) of all the linguistic variables, and it is mentioned in table 8.1.

Expressions for trapezoidal membership functions are shown in equation (8.3) (Jang et al., 1997).

$$\mu\text{Low}(x; 0.05, 0.1, 0.37, 0.38) = \begin{cases} 0 & x \leq 0.05 \\ (x - 0.05)/(0.1 - 0.05) & 0.05 \leq x \leq 0.1 \\ 1 & 0.1 \leq x \leq 0.37 \\ (0.38 - x)/(0.38 - 0.37) & 0.37 \leq x \leq 0.38 \\ 0 & 0.38 \leq x \end{cases}$$

$$(8.3)$$

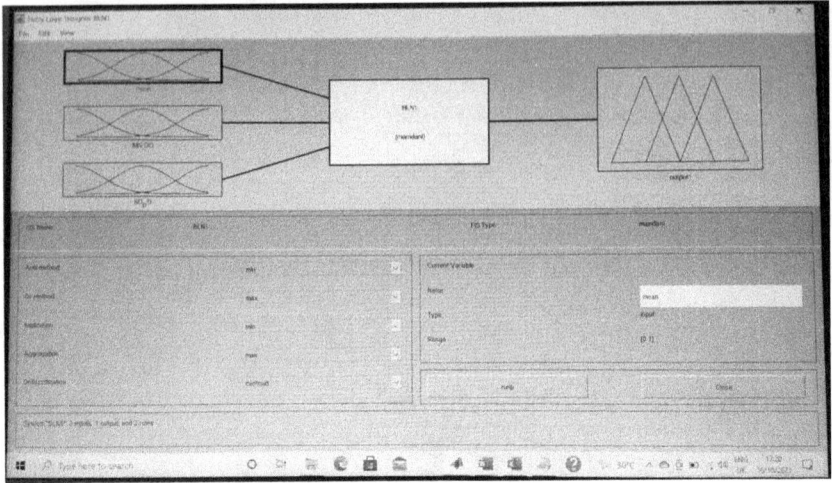

FIGURE 8.6 Snapshot of the fuzzy logic designer.

Source: Author's owner.

TABLE 8.1

Ranges and the Parameter Values for the MFs of the Linguistic Variables

I/O variables	Membership Function	MF Type	Parameters	Minimum	Maximum
Mean	Low	Trapezoidal	[0.05 0.1 0.37 0.38]	0.05	0.38
	High	Trapezoidal	[20 0.37 0.88]	0.2	1
Max norm of diagonal detail	Small	Generalized bell MF	[24.64 6.75 70]	40	100
coefficient	Large	Sigmoidal MF	[0.113 84.3]	50	150
Standard deviation	SL	Trapezoidal	[0.3 0.35 0.4 0.5]	0.3	0.5
of diagonal detail coefficient	SH	Trapezoidal	[0.41 0.44 0.5 0.7]	0.41	0.7
Categorized output	AD	Gaussian MF	[10.62 25]	0	50
	CN	Gaussian MF	[10.62 75]	50	100

Source: Author's owner.

The Gaussian, generalized bell, and sigmoidal MFs are represented by equations (8.4), (8.5), and (8.6), respectively. Gaussian MF and µAD are defined as

$$gaussian\,(x;\ 10.62,\ 25) = e^{-1/2\left(\frac{x-10.62}{25}\right)^2} \qquad (8.4)$$

Generalized bell MF and μSmall are defined as

$$\mu Small(x;\ 24.64,\ 6.75,\ 70) = \frac{1}{1 + [(x - 70)/24.64]^{2*6.75}}$$

$$= \frac{1}{1 + [(x - 70)/24.64]^{13.5}} \tag{8.5}$$

Sigmoidal MF and μLarge are defined as

$$\mu Large(x;\ 0.113,\ 84.3) = \frac{1}{1 + e^{[-0.113(x-84.3)]}} \tag{8.6}$$

Two optimized fuzzy rules were developed. The rule base of the FIS is given in table 8.2. By evaluating the three input variables (extracted textural features) using the developed fuzzy rules, categorized output values have been obtained.

In the future analysis of this study, it is suggested to increase the number of MRI samples for the analysis and use the VolBrain automated segmentation tool (Manjón & Coupé, 2016) to improve the system's performance as table 8.2.

Based on the categorized output values from the Mamdani FIS, AD, and CN subjects were classified, as mentioned in table 8.3.

TABLE 8.2
The Rule Base of the System

Rule Number	Mean	Max Norm of Diagonal Detail Coefficient	Standard Deviation of Diagonal Detail Coefficient	Categorized Output
Rule 1	Low	Large	SL	AD
Rule 2	High	Small	SH	CN

Source: Author's owner.

TABLE 8.3
Categorized Output of the FIS

MR Image Number	Subject's Actual Group Name	Mean	Max Norm of Diagonal Detail Coefficient	Standard Deviation of Diagonal Detail Coefficient	Categorized Output	Subject's Obtained Group Name
1	AD	0.15	104.5	0.394	25.2440	AD
2	CN	0.288	95	0.75	73.5856	CN
3	AD	0.12	60.5	0.36	26.8277	AD
4	CN	0.39	97.5	0.481	74.2815	CN

(Continued)

TABLE 8.3 (Continued)
Categorized Output of the FIS

MR Image Number	Subject's Actual Group Name	Mean	Max Norm of Diagonal Detail Coefficient	Standard Deviation of Diagonal Detail Coefficient	Categorized Output	Subject's Obtained Group Name
5	AD	0.2124	102.5	0.497	46.8652	AD
6	CN	0.88	68.5	0.499	74.7613	CN
7	AD	0.2115	130.5	0.312	25.5822	AD
8	CN	0.4343	90.5	0.596	74.7230	CN
9	AD	0.36	106.5	0.434	25.7548	AD
10	CN	0.208	50	0.415	59.8275	CN

Source: Author's owner.

8.5 CONCLUSION

In this proposed system, the mean of the ROI and 2D-wavelet textural features (max norms and standard deviation of the diagonal detail coefficient) were extracted using the Haar wavelet at level 2 from the ROI of the human MRI for a small group of subjects (Khanh & Khang, 2021).

Three extracted features were used for the classification of AD and CN with the Mamdani FIS classifier. It has been found that classification using FIS based on the 2D-DWT textural features improves the performance of the system (Tailor et al., 2022).

For the ten acquired samples of the MR images, 100% classification accuracy has been obtained in this semi-automated system (Hajimahmud et al., 2022).

In the future, by using a fully automated tool for the increased dataset, system performance will need to be evaluated (Rani et al., 2023).

REFERENCES

ADNI (2016). Alzheimer's disease Neuroimaging Initiative (ADNI). *Dataset of different research groups. ADNI site*, http://adni.loni.usc.edu/

Bhambri, P., S. Rani, G. Gupta & Khang, A. (2022). Cloud and Fog Computing Platforms for Internet of Things. ISBN: 978-1-032-101507, CRC Press. 10.1201/9781003213888

Hajimahmud, V. A., Khang, A. V. Hahanov, E. Litvinova, S. Chumachenko, & A. V. Alyar (2022). Autonomous Robots for Smart City: Closer to Augmented Humanity. *AI-Centric Smart City Ecosystems: Technologies, Design and Implementation* (1st Ed.). CRC Press. 10.1201/9781003252542-7

Jang, J. S. R., C. T. Sun & E. Mizutani (1997). Neuro-fuzzy and soft computing-a computational approach to learning and machine intelligence [Book Review]. *IEEE Transactions on automatic control*, 42(10), 1482–1484. https://www.researchgate.net/profile/Y-C-Ho/publication/2985273_Neuro-fuzzy_And_Soft_Computing_-_A_Computational_Approach_To_Learning_And_Machine_Intelligence_Book_Reviews/links/5df8e8-c3a6fdcc283728be1b/Neuro-fuzzy-And-Soft-Computing-A-Computational-Approach-To-Learning-And-Machine-Intelligence-Book-Reviews.pdf

Kar, S. & D. D. Majumder (2019). A novel approach of diffusion tensor visualization based neuro fuzzy classification system for early detection of Alzheimer's disease. *Journal of Alzheimer's disease Reports*, 3(1), 1–18. 10.3233/ADR-180082

Kavitha, A. R. & C. Chellamuthu. (2016). Brain tumour segmentation from MRI image using genetic algorithm with fuzzy initialisation and seeded modified region growing (GFSMRG) method. *The Imaging Science Journal*, 64(5), 285–297. 10.1080/13682199. 2016.1178412

Kavitha, S. & K. K. Thyagharajan (2018). Fuzzy Qualitative Reasoning Model for Astrocytoma Brain Tumor Grade Diagnosis. *Indian Journal of Science and Technology*, 11, 38. https:// sciresol.s3.us-east-2.amazonaws.com/IJST/Articles/2018/Issue-38/Article8.pdf

Khang, A., N. A. Ragimova, V. A. Hajimahmud & A. V. Alyar (2022). Advanced Technologies and Data Management in the Smart Healthcare System. *AI-Centric Smart City Ecosystems: Technologies, Design and Implementation* (1st Ed.). CRC Press. 10.1201/ 9781003252542-16

Khanh, H. H. & Khang, A. (2021). "The Role of Artificial Intelligence in Blockchain Applications," *Reinventing Manufacturing and Business Processes through Artificial Intelligence*, 20–40, CRC Press. 10.1201/9781003145011-2

Mallika, R. M., K. UshaRani & K. Hemalatha (2019). A fuzzy-based expert system to diagnose alzheimer's disease. *In Internet of Things and Personalized Healthcare Systems*, 65–74. Springer, Singapore. https://link.springer.com/chapter/10.1007/978-981-13-0866-6_6

Manjón, J. V. & P. Coupé (2016). volBrain: an online MRI brain volumetry system. *Frontiers in neuroinformatics*, 10, 30. https://www.frontiersin.org/articles/10.3389/fninf. 2016.00030/full

Manglam Publications. https://www.researchgate.net/profile/Maria-Lucas-8/publication/ 346017934_Contemporary_Research_in_Electronics_Computing_and_Mechanical_ Sciences/links/5fb637ec92851c933f3d6b70/Contemporary-Research-in-Electronics-Computing-and-Mechanical-Sciences.pdf#page=178

Pratt, W. K. (2007). Digital image processing: PIKS Scientific inside. *Image*, 89, 91. https:// onlinelibrary.wiley.com/doi/abs/10.1002/0470097434

Rajaei, A. & L. Rangarajan (2011). Wavelet features extraction for medical image classification. *Int. J. Eng. Sci*, 4, 131–141. https://core.ac.uk/download/pdf/35355853.pdf

Ramya, M. & M. Cyriac (2019). A Non Invasive Biomarkers for Alzheimer's disease Detection. *International Journal of Recent Technology and Engineering*, ISSN: 2277–3878, 8(2S5), 1–6. https://www.sciencedirect.com/science/article/pii/S0026265X22003782

Ramya, M. & A. R. Kavitha (2020a). Development of health care system for the prediction of Alzheimer's disease in the early stage. *Journal of Green Engineering*, IISN: 2245-4586, 10(9), 5138–5156. https://journals.sagepub.com/doi/abs/10.1177/095441192110 60989

Ramya, M. & A. R. Kavitha (2020b). Application of Soft computing techniques for Image analysis in Disease Diagnostic Systems in Contemporary Research in Electronics, *Computing and Mechanical Sciences*. ISBN 978-93-86123-75-6. https://researchgate. net/profile/Maria-Lucas-8/publication/346017934_Contemporary_Research_in_ Electronics_Computing_and_Mechanical_Sciences/links/5fb637ec92851c933f3d6b70/ Contemporary-Research-in-Electronics-Computing-and-Mechanical-Sciences.pdf# page=178

Rana, G., Khang, A. R. Sharma, A. K. Goel & A. K. Dubey (2021). Reinventing Manufacturing and Business Processes through Artificial Intelligence, (Eds.). CRC Press. 10.1201/9781003145011

Rani, S., M. Chauhan, A. Kataria & Khang A. (2021). IoT Equipped Intelligent Distributed Framework for Smart Healthcare Systems. *Networking and Internet Architecture*, (Eds.). CRC Press. 10.48550/arXiv.2110.04997

Rani, S., P. Bhambri, A. Kataria, Khang, A. & A. K. Sivaraman (Eds.). (2023). *Big Data, Cloud Computing and IoT: Tools and Applications* (1st Ed.). Chapman and Hall/CRC. 10.1201/9781003298335

Sørensen, L., C. Igel, N. Liv Hansen, M. Osler, M. Lauritzen, E. Rostrup ... & Alzheimer's Disease Neuroimaging Initiative and the Australian Imaging Biomarkers and Lifestyle Flagship Study of Ageing. (2016). *Early detection of Alzheimer's disease using M RI hippocampal texture. Human brain mapping*, 37(3), 1148–1161. https://ieeexplore. ieee.org/abstract/document/8857188/

Tailor, R. K., R. Pareek & Khang, A. (Eds.). (2022). Robot Process Automation in Blockchain. *The Data-Driven Blockchain Ecosystem: Fundamentals, Applications, and Emerging Technologies* (1st ed.), 149–164. CRC Press. 10.1201/9781003269281-8

Vrushank, S., T. Vidhi & Khang, A. (2023). Electronic Health Records Security and Privacy Enhancement using Blockchain Technology. *Data-Centric AI Solutions and Emerging Technologies in the Healthcare Ecosystem*. (1st ed.), (2023), P (1). CRC Press. 10.1201/9781003356189

9 Application of Machine Learning Algorithms in Diabetes Prediction

Muskan Singh, Anuradha Misra, and Praveen Kumar Misra

CONTENTS

9.1 INTRODUCTION

As we know, diabetes is caused because of an imbalance in the level of glucose in the patient. There is a decrease in the flow of the insulin hormone, which results in a higher glucose level, which causes diabetes. It is a major cause of death in the world. The number of patients are increasing day by day. Diabetes, with time, also affects other organs and leads to various types of health problems such as heart attack, kidney failure, low blood pressure, and many more (Dutta et al., 2018).

Diabetes mellitus is very common type diabetes which is caused by the abnormal amount of flow of insulin. Diabetes mellitus is further divided into two types: Type 1 and Type 2. This disease is a hereditary disease that is also one of the reasons for the

DOI: 10.1201/9781003356189-9

people to suffer from this disease. The symptoms for diabetes are weight loss, laziness, and higher glucose level.

Diabetes can be under-controlled if detected in the very early stage by maintaining and adopting a specific routine in one's lifestyle. The advancement in our technology has led to many such domains that are being used in such kinds of medical work.

Machine learning (ML) is that field which is been used in various fields and one such field in the healthcare sector. It's a subset of artificial intelligence (AI). Machine learning is the technique through which machines learn from their experiences by using certain algorithms to build models (Khang et al., 2022a).

9.2   MACHINE LEARNING (ML)

Machine learning is that branch of computer science which enables machines to learn from their own experiences, without programming in an exact manner. It focuses on making machines work smartly and efficiently (Rana et al., 2021). Its main aim is to make machines autonomous (Hajimahmud et al., 2022).

Machine learning is a subset of artificial intelligence. In the past few years, machine learning has been evolving rapidly day by day, becoming the leading technology around the world. We all know technology plays a very vital role in our society in today's generation (Babasaheb et al., 2023). Not only human beings are impacted by this but various types of public and private sectors have a great influence (VijiyaKumar et al., 2019).

Machine learning focuses on to development of computers and machines. It is a study of algorithms that build a mathematical model or code which is used in systems to input data. By using this data, they predict or make their own decisions from their working experience without explicitly programming. This learning makes the system automatic (Tailor et al., 2022).

The algorithms used in machines give them the ability to earn or access data from their surroundings and then analyze it for further research purposes. This process is iterative (Tiwari et al., 2019).

9.2.1   Machine Learning in Detecting Diabetes

Machine learning is the technique through which computers or machines are trained explicitly. ML plays a vital role in the healthcare sector for the last few years. There are various algorithms in machine learning that are applied on the data gathered from the patients to predict the disease (Khanh & Khang, 2021).

The algorithms are used to build up models that are used to study the data collected and then predict the results according to the datasets available (Rani et al., 2021).

Accumulated data from the patients are very useful in predicting the disease (Md. Faisal Faruque et al,. 2019).

9.2.2   Machine Learning Algorithms

When the data is ready for the further process in prediction of diabetes, machine learning algorithms are applied on the datasets.

Different techniques of machine learning algorithms have been used to build up the model to analyze the data and then for prediction of the results or consequences with great accuracy and precision (Joshi & Chawan, 2018).

9.2.3 SUPPORT VECTOR MACHINE (SVM)

It is used to solve linear and non-linear problems along with practical problems as well. This learning is used for classification and regression problems. It creates a line or hyperplane that separates the data into classes. The most popular technique of machine learning algorithms is SVM.

9.2.4 K-NEAREST NEIGHBOR (KNN)

KNN is used to solve classification as well as regression problems. This algorithm assumes that similar things are near to each other based on which it groups new work. For making a prediction for new data points, the algorithm finds out the closest neighbors in the datasets (Khang et al., 2023).

The drawback is the rate of working of the algorithm, the rate of working generally decreases when the dataset points are increased. So, it is considered to be as the lazy prediction technique. Here, K defines the number of nearest neighbors, which is always a positive integer (Naila & Sharma, 2016). The distance among the two close data points is defined by Euclidean distance.

9.2.5 LOGISTIC REGRESSION

This algorithm is a predictive analysis algorithm in machine learning. It also uses supervised learning technique. This algorithm is based on the concept of probability. Logistic regression is one of the simplest algorithms used in various classification problems such as cancer detection, heart disease, liver disease, spam detection, diabetes detection, and many more.

This algorithm assumes a linear relationship among the input variables and output variables. This algorithm is used when we have to classify or distinguish data items into categories. It classifies the data into binary form 0 and 1 only, logistic regression is based on the linear regression model. This algorithm uses sigmoid function to predict probability of positive and negative group of class (Sharma & Yadav, 2019).

9.2.6 RANDOM FOREST ALGORITHM

The random forest algorithm is also a machine learning technique that uses supervised learning. This is also used to solve regression and classification problems. It uses the method of ensemble learning that uses multiple learning algorithms together to solve any complex problem. This Learning provides better and accurate prediction or results comparative to other algorithms (Mathad & Khang, 2023).

The ensemble method is used to reduce the errors of noise and variance that usually occur in the model. Random forest algorithm is a type of ensemble learning method that is usually used in handling large amount of datasets. This algorithm was developed by Leo Bremen. The performance of a decision tree also improves using this random forest model.

The very first step in this model is to make correct choices and use the algorithm to create a decision tree for better prediction. The prediction result is stored and then voting is done for the result. The result or the prediction which has the highest number of votes is taken as preference.

9.3   STEPS OF DETECTION

- Data collection
- Data defining
- Data pre-processing
- Applying machine learning algorithms
- Analysis
- Result
- Conclusion

9.3.1   DATA COLLECTION

The very first process in the prediction of diabetes dataset is the accumulation of data from medical patients, which is required in the prediction of diabetes. The datasets include various body parameters, as shown below.

9.3.2   DATASET DEFINING AND DISTRIBUTION

The machine learning algorithm works upon datasets. The algorithm builds up a model that is used to classify the data and do comparative analysis for the accurate results (Bhambri et al., 2022).

For the model, different attributes of patient's health are required in the prediction of the disease. The attributes of the patient can be his age, sex, glucose level, body mass index (BMI), and many more body parameters useful for the detection of this disease.

The dataset that is being used in the paper is Pima Indian Diabetes Dataset imported from the unique client identifier (UCI) machine learning repository (Khang et al., 2022c). The raw information and facts is called data that is unprocessed and needs to be processed so that we can gain information useful for us from the data to be used in the situation wherever needed according to the environment, as shown in figure 9.1 and figure 9.2.

9.3.3   DATA PRE-PROCESSING

It is the most important process. Data pre-processing is the process of cleaning the data from unwanted data attributes and other impurities. Usually, datasets gathered from the medical patients have the null values or missing values and also other impurities which causes error in the computation of the data (Rani et al., 2023).

Also, the unwanted data affects the quality. So, data preprocessing process is done to improve data quality and its effectiveness. This process is necessary so that

```
data.head()
```

	Pregnancies	Glucose	BloodPressure	SkinThickness	Insulin	BMI	DiabetesPedigreeFunction	Age	Outcome
0	6	148	72	35	0	33.6	0.627	50	1
1	1	85	66	29	0	26.6	0.351	31	0
2	8	183	64	0	0	23.3	0.672	32	1
3	1	89	66	23	94	28.1	0.167	21	0
4	0	137	40	35	168	43.1	2.288	33	1

FIGURE 9.1 First 5 rows of the diabetes dataset.

Source: Author's owner.

```
data.tail()
```

	Pregnancies	Glucose	BloodPressure	SkinThickness	Insulin	BMI	DiabetesPedigreeFunction	Age	Outcome
763	10	101	76	48	180	32.9	0.171	63	0
764	2	122	70	27	0	36.8	0.340	27	0
765	5	121	72	23	112	26.2	0.245	30	0
766	1	126	60	0	0	30.1	0.349	47	1
767	1	93	70	31	0	30.4	0.315	23	0

FIGURE 9.2 Last 5 rows of the diabetes dataset.

Source: Author's owner.

machine learning algorithms could be applied effectively onto the datasets for accurate results and successful prediction. Data pre-processing is done in two steps on the available data (Khang et al., 2022b).

9.3.3.1 Missing Values Removal

In this process, the data that has the value of 0 (zero) as worth is eliminated. Other unwanted data are also removed in this process. Doing so helps to work faster and it also reduces the rate of error in the process of analyzing the data, as shown in figure 9.3.

```
data.isnull().sum()
Pregnancies                 0
Glucose                     0
BloodPressure               0
SkinThickness               0
Insulin                     0
BMI                         0
DiabetesPedigreeFunction    0
Age                         0
Outcome                     0
dtype: int64
```

FIGURE 9.3 Checking the null values in the dataset.

Source: Author's owner.

9.3.3.2   Splitting of Data

In the process, the data is split into a training dataset and a test dataset. The main aim of splitting is to compute all the attributes under same scale, as shown in figure 9.4.

The data in the training set is used in making the model based on the logic and algorithms and also the values provided in the dataset, as shown in figures 9.5 and 9.6.

```
from sklearn.model_selection import train_test_split
X_train, X_test, Y_train, Y_test = train_test_split(X, Y, test_size=0.4, random_state=101)

X_train.shape

(460, 8)

X_test.shape

(308, 8)

X.shape

(768, 8)
```

FIGURE 9.4   The training data dataset.

Source: Author's owner.

```
fig, ax = plt.subplots(figsize=(8,6))
sns.heatmap(liver_dataset.corr(), annot=True, fmt='.1g', cmap="viridis", cbar=False);
```

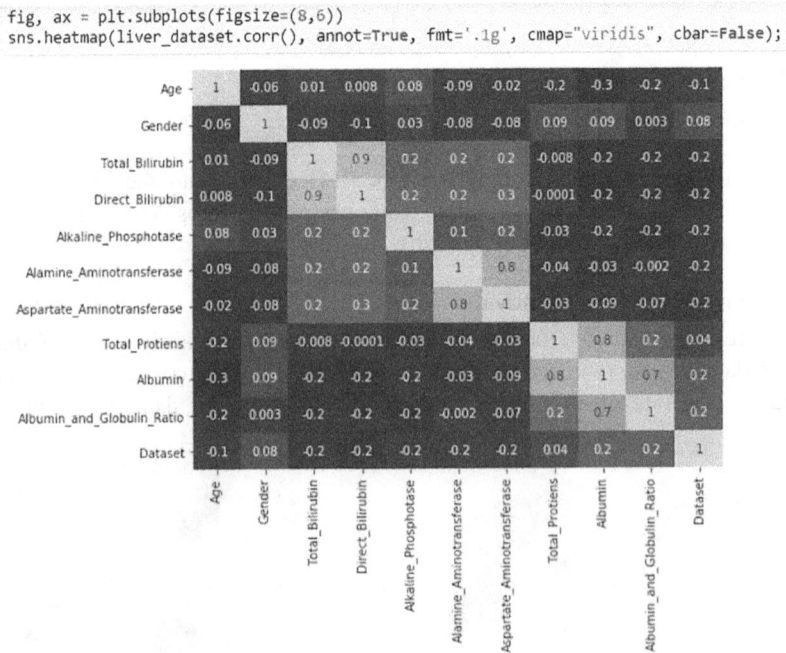

FIGURE 9.5   Correlation matrix of the dataset of diabetes.

Source: Author's owner.

9.3.4 OVERVIEW OF THE STEPS

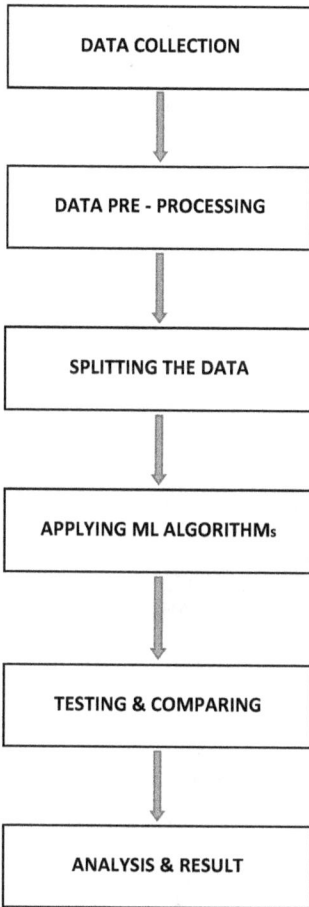

FIGURE 9.6 Overview of the steps.
Source: Author's owner.

9.4 TESTING AND COMPARING THE ALGORITHMS

After applying the algorithms, we will compute the accuracy of each and every model i.e., logistic regression, K-nearest neighbors, support vector machine, and random forest classifier. And after analyzing and comparing the accuracy for training and testing dataset, we will write the result in tabular format, as shown below.

And we can conclude that a random forest classifier model is the best algorithm for prediction of the diabetes disease, as shown in figures 9.7 and 9.8.

	Model	Training Accuracy %	Testing Accuracy %
0	Logistic Regression	78.478261	77.597403
1	K-nearest neighbors	79.782609	69.155844
2	Support Vector Machine	100.000000	65.584416
3	Random Forest Classifier	100.000000	74.025974

FIGURE 9.7 Accuracy results for diabetes prediction.

Source: Author's owner.

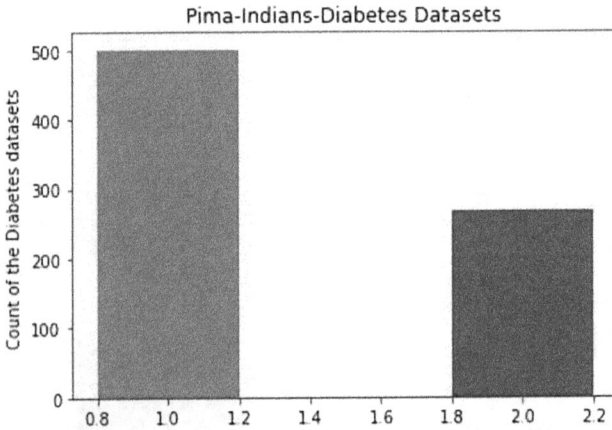

FIGURE 9.8 Result of diabetic and non-diabetic.

Source: Author's owner.

9.5 CONCLUSION

The main aim of this project is to discuss and study the machine learning algorithms technique that is being used to build a model for early diabetes prediction among the patients based on the datasets that are collected from the patients (Vrushank et al., 2023).

Algorithms such as SVM (support vector machine), KNN (K-nearest neighbor), and random forest are discussed in the paper, and, among the algorithms discussed in the paper, random forest is the best as the accuracy and precision is better than any other. These algorithms are used in building up the model for diabetes prediction (Khang et al., 2023a).

With the advancement of technology, machine learning will be very effective in our healthcare sector. It can help in saving humans' lives in any way. Early prediction in this type of disease will be a boon for our generation and upcoming generation. But people should also change their lifestyle and should adopt a proper routine in order to live a healthy life forever (Khang et al., 2023b).

REFERENCES

Babasaheb, J., B. Sphurti, Khang, A. "Industry Revolution 4.0: Workforce Competency Models and Designs," *Designing Workforce Management Systems for Industry 4.0: Data-Centric and AI-Enabled Approaches*, (1st Ed.), (2023), pp. 14–31. CRC Press. 10.1201/9781003357070-2

Bhambri, P., S. Rani, G. Gupta, Khang, A. "Cloud and Fog Computing Platforms for Internet of Things," ISBN: 978-1-032-101507, (2022), CRC Press. 10.1201/9781003213888

Dutta, D., D. Paul, P. Ghosh, "Analyzing Feature Importance's for Diabetes Prediction using Machine Learning," *IEEE*, (2018), pp. 928–942. https://ieeexplore.ieee.org/abstract/document/8614871/

Faruque, Md. Faisal, Asaduzzaman, Iqbal H. Sarker, "Performance Analysis of Machine Learning to Predict Diabetes Mellitus". *International Conference on Electrical, Computer and Communication Engineering* (ECCE), (7–9 February, 2019). https://ieeexplore.ieee.org/abstract/document/8679365/

Hajimahmud, V.A., Khang, A. V. Hahanov, E. Litvinova, S. Chumachenko, A.V. Alyar, "Autonomous Robots for Smart City: Closer to Augmented Humanity," *AI-Centric Smart City Ecosystems: Technologies, Design and Implementation* (1st Ed.), (2022). CRC Press. 10.1201/9781003252542-7

Joshi, Tejas N., Prof. Pramila M. Chawan, "Diabetes Prediction Using Machine Learning Techniques". *International Journal of Engineering Research and Application*, Volume 8, Issue 1, (Part–II) (January 2018), pp. 09–13. https://www.academia.edu/download/56913852/C0801020913.pdf

Khang, A., V. Hahanov, G.L. Abbas, V.A. Hajimahmud, "Cyber-Physical-Social System and İncident Management," *AI-Centric Smart City Ecosystems: Technologies, Design and Implementation* (1st Ed.), (2022a). CRC Press. 10.1201/9781003252542-2

Khang, A., S. Chowdhury, S. Sharma (Eds.), *The Data-Driven Blockchain Ecosystem: Fundamentals, Applications, and Emerging Technologies* (1st Ed.), (2022b). CRC Press. 10.1201/9781003269281

Khang, A., N.A. Ragimova, V.A. Hajimahmud, A.V. Alyar, "Advanced Technologies and Data Management in the Smart Healthcare System," *AI-Centric Smart City Ecosystems: Technologies, Design and Implementation* (1st Ed.), (2022c). CRC Press. 10.1201/9781003252542-16

Khang, A., S.K. Gupta, V.A. Hajimahmud, J. Babasaheb, G. Morris, (1st Ed.). *AI-Centric Modelling and Analytics: Concepts, Designs, Technologies, and Applications* (1st Ed.), (2023a). CRC Press. 10.1201/9781003400110

Khang, A., Vladimir Hahanov, Eugenia Litvinova, Svetlana Chumachenko, Triwiyanto, VA Hajimahmud, Ragimova Nazila Ali, Abuzarova Vusala Alyar, Anh P.T.N. The Analytics of Hospitality of Hospitals in Healthcare Ecosystem," *Data-Centric AI Solutions and Emerging Technologies in the Healthcare Ecosystem*. (1st Ed.), (2023b), P (4). CRC Press. 10.1201/9781003356189

Khang, A., G. Rana, R.K. Tailor, V.A. Hajimahmud, (Eds.), *Data-Centric AI Solutions and Emerging Technologies in the Healthcare Ecosystem* (1st Ed.), (2023c). CRC Press. 10.1201/9781003356189

Khanh, H.H., Khang, A. "The Role of Artificial Intelligence in Blockchain Applications," *Reinventing Manufacturing and Business Processes through Artificial Intelligence*, (2021), pp. 20–40, CRC Press. 10.1201/9781003145011-2

Mathad, K., Khang, A. 2023. "Hospital 4.0: Capitalization of Health and Healthcare in Industry 4.0 Economy," *Data-Centric AI Solutions and Emerging Technologies in the Healthcare Ecosystem*. (1st Ed.), (2023), P (4). CRC Press. 10.1201/9781003356189

Naila, A. Sharma, "Data Mining Application in Diabetes Diagnosis using biomedical Records of Pathological Attribute", *International Journal of Science and Research (IJSR)*, Volume 5 Issue 6, (2016), ISSN (Online): 2319-7064. http://192.248.57.140/handle/123456789/296

Rana, G., Khang, A. R. Sharma, A.K. Goel, A.K. Dubey, "Reinventing Manufacturing and Business Processes through Artificial Intelligence", (Eds.), (2021). CRC Press. 10.1201/9781003145011

Rani, S., M. Chauhan, A. Kataria, Khang, A. "IoT Equipped Intelligent Distributed Framework for Smart Healthcare Systems," *Networking and Internet Architecture*, (Eds.), (2021). CRC Press. 10.48550/arXiv.2110.04997

Rani, S., P. Bhambri, A. Kataria, Khang, A. A.K. Sivaraman (Eds.), *Big Data, Cloud Computing and IoT: Tools and Applications* (1st Ed.), (2023). Chapman and Hall/CRC. 10.1201/9781003298335

Sharma, A., P. Yadav, "The study of applications and trends of data mining", *Research Directions*, (May 2019), ISSN: 2321-5488. https://www.ingentaconnect.com/contentone/asp/jctn/2018/00000015/00000009/art00015

Tailor, R.K., R. Pareek, Khang, A. (Eds.), "Robot Process Automation in Blockchain," *The Data-Driven Blockchain Ecosystem: Fundamentals, Applications, and Emerging Technologies* (1st Ed.), (2022), pp. 149–164. CRC Press. 10.1201/9781003269281-8

Tiwari, S., N. Dhanda, A. Sharma, "A review on application of data mining in healthcare", *International Journal of Management, Technology and Engineering, Volume IX, Issue V*, MAY/2019, Volume IX, Issue V, (MAY/2019). https://google.com/books?id=LHQ5DwAAQBAJ

VijiyaKumar, K., B. Lavanya, I. Nirmala, S. Sofia Caroline, Proceeding of International Conference on Systems Computation Automation and Networking, (2019). IEEE. https://ieeexplore.ieee.org/abstract/document/8878802/

Vrushank, S., Vidhi T., Khang, A., 2023. "Electronic Health Records Security and Privacy Enhancement using Blockchain Technology," *Data-Centric AI Solutions and Emerging Technologies in the Healthcare Ecosystem.* (1st Ed.), (2023), P (1). CRC Press. 10.1201/9781003356189

10 An Improved Random Forest Model for Detecting Heart Disease

Avijit Kumar Chaudhuri, Sulekha Das, and Arkadip Ray

CONTENTS

10.1 INTRODUCTION

Human well-being is facing significant challenges as various virus-related diseases are increasing, as are cases of lifestyle disorders such as cardiovascular disease (CVD). Focused research and development to identify root causes as well as to develop cures are needed. CVD is the number one cause of death globally, with the World Health Organization (WHO) reporting 17.9 million deaths in 2016 (Babasaheb et al., 2023).

The situation warrants serious attention, especially in low- and middle-income countries, where CVD accounts for over three-quarters of deaths. CVD has behavioral risk factors; also, patients with hypertension and diabetes usually suffer from CVD.

Cardiologists typically interpret a patient's present diagnostic test results to diagnose CVD. The diagnosis becomes difficult when outcomes of tests conflict with each other, such as when a patient has high blood pressure (hypertension) but low cholesterol levels.

DOI: 10.1201/9781003356189-10

In this situation, the doctor may assess behavioral risk factors, such as smoking habits. In the absence of known risk factors, the diagnosis is especially challenging, and consistency of results among doctors is difficult to achieve. Human determination of the risks, or a diagnosis of CVD based on risk factors, is difficult (Khazaee, 2013).

The machine-learning (ML) approach is useful in this situation, given our increased ability to collect, store, and process data (Tailor et al., 2022), to reveal patterns and provide insights. Machine-learning techniques can predict risk at an early stage of CVD. The consequence of failure to predict the disease is especially severe (Rana et al., 2021).

In machine-learning applications (Khanh & Khang, 2021), besides accuracy, other performance measures, such as consistency, sensitivity, specificity, and area under the curve (AUC), are often equally important. Several machine learning approaches applied to the prediction of diseases in general and CVD in particular, fail to meet these additional performance criteria (Hajimahmud et al., 2022).

The success achieved in prediction depends on the type of techniques and datasets. Srinivas et al. (2010) use rule-based algorithms, decision tree (DT), Naive-Bayes (NB), and artificial neural network (ANN) to predict a heart attack (Khang et al., 2022a).

The authors introduce two new classifiers, ODANB and NCC2, and find NB techniques to achieve higher accuracy than other predictors.

- Soni et al. (2011) apply DT, NB, K-Nearest Neighbor, cluster-based classification, and neural network (NN) method, and find DT and NB to be relatively better predictors.
- Nahar et al. (2013) advocate the use of neural network and DT, while Thenmozhi & Deepika (2014) suggest the use of DT.
- Yazdani & Ramakrishnan (2015) develop a clinical decision support system based on an ANN to help doctors predict the CVD risk.
- Takci (2018) emphasize feature selection to improve accuracy. They recommended the use of the linear kernel SVM algorithm and the relief F method.
- Haq et al. (2018) evaluate seven standard machine-learning algorithms and three feature selection algorithms to predict heart disease.

However, feature selection leads to a loss of information (Khang et al., 2022b). Thus, the question remains: How can the accuracy level be improved without a reduction in features?

The above studies achieve accuracy between 80% and 90%. Other studies use associative classification and ensemble learning to improve the results (Fida et al., 2011).

- Singh & Kaur (2016) recommend an ensemble of genetic algorithm techniques and NN with fuzzy logic to achieve 99.97% accuracy.
- Liu et al. (2017), apply a rough-set-based technique on several CVD datasets, to achieve an accuracy as high as 93%.

- Abdar et al. (2019) apply the N2Genetic-nuSVM method to achieve an accuracy of 93.08% and F1-score techniques to achieve 91.51% accuracy.
- Shekar et al. (2019) develop a hybrid technique of ensemble machine-learning classifiers to predict CVD. This study builds a CVD prediction model for the Framingham Heart Study dataset (available on Kaggle). This data set consists of records of 4240 patients, with 15.2% patients suffering from CVD, the remaining without CVD, and 15 predictors of the CVD.

The data has an unequal distribution of classes, which results in classification bias towards the majority class. Most machine-learning techniques have poor prediction when the dataset is imbalanced (Khang & Sivaraman, 2022c).

Studies overcome this bias, which is notably higher when the number of variables exceeds the number of records, by identifying and using significant variables through feature selection approaches (Trivedi & Dey, 2013a). However, this leads to a loss of information as variables get left out of the study.

This study proposes an improved random forest (IRF) classifier. It compares it with several state-of-the-art machine-learning classifiers (logistic regression, NB, DT, support vector machine (SVM) with radial basis function kernel, and random forest) as well as previous studies on the same data set (Bhambri et al., 2022).

We base the comparison on several performance metrics and statistical tests (accuracy, sensitivity, specificity, AUC, Kappa statistic) on 50–50%, 66–34%, 80–20% splits of training and testing data, and use 10-fold cross-validation, as shown in figure 10.1. The aim is to answer the following research questions:

- RQ1: Is the proposed IRF classifier recommended for the prediction of CVD?
- RQ2: Does the proposed IRF classifier meet the additional criteria of AUC?
- RQ 3: Is the proposed IRF classifier consistent and statistically significant for the different levels of training and testing samples of the dataset?
- RQ4: What are the benefits of random over-sampling of the training dataset, and the consequences of (incorrect) over-sampling before splitting the dataset?

10.2 METHODOLOGY

10.2.1 DATASET

We use the Framingham Heart Study dataset, which is available at the kaggle.com website. This dataset comprises 4240 patient data, of which 15.2% were diagnosed with CVD, and the rest were without CVD. We provide a full description of the data in table 10.1, with 15 predictors of the CVD and two classes, i.e., patients with CVD and patients without CVD.

Before building the model, we examine the dataset. The output class of the data is highly imbalanced, with 84.8% positive (3596 patients without CVD) and 15.2% negative (644 patients with CVD).

Classification accuracy of approximately 85% (or an error rate of 15%) can be easily achieved, in such a domain, by considering each new patient to be without CVD.

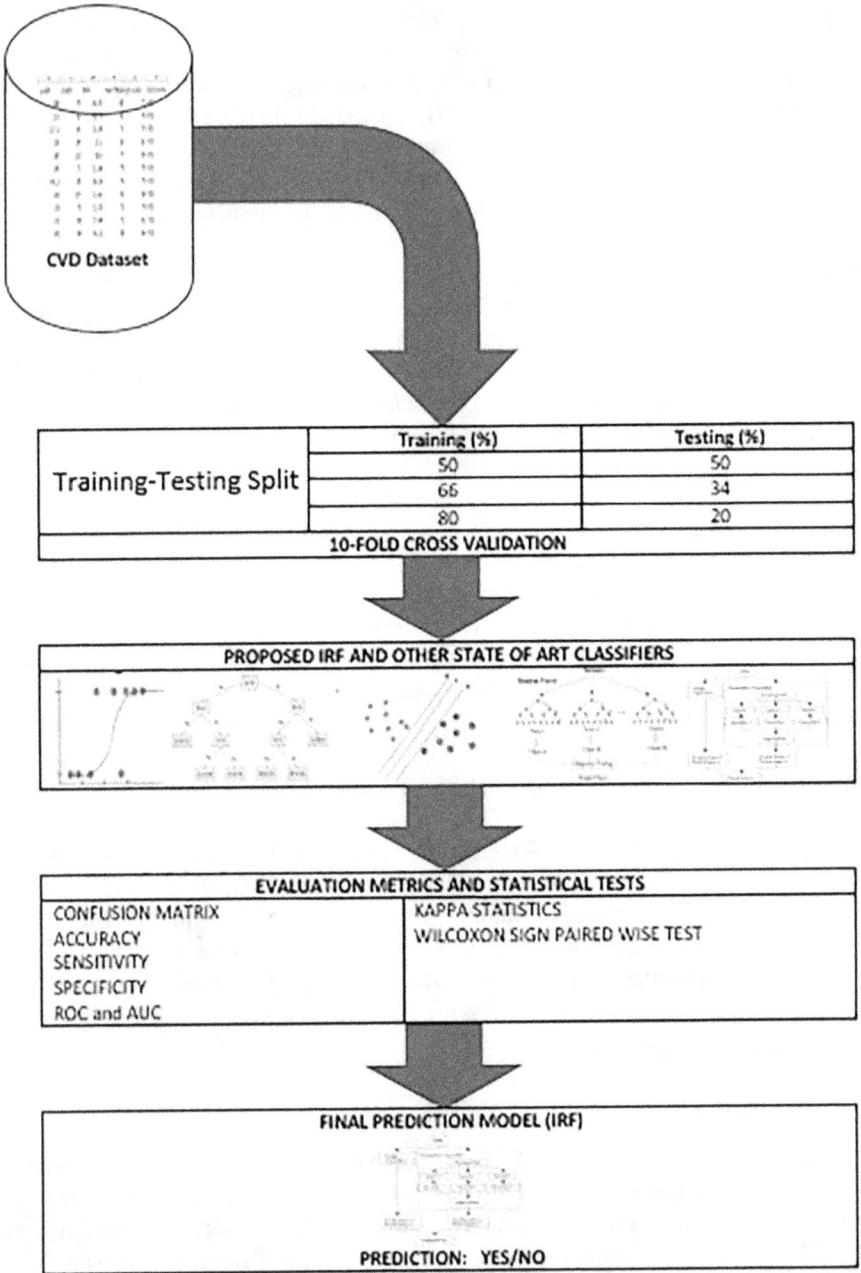

Training-Testing Split	Training (%)	Testing (%)
	50	50
	66	34
	80	20
10-FOLD CROSS VALIDATION		

PROPOSED IRF AND OTHER STATE OF ART CLASSIFIERS

EVALUATION METRICS AND STATISTICAL TESTS	
CONFUSION MATRIX ACCURACY SENSITIVITY SPECIFICITY ROC and AUC	KAPPA STATISTICS WILCOXON SIGN PAIRED WISE TEST

FINAL PREDICTION MODEL (IRF)

PREDICTION: YES/NO

FIGURE 10.1 Figure 10.1 displays the flowchart of the experimental design and CVD prediction model.

Source: Author's owner.

TABLE 10.1
Description of the Dataset

Sl. No	Attributes	Description	Range of Values	% of Categories	Mean	Std. Dev
1	Age	Age at exam time in years	Continuous		49.58	8.57
2	male	Male or Female	0 = Female 1 = Male	43% Male, 57% Female		
3	education	Education of the patient	= Some High School = High School or GED = Some College = College	11% Some High School 32% High School or GED 16% Some College 41% College		
4	currentSmoker	At present smoker or not	0 = non-smoker 1 = smoker	49% smoking; 51% non-smoking		
5	cigsPerDay	Smoking habits - Average no. of cigarettes/day	Continuous		9.01	11.92
6	BPMeds	Blood pressure medications	0 = not on medications; 1 = on medications	3% on medications; 97% not on medications		
7	prevalentStroke	Fasting blood sugar > 120 mg/dl	= false = true	0.6% with stroke; 99.4% no stroke		
8	prevalentHyp	Hypertension	= false = true	31.06% with 68.94% without		
9	diabetes	Diabetes present or not	= No = Yes	3% present; 97% not present		
10	totChol	Total amount of cholesterol present in blood	mg/dL		236.70	44.59

(Continued)

TABLE 10.1 (Continued)
Description of the Dataset

Sl. No	Attributes	Description	Range of Values	% of Categories	Mean	Std. Dev
11	sysBP	Systolic blood pressure	mmHg	132.35	22.03	
12	diaBP	Diastoloc blood pressure	mmHg	82.90	11.91	
13	BMI	Body mass index	Weight/Height (kg/m^2)	25.80	4.08	
14	heartRate	Beats/Min (Ventricular)	Continuous	75	12.03	
15	glucose		mg/dL	81.96	23.95	
16	TenYearCHD	Heart disease	0 = Not present 1 = Present			

Source: Author's owner.

The imbalance increases the chances of a sick patient being diagnosed as healthy (Type-2 error, which is especially severe in this case), and it reduces the likelihood of a healthy patient diagnosed as sick (Type-1 error, which is less severe and which we can correct in future exams). Moreover, the random splitting of the dataset to perform 10-fold cross-validation may result in the absence of negative instances from one or more subsets.

We balance the dataset using the over-sampling method and create approximately equal instances of each class. A comparison of over-sampling methods to balance data is provided by (Rani et al., 2023).

We compare the following three cases:

1. No over-sampling
2. Random over-sampling of the training data set
3. Over-sampling before splitting the data into training and testing sets

In Case (3), we replicate the negative instances to match the number of positive instances (Amin et al., 2016; Afzal et al., 2013; Trivedi & Dey, 2019). This replication results in 7136 records with 3596 positive and 3540 negative instances in the ratio 51:49.

We compare the proposed IRF classifier against the state-of-the-art classifiers in these three cases. The use of a simple over-sampling approach in Case (3) should indicate the minimum obtainable performance improvement. The use of the incorrect over-sampling approach in Case (3) should help differentiate its results from those of Case (1) and Case (2).

10.2.2   CHOICE OF MODELS

In this section, we describe the proposed IRF classifier and the state-of-the-art classifiers used in the comparative study.

10.2.2.1   Logistic Regression (LR)

LR allows the effect of several explanatory variables on a response variable to be analyzed simultaneously. It gives the linear combination of variables that predicts the probability of an event, such as the occurrence of CVD or no CVD. Thus, it estimates the contribution of a set of features to a binary outcome.

It is one of the most popular models, especially in clinical practice, since it enables the regression of dependent variables over broad types of variables. Its use in medical research has increased since the 1990s. Its interpretation is straightforward, and it helps in quick decision making. However, the problem with LR is its tendency to generate over-fitted models.

10.2.2.2   Naive-Bayes (NB)

The NB algorithm calculates a series of probabilities by counting the frequency and value combinations of a given dataset (Mostafa et al., 2019). It is known as a simple probabilistic classifier. The Bayes' algorithm employs conditional probability to determine the probability of a randomly selected feature selected as a classifier on a particular category.

NB assumes that any two randomly chosen features are statistically independent of each other, avoiding the problem from a large number of vectors in the Bayesian classifier (Trivedi & Dey, 2013b). This conditional presumption of independence seldom holds in real-world applications; hence, the characterization of this algorithm as "naive." The algorithmic rule, however, performs well and quickly learns numerous supervised classification problems (Dimitoglou et al., 2012).

The Bayes' theorem is one of the most common classification techniques applied to small datasets due to its simplicity, robustness, and accuracy. The performance of the NB classifier with large datasets and datasets with complex attribute dependencies is poor. Trivedi and Dey (2013b) showed that the Bayesian classifier performs better than NB on a dataset with 375 features.

10.2.2.3   Decision Tree (DT)

DT enables supervised classification and allows the processing of erroneous datasets and missing values. This method calculates the value of the dependent attribute, given the values of independent attributes (Shouman et al., 2012).

A DT classifier employs the C5.0 algorithm, which identifies the informative features based on the concept of entropy and forms a node in the tree if a split increases the information gain. It is an iterative process, and the classifier evaluates all features (Trivedi & Dey, 2013a). This method does not require any form of normalization or scaling of variables to set the relationship between dependent and independent attributes.

The results obtained from DT are not affected by outliers, as the classification is based on the proportion of samples with split ranges and not on absolute values. This method does not demand linearity in relationships between the dependent and independent attributes. DT explains the results well and is very intuitive.

A DT method works well in medical or healthcare databases (Khang et al., 2023a) and permits classification according to different labels, such as with or without the disease (Manikandan et al., 2020). This approach becomes difficult when the database is vast, leading to the use of the RF technique or the SVM model.

10.2.2.4   Support Vector Machine (SVM)

Vapnik created the SVM algorithm as a regulatory algorithm in 1995. The basis of this technique is to use exactness to generalize errors. This technique generates one 'hyperplane' and divides the data into classes to categorize the samples.

SVM shows good results for multi-domain or binomial applications in a big data environment. It performs faster after training (Cavallaro et al., 2015). However, this method is mathematically complicated and computationally expensive (Suthaharan, 2016).

A large dataset is likely to contain noise, and SVM yields poor results in such cases. This low performance is because SVM makes use of hyperplanes and support vectors that classify in higher-dimensional space.

Studies have overcome this drawback by combining SVM with other machine-learning techniques. The efficiency of SVM lies in its use of the appropriate kernel function and fine-tuning (Trivedi & Dey, 2013b).

10.2.2.5 Random Forest (RF)

RF, a supervised machine-learning algorithm, is a blended arrangement technique based on the statistical learning hypothesis. RF creates multiple DTs and combines them to give the best classification (Dauwan et al., 2016).

To generate the individual classifiers, it uses either a bagging or random selection of features (Trivedi & Dey, 2014). It uses a classifier strategy, called the unweighted majority of class votes, to minimize errors.

A large number of trees make an RF from the selected samples. Each tree votes and the most popular class gets chosen as the outcome in a classification problem. The introduction of the right kind of randomness impacts the accuracy of RF. The generation of the tree with minimal depth has an advantage as it is independent of how prediction error is measured.

10.2.2.6 Stacking and Proposed Classifier: Improved Random Forest (IRF)

Stacking aims to leverage several state-of-the-art classifiers' abilities to achieve prediction accuracy, which is an improvement over that of the individual classifiers in the ensemble. Stacking splits the training dataset into the same number of subsets as the classifiers in the ensemble and each classifier in the ensemble trains on a non-overlapping subset (Rani et al., 2023).

The method assigns a relative weight to each classifier based on achieved fit, to create a Meta RF classifier (Sikora, 2015; Bhasuran et al., 2016). The LR is usually the final meta-classifier. The proposed IRF method uses LR, SVM, and NB as the base classifiers, with RF as the final meta-classifier.

During the testing of a particular instance, a class distribution vector is created by individual base classifiers, which indicates the particular class of the instance. Let Δ_v denote the class distribution vector created by the vth base classifier. The class distribution vector for two classes is indicated as below:

$$\Delta_v = [\partial_{1v}\ \partial_{2v}] \quad \text{for } v = 1, 2, \dots n \qquad (10.1)$$

where,

$$0 \le \partial_{iv} \le 1 \quad \text{for } i = 1, 2; \ v = 1, 2, \dots, n$$
$$\sum_{i=1}^{2} \partial_{iv} = 1$$

We can represent the class vector for the 'n' base classifiers as follows:

$$\Delta = [\Delta_1\ \Delta_2 \dots \Delta_n]^T \qquad (10.2)$$

Finally, to create the meta-classifier the weight distribution vector is created to assign weight for each individual classifier. For the n classifier, the weight distribution vector is as follows:

$$\varnothing = [\theta_1\ \theta_2\ \theta_3 \dots \theta_n] \tag{10.3}$$

where,

$$0 \le \theta_v \le 1 \quad \text{for } v = 1, 2, \dots, n$$
$$\sum_{v=1}^{n} \theta_v = 1$$

With the help of the class distribution matrix (see equation 10.2) and the weight distribution matrix (see equation 10.3), the meta-classifier develops a $1 * 2$ distribution (see equation 10.4) to classify each instance in the test set.

$$\Delta' = \varnothing \Delta = [\partial_1^l\ \partial_2^l] \tag{10.4}$$

where,

$$\partial_i^l = \sum_{v=1}^{n} \varnothing_i \partial_{iv} \quad \text{for } i = 1, 2$$

The working of the proposed method is depicted in figure 10.2 (Wang et al., 2020; Dawngliani et al., 2019; Haq et al., 2018; Ransom et al., 2019).

10.3 ASSESSMENT OF PERFORMANCE OF MACHINE-LEARNING ALGORITHMS

In machine learning, we split the original dataset into a 'train' and 'test' dataset. We use the 'train' dataset to construct and tune the predictive model, and the 'test' data set to assess its generalizing (Trivedi & Dey, 2013a).

In this study, we applied this idea to split the balanced dataset into two subsets with the train: test ratio as 50–50, 66–34, and 80–20% as in table 10.2. We also perform 10-fold cross-validation.

After testing, we obtain a confusion matrix of each classifier, and accuracy, sensitivity, specificity, and AUC scores and Kappa statistics. Also, we perform the Wilcoxon sign rank-sum (WRS) test for pairwise data on the models (Khang et al., 2023b). Table 10.2 provides the confusion matrix and summarizes these metrics and statistical tests (table 10.3).

10.4 RESULTS AND DISCUSSION

In this study, we compared the performance of the proposed IRF classifier with five state-of-the-art machine-learning classifiers (LR, NB, SVM, DT, and RF) using the Python programming language.

We evaluated the model's performance in the case of (i) no over-sampling, (ii) random over-sampling of the training data set (which we refer to also as over-sampling after splitting), and (iii) over-sampling before splitting the data into training and testing sets.

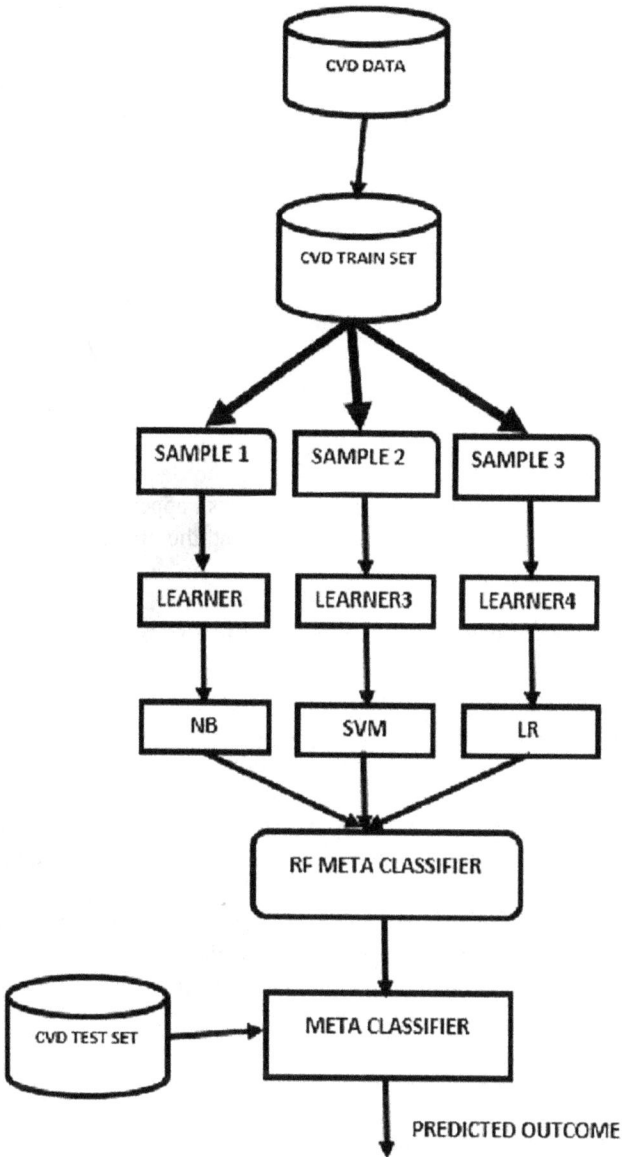

FIGURE 10.2 Working of the proposed classifier with n = 3.

Source: Author's owner.

The accuracy, sensitivity, specificity, AUC, and Kappa statistics are the basis of comparison and they are provided in tables 10.4–10.8, respectively.

As shown in table 10.4, the machine-learning approaches yielded different levels of accuracy. For the case of no over-sampling, all classifiers, except NB and DT, performed equally well. For the case of random over-sampling of the training data set, the accuracy of IRF, LR, and SVM reduced noticeably.

TABLE 10.2

Training and Testing Set of Patients

Train-Test	Over-Sampling	Over-Sampling	Before Splitting	After Splitting
B (C) % of Non-CVD (CVD) Patients in **A** – the no. of records in training set				
	A (B=C=50)	A	B	C
50–50	3596	3568	49.89	50.11
66–34	4748	4709	50.24	49.76
80–20	5754	5708	50.12	49.88
10-fold	6894	7136	50.39	49.61

Source: Author's owner.

In the case of over-sampling, before splitting the data into training and testing sets, several samples in the training and testing sets happen to be shared; this leads to highly optimistic results and does not reflect the model's actual predictive performance.

The accuracy of DT and RF increases dramatically. Due to over-sampling, the classification accuracy of patients with CVD is likely to improve, but the overall prediction accuracy may decrease. In this case, accuracy is not an ideal metric to assess predictive performance, and we also look at other metrics.

As shown in table 10.5, the results are for the comparison of sensitivity for (i) no over-sampling, (ii) over-sampling after splitting, and (iii) over-sampling before splitting.

As shown in table 10.6, the results are for the comparison of specificity for (i) no over-sampling, (ii) over-sampling after splitting, and (iii) over-sampling before splitting.

As shown in table 10.4 and table 10.5, the machine-learning approaches yielded different levels of sensitivity and specificity. For the case of no over-sampling, all classifiers, except DT, perform equally based on sensitivity. IRF, LR, and RF are the best performers, and DT is the worst performer based on specificity. For the case of random over-sampling of the training dataset, the sensitivity increases, and specificity decreases of IRF, LR, NB, and SVM. The magnitude of change is higher for IRF, LR, and SVM (Misra et al., 2023).

RF and NB are the best performers, and DT is the worst performer based on specificity. For the case of over-sampling, before splitting the data into training and testing sets, the sensitivity decreases, and specificity increases of SVM, noticeably, contradicting the results obtained by random over-sampling after of the training dataset as in table 10.7.

The composite metric ROC AUC score is often more useful for comparing models and providing clarity than accuracy, sensitivity, and specificity (Vandewiele et al. 2020).

We present the AUC values in table 10.6. AUC measures the degree to which the ROC curve is up in the northwest corner. For a balanced dataset, a score of 0.5 is

TABLE 10.3
Confusion Matrix and Performance Evaluation Metrics and Statistical Tests

S/N	Metrics	Formula/Description
1	Confusion Matrix	
		Actual
		Predicted Without CVD With CVD
		Without CVD True Positive (TP) False Positive (FP)
		With CVD False Negative (FN) True Negative (TN)
2	Accuracy	$\dfrac{TP+TN}{TP+TN+FP+FN} * 100$
3	Sensitivity	$\dfrac{TP}{TP+FN} * 100$
4	Specificity	$\dfrac{TN}{TN+FP} * 100$
5	Kappa statistics	$\dfrac{pa - pac}{1 - pac}$, 'pa' represents total agreement probability and 'pac'
6	Area under the curve (AUC)	Receiver operating characteristic (ROC) is plotted between Sensitivity and (1-Specificity). The area under the curve (AUC) measures the degree to which the curve is up in the northwest corner
7	Wilcoxon's Sign Rank-Sum (WRS)	The WRS test is used to determine whether two samples (AUC scores) vary considerably from each other

Source: Author's owner.

TABLE 10.4

The Comparison of Accuracies for (i) no Over-Sampling, (ii) Over-Sampling After Splitting, and (iii) Over-Sampling Before Splitting

	Accuracies (%)					
Train-Test	LR	NB	DT	SVM	RF	IRF
50–50	85,67,66	83,80,60	74,77,87	84,69,66	84,84,92	85,69,67
66–34	85,66,68	82,79,60	76,76,81	84,67,70	84,83,95	85,69,68
80–20	85,64,67	82,79,60	75,78,85	84,66,71	84,82,97	85,66,68
10-fold	85,66,67	82,80,63	74,76,92	84,65,75	84,84,98	85,67,66

Source: Author's owner.

TABLE 10.5

The Basis of Comparison of Accuracy, Sensitivity, Specificity, Area Under the Curve, and Kappa Statistics

	Sensitivity (%)					
Train-Test	LR	NB	DT	SVM	RF	IRF
50–50	85,92,67	83,87,90	75,86,67	85,90,69	85,85,87	85,90,70
66–34	85,91,68	83,87,90	76,85,69	84,90,70	84,85,92	85,90,70
80–20	85,91,66	82,86,89	76,85,72	85,89,71	85,81,100	85,90,72
10-fold	85,91,68	86,87,89	76,86,100	84,91,74	85,85,100	85,91,67

Source: Author's owner.

TABLE 10.6

The Basis of Comparison of Specificity for (i) no Over-Sampling, (ii) Over-Sampling After Splitting, and (iii) Over-Sampling Before Splitting

	Specificity (%)					
Train-Test	LR	NB	DT	SVM	RF	IRF
50–50	76,27,65	40,35,28	19,23,79	36,26,68	46,47,95	79,27,64
66–34	73,26,68	38,31,29	26,22,93	40,26,70	50,40,98	73,27,65
80–20	77,24,68	33,28,30	24,19,87	50,24,71	36,35,96	87,24,65
10-fold	67,26,67	36,33,36	21,21,86	30,25,76	50,41,96	65,26,67

Source: Author's owner.

TABLE 10.7

The Comparison of AUC for (i) no Over-Sampling, (ii) Over-Sampling After Splitting, and (iii) Oversampling Before Splitting

	AUC (%)					
Train-Test	LR	NB	DT	SVM	RF	IRF
50–50	52,67,66	58,60,60	52,54,87	50,64,66	51,54,92	52,66,67
66–34	52,67,67	57,58,53	57,53,82	50,64,68	51,53,92	52,65,68
80–20	52,64,61	55,56,54	56,51,93	51,62,69	51,50,98	52,63,68
10-fold	52,66,61	57,59,55	54,54,92	50,66,67	52,54,98	53,67,67

Source: Author's owner.

TABLE 10.8

The Comparison of Kappa Statistic for (i) no over-Sampling, (ii) Over-Sampling After Splitting, and (iii) Over-Sampling Before Splitting

	Kappa Statistic [−100,100]					
Train-Test	LR	NB	DT	SVM	RF	IRF
50–50	8,22,33	20,21,20	5,9,75	1,19,32	5,11,84	9,21,35
66–34	9,20,35	17,18,19	13,7,62	1,19,40	5,11,90	7,20,36
80–20	8,17,34	13,13,19	11,4,70	4,15,42	3,2,93	8,17,37
10-fold	8,20,35	17,20,26	7,8,84	0,19,50	6,12,96	11,21,33

Source: Author's owner.

considered no better than a random guess. A score of 0.6–0.7 is considered weak and 0.7 to 0.8 is considered acceptable. NB and DT (with the lowest accuracy) are the best performers, without over-sampling.

IRF, LR, SVM, and NB are the best performers for random over-sampling of the training dataset. IRF, LR, and SVM (whose accuracy and specificity reduces and sensitivity increase) by random over-sampling of the training data set, achieve approximately 30% improvement in AUC scores.

This improvement in the AUC score exceeds the average of 4–10% predicted as possible, with over-sampling, by Kovács. (2019), and Vandewiele et al. (2020). RF (DT), which performed well (poorly) based on accuracy, sensitivity, and specificity, shows poor performance based on AUC.

DT and RF achieve close to 100% improvement in the AUC score by over-sampling, before splitting the dataset into training and testing sets. The significant improvement in AUC agrees with the prediction of Vandewiele et al. (2020). In contrast, the performance of LR, NB, and SVM deteriorates, as shown in table 10.8.

Comparing the performances of different machine-learning classifiers might generate an ambiguous result if the comparison is based only on accuracy-based metrics. Cohen's Kappa Statistic (CKS) value assists in inspecting classifications that may be due to chance. The CKS takes a value between −1 and +1.

Kappa values of 0–0.20 are considered as slight, and of 0.21–0.40 are considered as fair. As the classifier's calculated Kappa value approaches 1, its performance is assumed to be more realistic than "by chance."

NB and DT are the best performers (also with the best AUC scores) for no over-sampling. IRF, LR, SVM, and NB are the best performers (also with the best AUC scores) for random over-sampling after of the training data set.

Class imbalance, in the presence of class overlap, increases the probability of classifying CVD patients as healthy (Rani et al., 2021). The SVM and NB method are known to show more performance than the DT method on reducing class overlap (Xiong et al. 2010).

DT and RF are poor performers (also with poor AUC scores) for no over-sampling and random over-sampling of the training dataset.

DT and RF achieve near-perfect results by oversampling before splitting the dataset into training and testing sets. The performance of IRF, LR, NB, and SVM also improves, as shown in table 10.9.

We also applied the non-parametric statistical WRS test to compare the performance of the different machine-learning algorithms used in this study (Wilcoxon, 1945). This hypothesis test evaluates the statistical differences among two AUC populations by comparing the median of a single column of numerical values against a hypothetical median.

Table 10.9 lists the p-values of the WRS test for the AUC scores recorded in the 10-fold cross-validation test, for case (ii) random over-sampling of the training data set.

The proposed IRF classifier produces a p-value less than 0.05 with RF, DT, and NB classifiers, which means the medians of these two distributions differ. Thus, the null hypothesis H0, for all these pairs can be rejected, which indicates that our proposed model yielded better results than these classification models.

Beunza et al., (2019) focused on the problem of imbalance of the Framingham Heart CVD dataset and tried to overcome this problem using feature engineering

TABLE 10.9

Wilcoxon Signed Rank-Sum Test for Over-Sampling After Splitting

LR	RF	IRF	NB	SVM	DT
LR	0.002	**0.769**	0.001	**0.193**	0.002
RF		0.001	0.001	0.001	**0.921**
IRF			0.001	**0.275**	0.008
NB				0.006	0.004
SVM					0.001

Source: Author's owner.

and oversampling methods. They selected eight features to include in the model and conducted over-sampling before splitting the dataset into training and testing sets.

They compared DT, boosted DT, RF, SVM, NN, and LR with optimized hyper-parameters. They found SVM to achieve the best AUC score of 68% using the R programming language. We achieved the same AUC value without feature engineering, without optimizing the value of hyper-parameters and random over-sampling only of the training dataset.

We recorded a significantly improved AUC only by over-sampling before splitting the dataset into training and testing sets.

10.5 CONCLUSION

CVD is one of the leading causes of death globally, especially in low- and middle-income countries. The detection of CVD requires several medical tests and their interpretation by doctors. In the case of conflict in the results of medical tests, the diagnosis becomes difficult, affecting the consistency.

Human determination of the risks, or a diagnosis of CVD based on risk factors, is difficult. Machine-learning techniques can predict risk at an early stage of CVD based on the features of regular lifestyles and results of a few medical tests.

We considered the Framingham Heart Study dataset (Khang et al., 2023a). This data set consisted of records of 4240 patients, with 15.2% patients suffering from CVD, the remaining without CVD, and 15 predictors of the CVD.

The dataset had an unequal distribution of classes. Such imbalanced datasets increase the likelihood of diagnosing sick patients as healthy (which is especially severe). We created approximately equal instances of each class by over-sampling.

We compared the three cases: (i) no over-sampling, (ii) random over-sampling of the training dataset, and (iii) over-sampling before splitting the dataset into training and testing sets. We applied 50–50%, 66–34%, and 80–20% train-test splits and 10-fold cross-validation.

We compared LR, NB, SVM, DT, and RF classifiers. A comparison of accuracy, sensitivity, specificity, ROC, AUC, and Kappa statistics highlighted the importance of the AUC metric. The best performers, for case (i), are NB and DT; for case (ii), are LR, SVM, and NB (due to reduction in class overlap); and for case (iii), are DT and RF (due to incorrect over-sampling). RF had more scope of improvement.

This chapter proposed an improved RF (IRF) model based on the ensemble learning technique, with RF as the meta-classifier and LR, SVM, and DT as the base classifiers. IRF exhibited a (above average) 30% improvement in the AUC score with random over-sampling of the training dataset. It also recorded a 20(10)% improvement in AUC score over RF and DT (NB) in case (ii) and was confirmed by the WRS test.

We can match the reported predictive performances on the same dataset, without using feature engineering and an optimal value of hyper-parameters, in case (ii). We could exceed it only in case (iii).

The proposed IRF is an ensemble of machine learning classifiers. Other classifiers could be tested and compared on the same dataset and used as base classifiers to improve the IRF results further.

The Framingham Heart Study data is secondary data collected from one location. CVD data from different regions and countries may be incorporated in the future to ensure the robustness and credibility of the IRF model.

The IRF model has been tested only on CVD classification, and it should further be evaluated on clinical datasets. The data used in this study is almost numeric. The IRF classifier can be tested on other applications where data nature is different, like text, image, audio, or video data (Vrushank, Vidhi & Khang, 2023).

REFERENCES

Abdar, M., Książek, W., Acharya, U.R., Tan, R.S., Makarenkov, V., & Pławiak, P. (2019). A new machine learning technique for an accurate diagnosis of coronary artery disease. *Computer Methods and Programs in Biomedicine*, 179, 104992. https://sciencedirect.com/science/article/pii/S0169260718314585

Afzal, Z., Schuemie, M.J., van Blijderveen, J.C., Sen, E.F., Sturkenboom, M.C., & Kors, J.A. (2013). Improving sensitivity of machine learning methods for automated case identification from free-text electronic medical records. *BMC Medical Informatics and Decision Making*. https://link.springer.com/article/10.1186/1472-6947-13-30

Amin, A., Anwar, S., Adnan, A., Nawaz, M., Howard, N., Qadir, J., Hawalah, A., & Hussain, A. (2016). Comparing over-sampling techniques to handle the class imbalance problem: *A customer churn prediction case study. IEEE Access*, 4, 7940–7957. https://ieeexplore.ieee.org/abstract/document/7707454/

Babasaheb, J., Sphurti, B., & Khang, A. (2023). Design of Competency Models in the Human Capital Management System. *Designing Workforce Management Systems for Industry 4.0: Data-Centric and AI-Enabled Approaches*, (1st ed.), (pp. 32–50). CRC Press. 10.1201/9781003357070-3

Beunza, J.J., Puertas, E., García-Ovejero, E., Villalba, G., Condes, E., Koleva, G., & Landecho, M.F. (2019). Comparison of machine learning algorithms for clinical event prediction (risk of coronary heart disease). *Journal of Biomedical Informatics*, 97, 103257. https://www.sciencedirect.com/science/article/pii/S1532046419301765

Bhambri, P., Rani, S., Gupta, G., & Khang, A. (2022) Cloud and Fog Computing Platforms for Internet of Things, ISBN: 978-1-032-101507, CRC Press. 10.1201/9781003213888

Bhasuran, B., Murugesan, G., Abdulkadhar, S., & Natarajan, J. (2016). Stacked ensemble combined with fuzzy matching for biomedical named entity recognition of diseases. *Journal of Biomedical Informatics*, 64, 1–9. https://www.sciencedirect.com/science/article/pii/S1532046416301216

Cavallaro, G., Riedel, M., Richerzhagen, M., Benediktsson, J.A., & Plaza, A. (2015). On understanding big data impacts in remotely sensed image classification using support vector machine methods. *IEEE Journal of Selected Topics in Applied Earth Observations and Remote Sensing*, 8(10), 4634–4646. https://opinvisindi.is/handle/20.500.11815/142

Dauwan, M., van der Zande, J.J., van Dellen, E., Sommer, I.E., Scheltens, P., Lemstra, A.W., Stam, C.J. (2016). Random forest to differentiate dementia with Lewy bodies from Alzheimer'ssease. *Alzheimer's & Dementia: Diagnosis, Assessment & Disease Monitoring*, 4, 99–106. https://www.sciencedirect.com/science/article/pii/S2352872916300392

Dawngliani, M.S., Chandrasekaran, N., Lalmuanawma, S., & Thangkhanhau, H. (2019, December). Prediction of Breast Cancer Recurrence Using Ensemble Machine Learning Classifiers. In International Conference on Security with Intelligent Computing and Big-data Services (pp. 232–244). Springer, Cham. https://link.springer.com/chapter/10.1007/978-3-030-46828-6_20

Dimitoglou, G., Adams, J.A., & Jim, C.M. (2012). Comparison of the C4.5 and a naïve Bayes classifier for the prediction of lung cancer survivability. arXiv preprint arXiv: 1206.1121. https://arxiv.org/abs/1206.1121

Fida, B., Nazir, M., Naveed, N., & Akram S. (2011). Heart disease classification ensemble optimization using genetic algorithm. *IEEE 14th International Multitopic Conference*, 19–24. https://ieeexplore.ieee.org/abstract/document/6151471/

Hajimahmud, V.A., Khang, A., Hahanov, V., Litvinova, E., Chumachenko, S., & Alyar, A.V. (2022). Autonomous Robots for Smart City: Closer to Augmented Humanity. *AI-Centric Smart City Ecosystems: Technologies, Design and Implementation* (1st Ed.). CRC Press. 10.1201/9781003252542-7

Haq, A.U., Li, J.P., Memon, M.H., Nazir, S., & Sun, R. (2018). A hybrid intelligent system framework for the prediction of heart disease using machine learning algorithms. *Mobile Information Systems*. https://www.hindawi.com/journals/MISY/2018/3860146/

Khang, A., Hahanov, V., Abbas, G.L., & Hajimahmud, V.A. (2022a). Cyber-Physical-Social System and İncident Management. *AI-Centric Smart City Ecosystems: Technologies, Design and Implementation* (1st Ed.). CRC Press. 10.1201/9781003252542-2

Khang, A., Rani, S., & Sivaraman, A.K. (2022). *AI-Centric Smart City Ecosystems: Technologies, Design and Implementation* (1st Ed.). CRC Press. 10.1201/9781003252542

Khang, A., Ragimova, N.A., Hajimahmud, V.A., & Alyar, A.V. (2022b). Advanced Technologies and Data Management in the Smart Healthcare System. *AI-Centric Smart City Ecosystems: Technologies, Design and Implementation* (1st Ed.). CRC Press. 10.1201/9781003252542-16

Khang, A., Hahanov, V., Litvinova, E., Chumachenko, S., Triwiyanto, Kadarningsih, A., Avromovic, Z., Ali, R.N., & Hajimahmud, A.V. (2023a). Cloud Platform and Data Storage Systems in Healthcare Ecosystem. *Data-Centric AI Solutions and Emerging Technologies in the Healthcare Ecosystem*. (1st Ed.), (2023), P (4). CRC Press. 10.1201/9781032398570-21

Khang, A., Rana, G., Tailor, R.K., & Hajimahmud, V.A., (Eds.). (2023b). *Data-Centric AI Solutions and Emerging Technologies in the Healthcare Ecosystem* (1st Ed.). CRC Press. 10.1201/9781003356189

Khang, A., Gupta, S.K., Dixit, C.K., & Somani, P. (2023c). Data-driven Application of Human Capital Management Databases, Big Data, and Data Mining. *Designing Workforce Management Systems for Industry 4.0: Data-Centric and AI-Enabled Approaches*, (1st Ed.), (pp. 113–133). CRC Press. 10.1201/9781003356189

Khanh, H.H., & Khang, A. (2021). The Role of Artificial Intelligence in Blockchain Applications. *Reinventing Manufacturing and Business Processes through Artificial Intelligence* (pp. 20–40). CRC Press. 10.1201/9781003145011-2

Khazaee, A. (2013). Heart beat classification using particle swarm optimization. *International Journal of Intelligent Systems and Applications*, 5(6), 25. https://www.researchgate.net/profile/Ali-Khazaee/publication/272853734_Heart_Beat_Classification_Using_Particle_Swarm_Optimization/links/577a548308aec3b743356612/Heart-Beat-Classification-Using-Particle-Swarm-Optimization.pdf

Kovács, G. (2019). An empirical comparison and evaluation of minority over-sampling techniques on a large number of imbalanced datasets. *Applied Soft Computing*, 83, https://www.sciencedirect.com/science/article/pii/S1568494619304429

Liu, X., Wang, X., Su, Q., Zhang, M., Zhu, Y., Wang, Q., & Wang, Q. (2017). A hybrid classification system for heart disease diagnosis based on the RFRS method. *Computational and Mathematical Methods in Medicine*. 2017. https://www.hindawi.com/journals/cmmm/2017/8272091/

Manikandan, R., Patan, R., Gandomi, A.H., Sivanesan, P., & Kalyanaraman, H. (2020). Hash polynomial two factor decision tree using IoT for smart health care scheduling. *Expert Systems with Applications*, 141, 112924. https://www.sciencedirect.com/science/article/pii/S0957417419306426

Misra, A., Shah, V., Khang, A., & Gupta, S.K., (Eds.). (2023). A*I-aided IoT Technologies and Applications in the Smart Business and Production* (1st Ed.). CRC Press. 10.1201/9781003392224

Mostafa, S.A., Mustapha, A., Mohammed, M.A., Hamed, R.I., Arunkumar, N., Ghani, M.K.A., & Khaleefah, S.H. (2019). Examining multiple feature evaluation and classification methods for improving the diagnosis of Parkinson's disease. *Cognitive Systems Research*, 54, 90–99. https://www.sciencedirect.com/science/article/pii/S1389041718308933

Nahar, J., Imam, T., Tickle, K.S., & Chen, Y.P.P. (2013). Computational intelligence for heart disease diagnosis: A medical knowledge driven approach. *Expert Systems with Applications*, 40 (1), 96–104. https://www.sciencedirect.com/science/article/pii/S0957417412008871

Prati, R.C., Batista, G.E., & Monard, M.C. (2004, April). Class Imbalances Versus Class Overlapping: An Analysis of a Learning System Behavior. In *Mexican International Conference on Artificial Intelligence* (pp. 312–321). Springer, Berlin. https://link.springer.com/chapter/10.1007/978-3-540-24694-7_32

Rana, G., Khang, A., Sharma, R., Goel, A.K., & Dubey, A.K. (2021). Reinventing Manufacturing and Business Processes through Artificial Intelligence, (Eds.). CRC Press. 10.1201/9781003145011

Rani, S., Chauhan, M., Kataria, A., & Khang, A. (2021). IoT Equipped Intelligent Distributed Framework for Smart Healthcare Systems. *Networking and Internet Architecture*, (Eds.). CRC Press. 10.48550/arXiv.2110.04997

Rani, S., Bhambri, P., Kataria, A., Khang A., & Sivaraman, A.K. (Eds.). (2023). *Big Data, Cloud Computing and IoT: Tools and Applications* (1st Ed.). Chapman and Hall/CRC. 10.1201/9781003298335.

Ransom, J., Galaznik, A., Buderi, R., McLean, C., Shilnikova, A., Lempernesse, B., & Berger, M. (2019). Pcn428 scalable prediction of cancer patient clinical events in real world clinical settings. *Value in Health*, 22, S519. https://www.valueinhealthjournal.com/article/S1098-3015(19)32999-7/abstract

Shekar, K.C., Chandra, P., & Rao, K.V. (2019). An Ensemble Classifier Characterized by Genetic Algorithm with Decision Tree for the Prophecy of Heart Disease. In *Innovations in Computer Science and Engineering* (pp. 9–15). Springer, Singapore. https://link.springer.com/chapter/10.1007/978-981-13-7082-3_2

Shouman, M., Turner, T., & Stocker, R. (2012). Applying k-nearest neighbour in diagnosing heart disease patients. *International Journal of Information and Education Technology*, 2(3), 220–223. https://www.academia.edu/download/13042698/Applying_k-Nearest_Neighbour_in__Diagnosing_Heart_Disease_Patients.pdf

Sikora, R. (2015). A Modified Stacking Ensemble Machine Learning Algorithm Using Genetic Algorithms. *In Handbook of Research on Organizational Transformations through Big Data Analytics* (pp. 43–53). IGI Global. https://www.igi-global.com/chapter/a-modified-stacking-ensemble-machine-learning-algorithm-using-genetic-algorithms/122748

Singh, J., & Kaur, R. (2016). Cardio vascular disease classification ensemble optimization using genetic algorithm and neural network. *Indian Journal of Science and Technology*, 9, S1. https://sciresol.s3.us-east-2.amazonaws.com/IJST/Articles/2016/Issue-Special/Article115.pdf

Soni, J., Ansari, U., Sharma, D., & Soni, S. (2011). Predictive data mining for medical diagnosis: An overview of heart disease prediction. *International Journal of Computer Applications*, 17(8), 43–48. https://chemical.journalspub.info/index.php?journal=JCME

Srinivas, K., Rani, B.K., & Govrdhan, A. (2010). Applications of data mining techniques in healthcare and prediction of heart attacks. *International Journal on Computer Science and Engineering* (IJCSE), 2(2), 250–255. https://www.researchgate.net/profile/Dr-Govardhan/publication/49617135_Applications_of_Data_Mining_Techniques_in_Healthcare_and_Prediction_of_Heart_Attacks/links/5435156d0cf2dc341daf6a8e/Applications-of-Data-Mining-Techniques-in-Healthcare-and-Prediction-of-Heart-Attacks.pdf

Suthaharan, S. (2016). Machine learning models and algorithms for big data classification. *Integrated Series in Information Systems*, 36, 1–12. https://link.springer.com/content/pdf/10.1007/978-1-4899-7641-3.pdf

Tailor, R.K., Pareek, R., & Khang, A., (Eds.). (2022). Robot Process Automation in Blockchain. *The Data-Driven Blockchain Ecosystem: Fundamentals, Applications, and Emerging Technologies* (1st Ed.), (pp. 149–164). CRC Press. 10.1201/9781003269281-8

Takci, H. (2018). Improvement of heart attack prediction by the feature selection methods. *Turkish Journal of Electrical Engineering and Computer Sciences*, 26(1), 1–10. https://journals.tubitak.gov.tr/elektrik/vol26/iss1/1/

Thenmozhi, K., & Deepika, P. (2014). Heart disease prediction using classification with different decision tree techniques. *International Journal of Engineering Research and General Science*, 2(6), 6–11. https://www.researchgate.net/profile/Deepika-Ponnusamy/publication/335259464_Heart_disease_prediction_using_classification_with_different_decision_tree_techniques/links/5dfb93a54585159aa48a1bcc/Heart-disease-prediction-using-classification-with-different-decision-tree-techniques.pdf

Trivedi, S.K., & Dey, S. (2013a). Effect of feature selection methods on machine learning classifiers for detecting email spams. *In Proceedings of the 2013 Research in Adaptive and Convergent Systems* (pp. 35–40). https://dl.acm.org/doi/abs/10.1145/2513228.2513313

Trivedi, S.K., & Dey, S. (2013b). Effect of various kernels and feature selection methods on SVM performance for detecting email spams. *International Journal of Computer Applications*, 66(21). https://www.academia.edu/download/45450741/pxc3886433_IJCA.pdf

Trivedi, S.K., & Dey, S. (2014). Interaction between feature subset selection techniques and machine learning classifiers for detecting unsolicited emails. *ACM SIGAPP Applied Computing Review*, 14(1), 53–61. doi:10.1145/2600617.2600622

Trivedi, S.K., & Dey, S. (2019). A modified content-based evolutionary approach to identify unsolicited emails. *Knowledge and Information Systems*, 60(3), 1427–1451. https://link.springer.com/article/10.1007/s10115-018-1271-1

Vandewiele, G., Dehaene, I., Kovács, G., Sterckx, L., Janssens, O., Ongenae, F., & VanHoecke, S. (2020). Overly Optimistic Prediction Results on Imbalanced Data: Flaws and Benefits of Applying Over-sampling. arXiv preprint arXiv:2001.06296.

Vrushank, S., Vidhi, T., & Khang, A. (2023). Electronic Health Records Security and Privacy Enhancement using Blockchain Technology. *Data-Centric AI Solutions and Emerging Technologies in the Healthcare Ecosystem*. (1st Ed.), (2023), P (1). CRC Press. 10.1201/9781003356189

Wang, L., Zhao, Z., Luo, Y., Yu, H., Wu, S., Ren, X., & Huang, X. (2020). Classifying 2-year recurrence in patients with DLBCL using clinical variables with imbalanced data and machine learning methods. *Computer Methods and Programs in Biomedicine*, 105567. https://www.sciencedirect.com/science/article/pii/S0169260719320024

Wilcoxon, F. (1945). Individual comparisons by ranking methods. *Biometrics Bulletin*, 1(6), 80–83. http://www.jstor.org/stable/3001968, 1945.

Xiong, H., Wu, J., & Liu, L. (2010, December). Classification with classoverlapping: A systematic study. *In Proceedings of the 1st International Conference on E-Business Intelligence (ICEBI2010)*, Atlantis Press. https://www.atlantis-press.com/article/2053.pdf

Yazdani, A., & Ramakrishnan, K. (2015). Performance Evaluation of Artificial Neural Network Models for the Prediction of the Risk of Heart Disease. In *International Conference for Innovation in Biomedical Engineering and Life Sciences* (pp. 179–182). Springer, Singapore. https://link.springer.com/chapter/10.1007/978-981-10-0266-3_37

11 A Hybrid Feature Selection and Stacked Generalization Model to Detect Breast Cancer

Avijit Kumar Chaudhuri, Sulekha Das, and Arkadip Ray

CONTENTS

11.1 INTRODUCTION

Cancer resulted in approximately 9.6 million deaths globally in 2018 and is the second primary reason for death. Breast cancer is prevalent among women and accounts for 0.5 million deaths yearly. In most cases, the diagnosis of breast cancer is at an advanced stage of the disease. The delayed diagnosis is usually due to a lack of awareness and resources (Khang et al., 2023a). The chances of survival in the early diagnosis of localized breast cancer exceed 80%.

DOI: 10.1201/9781003356189-11

The diagnosis of a disease requires tests performed upon the patient. A mass on the breast is diagnosed as cancer by mammography. The radiologists' interpretations of mammograms usually vary, resulting in low accuracy of prediction. In fine-needle aspiration cytology (FNAC) fluid is extracted from the breast mass.

The cell nucleus analysis determines for every trait, the mean, the standard error, and the worst (mean of the three largest values). For example, in the Wisconsin (Diagnostic) Dataset of Breast Cancer (WBC1), ten traits result in 30 features.

Physicians find it challenging to learn relevant cancer features due to the significant volume of cancer cases. The technological advancement for collecting, storing, and analyzing data has been notable in recent years. Machine learning (ML) methods help the physician make sense of the wealth of data and diagnosis of cancer. This problem is treated as a classification problem (Khanh & Khang, 2021).

The machine learning classifier is trained on an FNAC feature dataset classified into two sets: malignant and benign. The classifier can then generalize and predict a tumor as cancerous or benign, given its feature values.

The computerized diagnostic tool should generalize well and diagnose new patients, especially those with cancer, correctly. Misdiagnosing a few healthy patients' as having cancer can be rectified with additional tests. Additional, this system can provide insight into why the outputs (exhibiting interpretability).

Usually, the medical tests required to assess a patient's illness correctly result in many features. As features increase in number, they make the classification and human interpretation more challenging. In some instances, features number more than the patients (the curse of dimensionality).

Certain features cause the machine learning method to over fit the data and reduce its ability to generalize. The solution is to identify the most relevant features by reducing redundancy. Besides reducing the computational effort, this improves the classifier's performance and interpretations of the physician's results (Khang et al., 2022a).

Filter and wrapper approaches are two popular methods to reduce feature subspace. The filter approach identifies relevant features by studying their statistical properties and two types: univariate and multivariate methods.

The univariate methods ignore the possibility of dependency among features, and these methods differ based on the choice of the feature evaluation criterion. One such widely used feature evaluation criterion is information gain, which indicates its information quantity and security (Khang et al., 2022c). The multivariate methods provide better performance by evaluating dependency among features but require more computational effort (Breast Cancer Wisconsin (Diagnostic) Data Set, 2023).

There are again many multivariate feature selection methods. One such method evaluates each feature's ability to predict and the redundancy among features. The wrapper method evaluates a subset of features using a classifier algorithm. Therefore, it requires higher computational effort, especially when features are several in number.

Most studies on the WBC dataset focus on the reduction in features. Stoean and Stoean (2013) propose an approach that uses the support vector machine (SVM), precisely the relabeled samples or the support vectors, to train the cooperative co-evolution classifier. A hill climbing method embedded in the cooperative co-evolution classifier identifies the significant features (Khang et al., 2022a).

Astudillo and Oommen (2013) train tree-based topology-oriented self-organizing maps and label each node in the neural network using a Euclidean criterion. To classify the test data, the closest neuron and its class are determined.

Koloseni et al. (2013) use a generalized differential evolution classifier approach. Instead of evaluating only one distance measure, they consider distance measures for each feature. Three approaches to optimize the free parameters of each distance measure are considered.

The distance measures are summed for the final classification decisions. Tabakhi et al. (2014) propose an unsupervised ant colony filter approach for feature selection. They evaluate the redundancy among features using the absolute value of the cosine.

Feature extraction tends to focus on data transfer into a quantified form. Zheng et al. (2014) use the K-mean algorithm to identify patterns in the dataset and reduce its dimensionality. The new pattern thus obtained serves as extracted features of tumors. Chen et al. (2014) select parameter values and features for SVM using a parallel time-variant particle swarm optimization (PSO) algorithm.

PSO's objective function is a weighted function of the average classification accuracy rates, the number of support vectors, and the selected features. Saez et al. (2014) compare the nearest-neighbor classifier's performance using several features weighing algorithms. Lim and Cha (2015) incorporate feature weights in the Bandler–Kohout (BK) sub-product and propose an approach to automatically train the BK sub-product (without the use of predefined rules or experts knowledge) (Hajimahmud et al., 2022).

Aličković and Subasi (2017) propose a genetic algorithm, with fitness evaluation using rotation forest, to eliminate irrelevant features. Abdar et al. (2018) evaluate the performance of four two-layered nested ensemble classifiers.

The base-classifiers are logistic model tree and stochastic gradient descent (SGD), along with either BayesNet or Naïve-Bayes. The meta-classifiers are SGD and J48, with or without reduced error pruning tree, as shown in table 11.1.

This chapter proposes a hybrid filter-wrapper feature selection method, which in Phase I utilizes a greedy step-wise search and multivariate-feature evaluator.

- **Phase** 1 achieves an approximate solution with low computational effort.
- **Phase** 2 utilizes a best-first search and logistic regression learning algorithm to evaluate the features. The wrapper approach's computational effort in Phase 2 is reduced due to the reduced feature sub-space in Phase 1. This method attempts to select features iteratively. Its greedy nature requires lower computational effort and is preferred when features are several in number.
- In **Phase** 3, several frequently used machine learning classifiers and a stacked generalization approach are used in the reduced feature sub-space to identify patients with or without cancer. Ten-fold cross-validations and different splits of datasets as training and testing are used.

The experimental, which compares predictions with all features, the feature subset obtained in Phase 1, and the feature subset obtained in Phase 2 demonstrate the proposed hybrid feature selection method's efficiency and effectiveness.

TABLE 11.1

Summary of Studies on the Dataset of Breast Cancer Studies on Wisconsin (Diagnostic) Dataset of Breast Cancer

Study	Classification Method	Feature Selection Method
Stoean & Stoean (2013)	Hybrid of support vector machine (SVM) and cooperative coevolution	Hill climbing method embedded in cooperative co-evolution
Astudillo & Oommen (2013)	Tree-based topology-oriented self-organizing maps	–
Koloseni et al. (2013)	Generalized differential evolution classifier	–
Tabakhi et al. (2014)	Naïve-Bayes (NB)	Ant colony optimization (filter based and unsupervised approach)
Zheng et al. (2014)	SVM	K-means algorithm (feature extraction and selection)
Chen et al. (2014)	Parallel time Variant particle swarm optimization (PTVPSO)-SVM	PTVPSO-SVM
Saez et al. (2014)	Mutual Information feature weighing method with k-NN	Weights determined for features
Lim & Cha (2015)	Bandler–Kohout with interval valued fuzzy set	Weights determined for features
Aličković & Subasi (2017)	Rotation forest	Genetic algorithm with rotation forest to evaluate fitness
Abdar et al. (2018)	Nested ensemble of 3 base classifiers (NB, logistic model tree, stochastic gradient descent (SGD)) and 3 meta-classifiers SGD, C4.5, reduced error pruning tree	–

Source: Author's owner.

It reveals an enhancement in performance when compared with previous works. The architecture for the proposed classifier for breast cancer prediction has been depicted in figure 11.1 below.

11.2   DESCRIPTION OF THE DATASET

This study incorporates the publicly available Wisconsin (Diagnostic) Dataset of Breast Cancer, from UCI Machine Learning Online Repository. This dataset consists of 569 patients' records with 212 that are "malignant" and the rest (357) are benign with a 37.2 and 62.7% ratio. The dataset consists of 30 real-valued input predictors of the diagnosis results, i.e., benign or malignant, as described in table 11.2.

The different aspects of the cell nucleus image of an FNA of a breast mass are measured. If we relate two images of the elongated and circular nucleus by their characteristic values, then the mean nucleus radius alone cannot distinguish them.

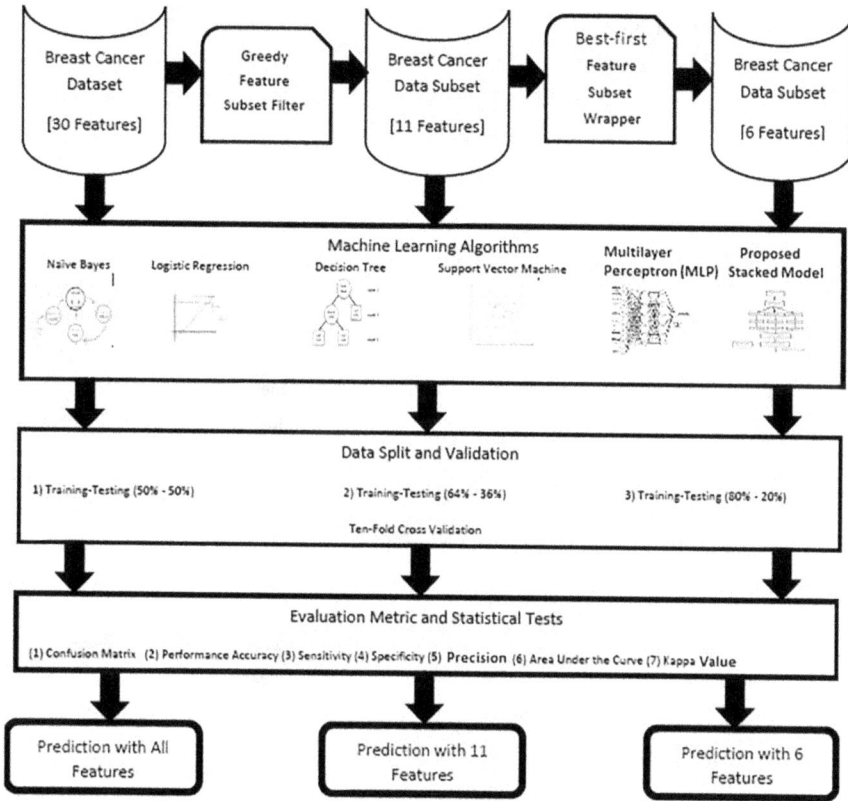

FIGURE 11.1 Breast cancer prediction framework.

Source: Author's owner.

TABLE 11.2
Description of the Dataset

S.N.	Feature	Description	Status	Range	
				Min	Max
	diagnosis	The diagnosis of breast tissues M = malignant, B = benign; B - 63%, M - 37%			
1	radius	Mean of distances from center to perimeter points	mean	6.98	28.11
			se	0.112	2.873
			worst	7.93	36.04
2	texture	Standard deviation of the magnitude of the gray scale	mean	9.71	39.28
			se	0.36	4.89
			worst	12.02	49.54

(Continued)

TABLE 11.2 (Continued)
Description of the Dataset

S.N.	Feature	Description	Status	Range	
				Min	Max
3	perimeter		mean	43.79	188.5
			se	0.76	21.98
			worst	50.41	251.2
4	area		mean	143.5	2501.0
			se	6.8	542.2
			worst	185.2	4254.0
5	smoothness	Local difference in radius length	mean	0.053	0.163
			se	0.002	0.031
			worst	0.071	0.223
6	compactness	$(perimeter)^2/$ area $- 1.0$	mean	0.019	0.345
			se	0.002	0.135
			worst	0.027	1.058
7	concavity	Severity of concave sections of contour	mean	0.0	0.427
			se	0.0	0.396
			worst	0.0	1.252
8	concave points	Number of concave portions of the contour	mean	0.0	0.201
			se	0.0	0.053
			worst	0.0	0.291
9	symmetry		mean	0.106	0.304
			se	0.008	0.079
			worst	0.157	0.664
10	fractal dimensions	'Coastline approximation' $- 1$	mean	0.05	0.097
			se	0.001	0.03
			worst	0.055	0.208

Source: Author's owner.

The dataset contains the mean of the assessed features from each image and the standard error (se) and the highest (worst) value to ensure that the averaging process does not ignore even rare anomalies (Rani et al., 2021).

11.3 HYBRID FILTER-WRAPPER FEATURE SELECTION

We propose a two-step feature selection method. In the first stage, WBC data with all the 30 features undergo greedy stepwise feature selection with a multivariate evaluator. The greedy algorithm adds the best feature in forwarding search at each round.

The multivariate filter approach selects a subset of features well correlated with the class but not among themselves. Features with high prediction ability and low redundancy are considered, thereby overcoming the Univariate-filter approach's shortcomings. Stage 1 results in 11 of the most informative features.

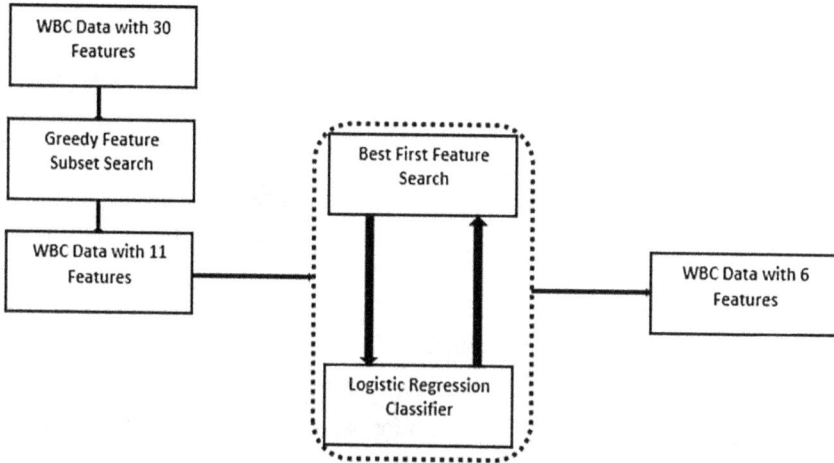

FIGURE 11.2 Hybrid Filter-wrapper feature selection.

Source: Author's owner.

The 11 features' sub-space is further reduced in the second stage using best-first search and wrapper feature selection. The best-first search starts by creating N (=11) models, each using only one of the N features obtained in Stage 1 as an input.

The feature that yields the model with the best classification accuracy (evaluated using logistic regression classifier) is selected. In the next iteration, it creates another set of N-1 models with two input features: the one selected in the previous iteration and another of the N-1 remaining features.

Again, the combination of features that gives the best performance is selected. Stage 2 results in the six most informative features. The feature selection method is depicted in Figure 11.2 below.

11.4 MACHINE LEARNING MODELS

We also propose a stacked classifier as a prediction model for breast cancer. The model is evaluated against several popular classifiers such as logistic regression (LR), Naïve-Bayes (NB), Hoeffding tree (HT), SVM, and multilayer perceptron network (MLN). This section describes these classifier models briefly.

11.4.1 LOGISTIC REGRESSION

Logistic regression is a popular approach for problems with two class values. The logistic function is a sigmoid function (an S-shaped curve). The function takes any real-valued number and maps it into a value between (but never exactly) 0 and 1.

The logistic regression equation is a linear combination of input values and uses coefficient values (weights) to predict an output value. The weights are determined by minimizing the sum of (negative) multinomial log-likelihood function and a ridge estimator (Khang et al., 2023b).

11.4.2   Naïve-Bayes

The Naïve-Bayes classifier is motivated by the Bayes' theorem and assumes that each feature makes an independent and equal contribution to the outcome. These assumptions are, especially the independence assumption is, generally incorrect in practice.

The approach, despite being "naïve," often perform well on several real-world problems. The method determines the probability of feature values for different class outcomes and selects the most probable outcome.

11.4.3   Decision Tree (Hoeffding Tree)

A decision tree is a popular classifier. It splits the original feature set into subsets at each node in response to a feature test. We use information gain as the splitting criterion.

Each subsequent subset is further split recursively until the subset at a node has a shared value of the outcome variable or no further improvement in predictions. Hoeffding trees use a small sample to select a splitting feature and provide good performance (Khang et al., 2022c).

11.4.4   Support Vector Machine

A support vector machine transforms the data points and identifies a hyperplane (which in two dimensions is a line) to separate the classes. This line, or decision boundary, is so chosen that its distance to each class's nearest element is the largest. In the absence of a linear decision boundary, SVM maps the space to a higher dimension using the Kernel function.

We use the polynomial kernel, which considers the similarity of the given features and their combinations. The SVM is trained by solving a quadratic programming problem, for which the sequential minimal optimization algorithm is employed.

11.4.5   Multilayer Perceptron

Artificial neural networks (ANNs) are a biologically inspired method and multilayer perceptron (MLP), a feedforward ANN, is the most commonly used ANN. An MLP consists of an input layer, an output layer, and one or more hidden layers (Rana et al., 2021).

We chose the number of hidden layers as a value, half the sum of the number of features and classes. All nodes use a sigmoid activation function, other than the input nodes and backpropagation is used for training. MLP does not require the data to be linearly separable.

11.4.6   Stacked Model

Stacking utilizes the output of base classifiers to train a meta-classifier, which is responsible for the final prediction. Stacking thus leverages the capabilities of individual base classifiers to learn a part of the problem.

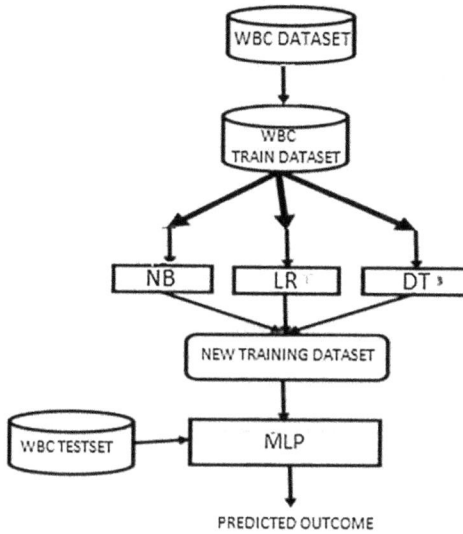

FIGURE 11.3 Proposed stacked model.

Source: Author's owner.

We propose a stacked model with three base classifiers of different types: logistic regression, Naïve-Bayes, and Hoeffding trees, with multilayer perceptron as the meta-classifier. The three base classifiers are selected because they demonstrate improved performance with a reduction in feature sub-space (please refer to Section 11.4.6).

Multilayer perceptron performs well both in the original and the reduced feature space (please refer to Section 11.4.6). The pictorial diagram of the proposed stacked model is depicted in figure 11.3.

11.5 ASSESSMENT OF MODEL PERFORMANCE

The classification performance of models is evaluated using the metrics and summarized in table 11.3.

The training and testing set partitions used are summarized in table 11.4.

High precision indicates that the method misclassifies only a few healthy patents as having cancer. Sensitivity values are the percent of real cancer patients detected correctly, and we should aim for high sensitivity and avoid misclassifying any cancer patient as healthy (Khang et al., 2023a).

The error due to a few healthy patients' misclassifications as having cancer can be easily corrected in further tests. Specificity is the percent of patients correctly detected as not having cancer. AUC is the area under the ROC curve and is directly correlated with a given classifier's overall accuracy.

It takes values from 0 to 1, and the values 0, 1, and 0.5 imply an entirely inaccurate test, a perfectly accurate test, and no discrimination, respectively. An acceptable value, an excellent value, and an outstanding value lie in the range of 0.7 to 0.8, 0.8 to 0.9, and 0.9–1.

TABLE 11.3

Confusion matrix and Performance Evaluation Metrics and Statistical Tests

S/N	Metrics	Formula/Description			
1	Confusion Matrix			Actual	
		Predicted		Malignant (Positive)	Benign (Negative)
			Malignant (Positive)	True Positive, T_P	False Positive, F_P
			Benign (Negative)	False Negative, F_N	True Negative, T_N
				Sensitivity $= \dfrac{T_p}{(T_p + F_N)}$	Sensitivity $= \dfrac{T_N}{(F_p + T_N)}$
2	Accuracy	$\dfrac{T_p + T_N}{(T_P + F_N)(T_P + F_N)}$			
3	Precision	$\dfrac{T_P}{T_P + F_p}$			
4	AUC (area under the curve)	A curve plotted between sensitivity and (1-specificity) is called a receiver operating characteristic (ROC). AUC measures the degree to which the curve is up in the northwest corner.			
5	Kappa Statistic	$(P_c - P_b) / (1 - P_b)$ P_c is complete agreement probability, and P_b represents likelihood 'by chance'. Its range is (−1, 1).			

Source: Author's owner.

TABLE 11.4

Training and Testing Set Partition

Training-Testing Partition	Total Training Records	Positive Records in Training Set	Negative Records in Training Set
50–50	284	111(39%)	173(61%)
66–34	364	135(37%)	229(63%)
80–20	455	169(37%)	286(63%)
10-fold cross-validation	569	212(37%)	357(63%)

Source: Author's owner.

The Kappa value evaluates the observed accuracy against the expected accuracy (random chance). An observed accuracy of 80% with an expected accuracy of 50% is preferable over 75%. A higher value of Kappa is sought.

TABLE 11.5
Features Selected Using Hybrid Filter-Wrapper Approach

Approach	Selected Features
Phase 1: Greedy stepwise and Filter (11 features)	texture_mean, concavity_mean, concave points_mean, area_se, symmetry_se, radius_worst, perimeter_worst, area_worst, smoothness_worst, concavity_worst, concavity points_worst
Phase 2: Best-first and Wrapper (6 features)	texture_mean, symmetry_se, perimeter_worst, area_worst, smoothness_worst, concavity_worst

Source: Author's owner.

11.6   RESULTS AND DISCUSSION

The selected features in Phase 1 and Phase 2 of the hybrid filter-wrapper approach are provided in table 11.5.

Three different setups of experiments are used:

1. the complete dataset with all 30 features,
2. the dataset with only 11 features obtained in Phase 1,
3. the dataset with only six features obtained in Phase 2.

A comparative analysis of LR, NB, SVM, HT, MLP, and the stacked model was performed in the three settings using 50–50, 66–34, and 80–20 train-test split of the dataset, and the results validated using 10-fold cross-validation (c.v).

The classification accuracy, sensitivity, precision, and specificity values are provided in table 11.6–11.9, respectively.

The AUC and Kappa values are provided in table 11.10 and table 11.11, respectively. All results are obtained using Weka 3.8.4 and multiplied by 100.

11.6.1   RESULTS WITH ALL FEATURES

The SVM and MLP method provides the best accuracy, SVM, MLP, and stacked provide the best sensitivity, and LR, SVM, and MLP provide the best precision in the original feature space.

TABLE 11.6
Comparison of Accuracies with All Features, 11 Features and 6 Features

Train-Test Split	LR	NB	SVM	HT	MLP	STACKED
50–50	91, 96, 98	92, 94, 96	97, 97, 96	92, 94, 96	97 ,97, 98	92, 97, 98
66–34	96, 95, 97	92, 94, 95	98, 96, 96	93, 94,95	96, 96, 97	94, 96, 97
80–20	94, 95, 96	93, 93, 96	96, 95, 95	93, 94, 95	97, 96, 96	96, 96, 98
10-fold c.v	95, 96, 97	93, 94, 94	97, 96, 96	93, 94, 95	95, 96, 97	94, 96, 97

Source: Author's owner.

TABLE 11.7

Comparison of Sensitivity with All Features, 11 Features and 6 Features

Train-Test Split	LR	NB	SVM	HT	MLP	STACKED
50–50	89, 96, 98	94, 96, 97	100, 98, 98	93, 96, 97	96, 98, 99	95, 99, 98
66–34	97, 98, 98	94, 96, 99	99, 99, 99	95, 96, 98	97, 96, 98	100, 99, 98
80–20	94, 98, 97	94, 96, 98	98, 98, 98	94, 96, 96	98, 98, 97	100, 100, 98
10-fold c.v	95, 97, 98	95, 96, 96	99, 99, 99	95, 96, 96	96, 97, 98	96, 99, 98

Source: Author's owner.

TABLE 11.8

Comparison of Precision with All Features, 11 Features and 6 Features

Train-Test Split	LR	NB	SVM	HT	MLP	STACKED
50–50	96, 97, 98	94, 94, 96	96, 96, 96	95, 95, 96	98, 97, 97	94, 97, 98
66–34	97, 95, 97	93, 94, 94	98, 96, 96	94, 95, 95	96, 97, 97	92, 95, 97
80–20	97, 95, 97	96, 94, 96	96, 95, 95	96, 96, 97	97, 96, 97	95, 95, 98
10-fold c.v	96, 96, 96	93, 94, 95	97, 95, 95	93, 95, 95	96, 96, 97	95, 95,97

Source: Author's owner.

TABLE 11.9

Comparison of Specificity with All Features, 11 Features and 6 Features

Train-Test Split	LR	NB	SVM	HT	MLP	STACKED
50–50	94, 95, 98	90, 90, 94	93, 94, 93	91, 91, 94	98, 95, 96	89, 95, 98
66–34	95, 91, 95	88, 89, 89	97, 92, 92	89, 91, 91	94, 95, 95	85, 91, 95
80–20	94, 88, 94	91, 88, 91	91, 88, 88	91, 91, 94	94, 91, 94	88, 88, 97
10-fold c.v	93, 94, 94	89, 90, 91	94, 91, 91	89, 91, 92	93, 94, 95	91, 92, 96

Source: Author's owner.

TABLE 11.10

Comparison of AUC Value with All Features, 11 Features and 6 Features

Train-Test Split	LR	NB	SVM	HT	MLP	STACKED
50–50	97, 98, 99	97, 98, 98	96, 96, 96	98, 99, 99	99, 99, 99	98, 99, 99
66–34	97, 99, 99	97, 97, 98	98, 95, 95	98, 99, 99	99, 99, 99	98, 99, 98
80–20	96, 99, 99	95, 95, 96	95, 93, 93	98, 98, 99	99, 99, 98	99, 99, 98
10-fold c.v	97, 99, 99	98, 98, 98	97, 95, 95	98, 98, 98	99, 98, 98	96, 97, 98

Source: Author's owner.

TABLE 11.11

Comparison of Kappa Statistic with All Features, 11 Features and 6 Features

Train-Test Split	LR	NB	SVM	HT	MLP	STACKED
50–50	81, 91, 96	84, 87, 92	94, 93, 92	83, 88, 91	93, 94, 96	84, 95, 96
66–34	93, 90, 94	82, 87, 90	96, 93, 93	85, 88, 90	91, 92, 94	88, 91, 94
80–20	88, 89, 91	85, 85, 91	91, 89, 89	85, 87, 89	93, 91, 91	91,91,95
10-fold c.v	89, 92, 93	85, 87, 88	95, 92, 91	85, 88, 89	90, 92, 94	89, 93, 94

Source: Author's owner.

LR, NB, HT, and stacked provide relatively smaller accuracy value; NB and HT provide relatively smaller sensitivity value; and NB, HT, and stacked provide relatively smaller precision value.

LR, SVM, and MLP provide the best specificity value, and NB, HT, and stacked method provide relatively smaller specificity value.

HT, MLP, and stacked methods provide AUC values of 9899% with 30 features, while LR, NB, and SVM providing AUC values of 95–98%.

SVM and MLP record a 0.9–0.96 Kappa value, while NB and HT record a relatively smaller 0.82–0.85 value.

11.6.2 Results with Six Features

The stacked method provides the best accuracy, precision, and specificity with six features, followed by MLP and LR methods. The NB, SVM, and HT models provide relatively smaller accuracy, precision, and specificity values.

With six features, the sensitivity values of all tested classifiers are relatively indistinguishable.

LR, HT, MLP, and stacked method provide AUC values of 98–99% with six features, while NB and SVM provide AUC values of 95–98%. LR, MLP, and stacked have 0.91–0.96 Kappa value with six features, while NB and HT have 0.88–0.91 value, as table 11.11 and table 11.12 display groups of the classifiers based on relative performance.

LR records a sensitivity of 89–97% and a Kappa value of 0.81–0.93, with all features. The stacked model records a Kappa value of 0.84–0.91, with all features. SVM records a Kappa value of 0.89–0.93, with six features. We chose to group them along with classifiers with relatively smaller values.

11.6.3 Effect of Feature Reduction

The reduction in feature sub-space from 30 to 6, through feature selection, improves LR, NB, and HT methods' performance.

TABLE 11.12

Grouping of Classifiers Based on Relative Performance

	All Features		6 Features	
	High value	Relatively smaller value	High value	Relatively smaller value
Accuracy	SVM, MLP (96–98)	LR, NB, HT, Stacked (91–96)	LR, MLP, Stacked (96–98)	NB, SVM, HT (94–96)
Sensitivity	SVM, MLP, Stacked (95–100)	NB, HT (93–95) LR (89–97)	All are indistinguishable (96–99)	
Precision	LR, SVM, MLP (96–98)	NB, HT, Stacked (93–96)	LR, MLP, Stacked (96–98)	NB, SVM (94–96) HT (95–97)
Specificity	LR, SVM, MLP (91–98)	NB, HT, Stacked (85–91)	LR, MLP, Stacked (94–98)	NB, SVM, HT (88–94)
AUC	HT, MLP, Stacked (98–99)	LR, NB, SVM (95–98)	LR, HT, MLP, Stacked (98–99)	NB, SVM (95–98)
Kappa	SVM, MLP (90–96)	NB, HT (82–85) LR (81–93) Stacked (84–91)	LR, MLP, Stacked (91–96)	NB, HT (88–91) SVM (89–93)

Source: Author's owner.

TABLE 11.13

Percentage Improvement in Performance (minimum, Maximum) Due to Feature Reduction from 30 to 6

	LR	NB	SVM	HT	MLP	STACKED
Accuracy	1.0,7.6	1.0,4.3	−2.0,−1.0	2.1,4.3	−1.0,2.1	2.0,5.4
Sensitivity	1.0,10.1	1.0,5.3	−2.0,0	1.0,4.3	−1.0,3.1	−2.0,3.1
Precision	0,2.0	0,2.1	−2.0,0	1.0,2.1	−1.0,1.0	2.1,5.4
Specificity	0,4.2	0,4.4	−5.1,0	2.2,3.3	−2.0,2.1	5.4,11.7
AUC	2.0,3.1	0,1.0	−3.0,0	0,1	−1,0	−1,2
Kappa	1,15	3.5,9.7	−4.2,−2.1	2.3,9.6	−2.1,4.4	4.3,14.2

Source: Author's owner.

1. The accuracy, sensitivity, and Kappa value of the three methods increases.
2. The precision and specificity values of LR and NB are non-decreasing, while that of HT increases.
3. The AUC values of NB and HT are non-decreasing, while that of LR increases. In contrast, SVMs' accuracy and Kappa value decrease, and its sensitivity, precision, specificity, and AUC value are non-increasing. The accuracy, precision, specificity, and Kappa value of the stacked method increases, while the change in its sensitivity and AUC values is indeterminate. The change in the performance of the MLP method is similarly indeterminate. MLP performs well in both the original feature space and six features (please refer to Table 11.12). The minimum and maximum percentage improvement in performance due to feature reduction are provided in table 11.13.

11.6.4   COMPARISON OF RESULTS WITH THOSE IN PREVIOUS RESEARCH WORKS

Table 11.14 compares the stacked, LR, and MLP models' accuracy with six features with the SVM model in the original feature space and other research work on the same dataset (Bhambri et al., 2022). The SVM model performs slightly better than stacked, LR, and MLP models in terms of accuracy, but the additional features make it harder to interpret.

Chen et al. (2014) and Aličković and Subasi (2017) also record a higher accuracy, but with several additional features. Unlike the SVM, MLP, and LR methods, the stacked model provides good accuracy with both 50–50 and 80–20 split of the dataset and is, therefore, more reliable.

TABLE 11.14

Comparison of Number of Features Selected and Classification Accuracies with Previous Studies

Study	No. of Features Selected	Accuracy (%)	Study	No. of Features Selected	Accuracy (%)
Stoean & Stoean (2013)	15.43 (average)	97.23	Chen et al. (2014)	13.4	**99.87**
Astudillo & Oommen (2013)	–	93.32	Saez et al. (2014)	–	96.14
Koloseni et al. (2013)	–	93.64	Lim & Cha (2015)	–	95.26
Tabakhi et al. (2014)	5	92.42	Aličković & Subasi (2017)	14	**99.48**
Zheng et al. (2014)	6 (new subspace)	97.38	Abdar et al. (2018)	–	98.07
This Study Stacked (80–20 train-test split)	6	98.245	**This Study** SVM (66–34 train-test split)	–	98.445
This Study LR, MLP, Stacked (50–50 train-test split)	6	98.239			

Source: Author's owner.

11.7 CONCLUSION

Cancer is responsible for many deaths worldwide, and yearly a half-million women die of breast cancer alone. Early diagnosis of breast cancer improves the survival rate, which can exceed 80%.

The mammograms are often challenging to interpret, and so are the features (which are several in number) of the cell nucleus of the fluid extracted from the breast mass. For example, the Wisconsin (Diagnostic) Dataset of Breast Cancer (WBC) has 30 features.

The cost of collecting, storing, and analyzing data has been reducing at an increasing rate. Machine learning methods help the physician make sense of the large volume of data, identify relevant features, and diagnose cancer.

A small number of features help the physician understand the reason for the diagnosis. A correct diagnosis of new patients, especially those with cancer, is essential. An error in diagnosing a few healthy patients' as having cancer is rectified with additional tests.

We proposed a two-phase hybrid filter-wrapper feature selection method and evaluated it using the WBC dataset.

- Phase 1 uses a greedy step-wise search and multivariate-feature evaluator and results in 11 features. The multivariate filter approach identifies features well correlated with the class but not among themselves.
- Phase 2 utilizes a best-first search and Logistic regression learning algorithm (in a wrapper approach) to evaluate the features and results in six features.
- In Phase 3, logistic regression (LR), Naïve-Bayes (NB), Hoeffding tree (HT), support vector machine (SVM) with the polynomial kernel, and multilayer perceptron network (MLN) are used in the reduced feature subspace to identify patients with or without cancer.

Ten-fold cross-validations and 50–50, 66–34, and 80–20 train-test splits of the datasets are used. We also propose a stacked model, with LR, NB, and HT as the base classifiers and MLP as the meta-classifier.

Three different setups of the experiment: (1) with the complete dataset of all 30 features, (2) with the dataset of only 11 features obtained in Phase 1, and (3) with the dataset of only six features obtained in Phase 2, leads to the following conclusions:

1. The SVM model performs best in the original feature space and records 98.445% accuracy with 66–34 split.
2. The LR and MLP models perform best with six features and record 98.239% accuracy with a 50–50 split.
3. The LR, NB, and HT demonstrate improvement in accuracy, sensitivity, precision, specificity, AUC, and Kappa values, with the reduction in features to six.
4. The MLP method performs well in both the original feature space and with six features.

5. The stacked model performs well with six features and records 98.239% accuracy with a 50–50 split and 98.245% accuracy with a 80–20 split.
6. The LR, MLP, and the proposed stacked model record a higher accuracy with six features than most previous works. Chen et al. (2014) and Aličković and Subasi (2017) record a higher accuracy, but with several additional features and more sophisticated methodologies, which negatively impacts interpretation (Khang et al., 2023c).

The WBC data is secondary data collected from one location. Breast cancer data from different regions and countries may be incorporated in the future to ensure the robustness and credibility of the proposed hybrid feature selection approach and stacked model (Vrushank et al., 2023).

The proposed methodology has been tested only on breast cancer classification, and it should further have evaluated clinical datasets. The data used in this study is almost numeric. The proposed methodology can be tested on other applications where data nature is different (Eugenia Litvinova et al., 2023).

REFERENCES

Abdar, M., Zomorodi-Moghadam, M., Zhou, X., Gururajan, R., Tao, X., Barua, P. D., & Gururajan, R. (2018). A new nested ensemble technique for automated diagnosis of breast cancer. *Pattern Recognition Letters*. https://www.sciencedirect.com/science/article/pii/S0167865518308766

Alickovic, E., & Subasi, A. (2017). Breast Cancer Diagnosis Using GA Feature Selection and Rotation Forest. *Neural Computing and Applications*, 28 (4), 753–763. https://link.springer.com/article/10.1007/s00521-015-2103-9

Astudillo, C. A., & Oommen, B. J. (2013). On achieving semi-supervised pattern recognition by utilizing tree-based SOMs. *Pattern Recognition*, 46 (1), 293–304. https://www.sciencedirect.com/science/article/pii/S0031320312003226

Breast Cancer Wisconsin (Diagnostic) Data Set, (2023). Retrieved from https://archive.ics.uci.edu/ml/datasets/Breast+Cancer+Wisconsin+(Diagnostic)

Bhambri, P., Rani, S., Gupta, G., & Khang, A. (2022). *Cloud and Fog Computing Platforms for Internet of Things*. ISBN: 978-1-032-101507. CRC Press. 10.1201/9781003213888

Chen, H., Yang, B., Jing Wang, S., Wang, G., Zhong Li, H., & bin Liu, W. (2014). Towards an optimal support vector machine classifier using a parallel particle swarm optimization strategy. *Applied Mathematics and Computation*, 239, 180–197. https://sciencedirect.com/science/article/pii/S0096300314005724

Hajimahmud, V. A., Khang, A., Hahanov, V., Litvinova, E., Chumachenko, S., & Alyar, A. V. (2022). Autonomous Robots for Smart City: Closer to Augmented Humanity. *AI-Centric Smart City Ecosystems: Technologies, Design and Implementation* (1st Ed.). CRC Press. 10.1201/9781003252542-7

Khang, A., Ragimova, N. A., Hajimahmud, V. A., & Alyar, A. V. (2022a). Advanced Technologies and Data Management in the Smart Healthcare System. *AI-Centric Smart City Ecosystems: Technologies, Design and Implementation* (1st Ed.). CRC Press. 10.1201/9781003252542-16

Khang, A., Hahanov, V., Abbas, G. L., & Hajimahmud, V. A.. (2022b). Cyber-Physical-Social System and İncident Management. *AI-Centric Smart City Ecosystems: Technologies, Design and Implementation* (1st Ed.). CRC Press. 10.1201/9781003252542-2

Khang, A., Vladimir Hahanov, Eugenia Litvinova, Svetlana Chumachenko, Triwiyanto, Ana Kadarningsih, Zoran Avromovic, Ragimova Nazila Ali, Abdullayev Vugar Hajimahmud (2023a). Cloud Platform and Data Storage Systems in Healthcare Ecosystem. *Data-Centric AI Solutions and Emerging Technologies in the Healthcare Ecosystem.* (1st ed.), (2023), P (4). CRC Press. 10.1201/9781032398570-21

Khang, A., Rani, S., Gujrati, R., Uygun, H., & Gupta, S. K., (Eds.). (2023b). *Designing Workforce Management Systems for Industry 4.0: Data-Centric and AI-Enabled Approaches* (1st Ed.). CRC Press. 10.1201/99781003357070

Khang, A., Rana, G., Tailor, R. K., & Hajimahmud, V. A., (Eds.). (2023c). *Data-Centric AI Solutions and Emerging Technologies in the Healthcare Ecosystem* (1st Ed.). CRC Press. 10.1201/9781003356189

Khanh, H. H., & Khang, A. (2021) The Role of Artificial Intelligence in Blockchain Applications. *Reinventing Manufacturing and Business Processes through Artificial Intelligence*, 20–40. CRC Press. 10.1201/9781003145011-2

Koloseni, D., Lampinen, J., & Luukka, P. (2013). Differential evolution based nearest prototype classifier with optimized distance measures for the features in the data sets. *Expert Systems with Applications*, 40 (10), 4075–4082. https://www.sciencedirect.com/science/article/pii/ S0957417413000535

Lim, C. K., & Chan, C. S. (2015). A weighted inference engine based on interval-valued fuzzy relational theory. *Expert Systems with Applications*, 42 (7), 3410–3419. https://www.sciencedirect.com/science/article/pii/S0957417414008045

Rana, G., Khang, A., Sharma, R., Goel, A. K., & Dubey, A. K. (2021). *Reinventing Manufacturing and Business Processes through Artificial Intelligence*, (Eds.). CRC Press. 10.1201/9781003145011

Rani, S., Chauhan, M., Kataria, A., & Khang, A. (2021). IoT Equipped Intelligent Distributed Framework for Smart Healthcare Systems. *Networking and Internet Architecture*, (Eds.). CRC Press. 10.48550/arXiv.2110.04997

Saez, J. A., Derrac, J., Luengo, J., & Herrera, F. (2014). Statistical computation of feature weighting schemes through data estimation for nearest neighbor classifiers. *Pattern Recognition*, 47 (12), 3941–3948. https://www.sciencedirect.com/science/article/pii/ S0031320314002349

Stoean, R., & Stoean, C. (2013). Modeling medical decision making by support vector machines, explaining by rules of evolutionary algorithms with feature selection. *Expert Systems with Applications*, 40 (7), 2677–2686. https://www.sciencedirect.com/science/article/pii/S0957417412012171

Tabakhi, S., Moradi, P., & Akhlaghian, F. (2014). An unsupervised feature selection algorithm based on ant colony optimization. *Engineering Applications of Artificial Intelligence*, 32, 112–123. https://www.sciencedirect.com/science/article/pii/S0952197614000621

Vrushank, S., Vidhi, T., & Khang, A. (2023). Electronic Health Records Security and Privacy Enhancement using Blockchain Technology. *Data-Centric AI Solutions and Emerging Technologies in the Healthcare Ecosystem.* (1st ed.), (2023), P (1). CRC Press. 10.1201/9781003356189

Zheng, B., Yoon, S. W., & Lam, S. S. (2014). Breast cancer diagnosis based on feature extraction using a hybrid of K-means and support vector machine algorithms. *Expert Systems with Applications*, 41 (4), 1476–1482. https://www.sciencedirect.com/science/article/pii/S0957417413006659

Khan, A., Vladimir [illegible], [illegible] Larionova, Svetlana Chumachenko, [illegible], [illegible], Zenat [illegible], Bagimova [illegible], A.K. [illegible] Vugar [illegible] (2023). Cloud Platform and Data Storage Systems in Healthcare Ecosystem [illegible] Centric AI Solutions and Emerging Technologies in the Healthcare Ecosystem [illegible] (2023), [illegible] CRC Press. [illegible] 10.1201/[illegible]

Khang, [illegible] Gupta, [illegible] Gupta, H. & Gupta [illegible] (2023). [illegible] Workforce [illegible] Approaches [illegible], CRC Press. 10.1201/9781003357070

Khang, A., Rana, G., Tailor, R. K., & Hajimahmud, V. A. (Eds.). (2023). Data-Centric AI Solutions and Emerging Technologies in the Healthcare Ecosystem (1st Ed.). CRC Press. 10.1201/9781003356189

Khatib, [illegible] H. [illegible] (2016). [illegible] Intelligence, 21, [illegible]

[illegible]

[illegible] A [illegible] inference engine [illegible] based [illegible] Applications [illegible]

[illegible] Khang, A., Sharma, [illegible] Big Data, [illegible] 50 [illegible]

Rani, [illegible], Khang, A. (2021). [illegible] Networking and [illegible] (Eds.) [illegible]

Saez, [illegible], Herrera, F. (2013). Statistical computation [illegible] nearest neighbor classification [illegible] 2013 [illegible] https://www.sciencedirect.com/science/article/pii/S003 [illegible]

Tiegan, S. [illegible] for breast cancer diagnosis based on [illegible] support vector machine [illegible] feature selection [illegible] Systems [illegible] https://www.sciencedirect.com/science/article/pii/[illegible]

[illegible], Hossain [illegible] (2018). An improved feature selection algorithm based on [illegible] Engineering Applications of Artificial Intelligence, 72, 112–123. https://www.sciencedirect.com/science/article/pii/S0952197618300629

Vrushank, S., [illegible], Khang, A. (2023). Electronic Health Records [illegible] using Blockchain Technology. Data-Centric AI Solutions and Emerging Technologies in the Healthcare Ecosystem (1st Ed.). CRC Press. 10.1201/[illegible]

Zheng, B., Yoon, S. W., & Lam, S. S. (2014). Breast cancer diagnosis based on feature extraction using a hybrid of k-means and support vector machine algorithms. Expert Systems with Applications, 41(4), 1476–1482. https://www.sciencedirect.com/science/article/pii/S0957417413006350

12 Hepatocellular Carcinoma Patients Survival Forecasting Model Using Ensemble Learning Approach

*Samuel Faluyi, Kofoworola Fapohunda,
Temitayo Balogun, and Olufunke Oluwabusayo*

CONTENTS

DOI: 10.1201/9781003356189-12

12.1   INTRODUCTION

The primary type of liver cancer, hepatocellular carcinoma, is one of the leading cancerous growths that cause human death. Hepatocellular carcinoma (HCC) is the third most prevalent cause of mortality globally as the fifth most prominent malignancy, according to Chiu et al. (2013).

Unlike the secondary type of liver cancer that is transferable among other human organs, hepatocellular carcinoma is not transferable; it is only from the organ of the liver and is usually caused as a result of unmanaged decompensation stage of liver cirrhosis.

According to widespread consensus, chronic liver inflammation is brought on by aflatoxin, alcoholism non-alcoholic liver cirrhosis, hepatitis virus infection, and other factors that lead to hepatocellular carcinoma.

Patients still have a significant chance of dying even after major resection (Bertuccio et al., 2017; Zhu et al., 2022). For years, liver surgeons have struggled with the question of how to increase the chance of survival of HCC patients who have had the hepatitis B virus.

To increase the survivability of these patients as well as the therapeutic effect on hepatocellular carcinoma, it is necessary to identify risk factors influencing the prognosis of these individuals after radical resection of the hepatitis B virus related to hepatocellular carcinoma. However, in an effort to maintain the remaining liver size to the greatest extent possible, leftover cancer cells may develop during surgery.

Additionally, after extensive resection of hepatocellular carcinoma, liver cirrhosis increases the chance of late resurgence (Cheng et al., 2015). Hepatocellular carcinoma resurgence due to liver cirrhosis may compromise a patient's long-term survival.

The long-term survival of these individuals is further impacted by complications from liver cirrhosis, such as portal hypertension and gastroduodenal hemorrhage brought on by esophagus and gastric varices (Zhu et al., 2022).

More so Sato et al. (2021) mentioned that within five years of receiving radiofrequency ablation (RFA) therapy, up to 70% of patients experience a recurrence of their HCC, including local tumor growth and distant recurrence brought on by intrahepatic metastasis or de novo primary cancer development (Sato et al., 2021; Shiina et al., 2012).

The likelihood of HCC recurrence varied considerably amongst individuals and was demonstrated to be influenced by both underlying chronic liver cirrhosis conditions, such as the scarring or inflammation, as well as the tumor characteristics, such as tumor size, quantity, or biomarkers.

All of these influence the growth of HCC (Lee et al., 2015; Sato et al., 2021; Shiina et al., 2012). The prognosis of hepatocellular carcinoma has been proven to be tedious in achieving with higher accuracy, with the aid of an ensemble learner that could help improve the forecast of survivability of patients based on historical dataset.

The part of artificial intelligence which allows computer to learn pattern, trends, and insight from historical dataset to perform tasks independently with little or no human involvement can be regarded as machine learning (ML) (Rana et al., 2021).

According to IBM, "Machine learning is a branch of artificial intelligence (AI) and computer science which focuses on the use of data and algorithms to imitate the way that humans learn, gradually improving its accuracy. Machine learning is an important component of the growing field of data science (Khanh & Khang, 2021).

Through the use of statistical methods, algorithms are trained to make classifications or predictions, and to uncover key insights in data mining projects (Rani et al., 2021). These insights subsequently drive decision-making within applications and businesses, ideally impacting key growth metrics" (IBM, 2022).

Using several alternative models rather than simply one increases reliability. An ensemble is a group of various models cooperating on a single set (Howal, 2018).

Furthermore, Dyakonov (2021) stated that an ensemble, which is often referred to as a "multiple classifier system," can be described as an algorithm made up of several machine learning techniques, and the creation of an ensemble is known as ensemble learning.

Motivation: Hepatocellular carcinoma (HCC), which accounts for over 75% of all types of liver cancer cases across the world, is the most prevalent kind. In every region of the world, the prediction for HCC is dismal. As a result, the rates of incidence and death are about equal (McGlynn et al., 2021).

Furthermore, among hepatitis B virus (HBV) carriers, the chance that they will develop HCC is between 10% and 25%. However, incidence varies depending on whether a person had cirrhosis and/or an active HBV infection.

Demographic factors (such as male sex, older age, Asian or African ancestry, and family history of HCC), viral factors (such as high HBV replication levels, HBV genotype, infection duration, and coinfection with HCV or HIV), and environmental exposures (such as aflatoxin, alcohol, tobacco, obesity, and diabetes) are cofactors that also increase risk among HBV carriers.

Certain risk variables have been taken into account when developing scoring systems or surveillance guidelines. However, it is possible that these suggestions do not accurately predict HCC risk in HBV carriers who receive antiviral medication.

Also, chronic HCV infection raises risk by 10–20 fold. Since HCV is an RNA virus and does not integrate into the host's genome, it is unlikely that it will be the main factor in the development of tumors. As cirrhosis occurs before over 90% of HCC cases associated with HCV, it is more plausible that HCV encourages carcinogenesis through repeated damage, regeneration, and fibrosis (McGlynn et al., 2021).

The prognosis of hepatocellular carcinoma oftentimes has been said to be difficult, but the adoption of ensemble learners on a dataset containing relevant attributes along with risk factors could improve predictions, which necessitate this study (Khang et al., 2023a).

Aim and Objectives: The aim of this research work is to adopt ensemble learning approach of machine learning (ML) to develop a comparative survival forecasting model for hepatocellular carcinoma patients. The specific objectives of the study include:

   i. to collect dataset from secondary source
   ii. pre-process and filter the collected dataset;

iii. carryout exploratory data analysis (EDA) on the dataset;
iv. formulate the model;
v. simulate the model and validate the model.

The remaining sections are arranged as follows: section 2 (related work), section 3 (methods and materials), section 4 (result presentation), and section 5 (conclusion).

12.2   RELATED WORK

12.2.1   CONCEPTUAL FRAMEWORK

Ensemble learning is considered as subset of machine learning techniques, which apply general meta method by merging multiple models to acquire better performance for predictions. Situations when there are uncertainties in data representation, solution objectives, modeling methodologies, or the presence of random beginning seeds in a model are all good reasons for adoption of ensemble learning approach (Khang & Hajimahmud, 2022a).

The individual traditional model or candidate techniques are referred to as base learner methods (Anifowose, 2020). Each base learner operates independently, as in a standard machine learning method, and the results are eventually integrated to generate a single robust output.

In the case of regression and classification approaches, the combination could be carried out by applying either of the averaging (simple or weighted) approaches and voting (majority or weighted) methods. It assumes that each base learner is an "expert," and the output is an "expert opinion." Ensemble learner approaches are also known as "committee of machines" or "committee of experts" (Anifowose, 2020).

12.2.2   XGBOOST

XGBoost (also known as extreme gradient boosting) is an ensemble machine learning approach based on the gradient boosting principle and built on the basis of a decision tree model. It is used to optimize gradient boosting approaches through parallel processing, decision tree pruning, missing value handling, and lowering the risk of bias or overfitting in a model. It uses first- and second-order gradient of loss function when calculating the tree of each iteration, and also uses shrinkage parameter to reduce the optimal node predictions performed in each iteration and add the predictions to the current function.

XGBoost also uses row and column resampling; all the techniques are adopted to avoid overfitting in XGBoost algorithm (Gomez-Rios et al., 2017). It implements lots of features to give a fast and scalable algorithm, parallel and distributed computing, a tree learning algorithm for handling sparse data, and an approximate algorithm for split finding when the data does not fit into memory (Gomez-Rios et al., 2017).

XGBoost is a powerful and dynamic algorithm that may be used to tackle a variety of issues such as classification and regression, forecasting, and ranking.

The main goal of the XGB model is to ensure that machines are performing at their best in terms of accuracy, scalability, and mobility. Extreme gradient boosting (XGB), on the other hand, is noted for its thoroughness in optimization to produce superior results with fewer resources while also being efficient (Khang et al., 2023b).

Gradient boosting is famous for its error mitigation through gradient descent algorithm. The algorithm uses an exact greedy search technique to elicit the best tree-like configuration with the addition of a split to the prevailing leaf nodes in every attempt and their gain index can be calculated as equation 12.1 follows:

$$Gain\ Index = \frac{1}{2}\left[\frac{G_{Le}^2}{H_{Le} + \lambda} + \frac{G_{Ri}^2}{H_{Ri} + \lambda} - \frac{(G_{Le} + G_{Ri})^2}{H_{Le} + H_{Ri} + \lambda}\right] - \gamma \quad (12.1)$$

Where γ is the cost of complexity when a leaf is added (He et al., 2018; Chen & Guestrin, 2016).

A threshold is set to limit tree growth, and when the gain surpasses the threshold, node splits occur. When XGBoost is also pre-pruned, the objective function is optimized because it is a threshold in the equation above that specifies the coefficient of the leaf node in regularization terms (Chen & Guestrin, 2016).

12.2.3 AdaBoost

AdaBoost (Adaptive boosting) is a famous boosting algorithm suitable for handling distribution, representing weights of each instance. An AdaBoost classifier first fits a classifier on the original data set, and then fits a copy of the same classifier on an updated dataset with the inaccurate and error-prone data points balanced out so that the subsequent classifiers can focus on the situations that cause the most inaccuracy (Bobkov et al., 2016).

The distribution changes in every iteration; that is, each time it calls the weak classifier (Freund & Schapire, 2012). The weights tell AdaBoost which instances have to be in more consideration than others; higher weight in an instance implies that instance has been misclassified, and, thus, close attention in the next call to the weak classifier (the weights will be set equally for all the instances at the initial stage).

It is said every time AdaBoost endeavors to train a weak classifier, it returns a weak hypothesis and brings about selecting a hypothesis that minimizes the weighted error (Freund & Schapire, 2012; Gomez-Rios et al., 2017).

On this note, AdaBoost selects a parameter, which measures the weak hypothesis importance. Thus, the more accuracy it gets, corresponds the importance assigned to it. An AdaBoost computation is performed by altering the information flow, as indicated by the order modification of the preparation set's test, as well as the final precision of the universal arrangement to determine the weight of each example.

The masses of the altered novel information are then sent to the lower classifier for preparation, and each preparation classifier is then merged as an official conclusion classifier. As a result, AdaBoost concentrates on the incorrectly identified points by boosting the weights of the misclassified input, reducing error, and increasing accuracy (Azmi & Baliga, 2020).

12.3 METHODS AND MATERIALS

For the purposes of this study, a comparative examination of various different ensemble learning methodologies was used. The methods employed included gathering data from a secondary source (Kaggle), choosing appropriate properties for the creation of models, training the model, and evaluating it to determine its performance (Bhambri et al., 2022).

Ensemble machine learning approaches, XGBoost and AdaBoost, were chosen for this investigation. Python-3 was utilized as the simulation environment, and it was used to create a survival model based on the data gathered using particular ensemble learning methods. Therefore, precision, f1-score, ROC score, and other evaluation metrics are used to validate the models and to conduct a comparative examination.

12.3.1 IDENTIFICATION AND COLLECTION OF THE DATASET

The data used for this study was obtained via a secondary source (Kaggle data repository). The data consisted of 50 attributes that made up the risk factors of hepatocellular carcinoma (such as alcoholism, genetics, hepatitis B virus, hepatitis C virus, diabetes, obesity, liver cirrhosis, non-alcohol fat, etc.), and suitable for the classification of the hepatocellular carcinoma survival model.

Observations of 165 patients were taken with respect to the 50 attributes, where the last column represents the class (0 and 1), where 0 means non-survival and 1 means survival.

12.3.2 MODEL FORMULATION

Data were gathered from the Kaggle data repository, after which the dataset was filtered to remove redundancy and fill the missing value present in the dataset. However, pre-process, which includes statistical analysis and exploratory data analysis (EDA), was performed on the data, and a correlation coefficient along with correlation matrix was determine to identify the statistically important characteristics of the dataset (Rani et al., 2023).

Two-way split were then performed on the dataset, which were split into a train dataset and a test dataset, with a proportion of 80% and 20% split between the two. Before fitting of the model, a 10-fold cross-validation was carried out on a trained dataset to avoid overfitting and under-fitting. Then the model was fit using ensemble learning techniques: random forest algorithm, XGBoost algorithm, AdaBoost, and CatBoost algorithm.

12.3.3 SIMULATION ENVIRONMENT FOR MODELING

Following the identification of the required classifiers for the formulation of hepatocellular carcinoma survival models, simulation of the model was carried out using a dataset obtained from a secondary source ('Kaggle'), which consisted of 165 patient observations along with 50 relevant attributes suitable for classification. The Jupyter notebook of the Python 3 software program was utilized as the simulation environment for developing the model.

12.3.4 ANALYSIS AND VALIDATION OF THE MODEL

Various indicators were utilized to analyze and to validate the survival model's performance during the evaluation phase. Many parameters must be identified from the results of the classifiers during model testing in order to calculate these metrics. Positive and negative rates, as well as other characteristics, are included in the statistics.

Negatives (zero) signify non-survival, while positives (one) represent survival from hepatocellular carcinoma. The following parameters were utilized for compare performance: accuracy, precision, F1, recall, AUC, and ROC.

Performance metrices used in this study include confusion matrix, classification report (precision, recall, f1-score), ROC curve, ROC, and AUC score. Confusion matrix is one way to determine how effective a model has performed in machine (ensemble) learning classifier. It shows the extent at which model is able to classified correctly.

A confusion matrix is typically made up of true positive rate (TPR), false positive rate (FPR), false negative rate (FNR) and true negative rate. True positive rate and true negative rate can be regarded as the correct classification, while the false positive rate and true negative rate are the incorrect classification or misclassification.

The precision of equation 12.2, recalled as equation 12.3, and f1-score in equation 12.4 are derived from a confusion matrix. They can be obtained as follows:

$$Precision\,(P) = \frac{TPR}{TPR + FPR} \tag{12.2}$$

$$Recall\,(R) = \frac{TPR}{TPR + FNR} \tag{12.3}$$

$$F1 - score = \frac{2 * R * P}{R + P} \tag{12.4}$$

F1-score is used to measure and compare precision and recall of the model. It provides the harmonica average of precision and recall.

The AUC-ROC curve is a performance metric for classification issues at different threshold levels, where AUC is the level of separability and ROC is the probability curve. This indicates how well the model can distinguish between different classes.

The AUC indicates how well the model predicts correctly. The higher the AUC, the better the model can predict a future event (valid and fraud transaction). The ROC curve is plotted with TPR on the y-axis and FPR on the x-axis of the graph.

12.4 IMPLEMENTATION AND RESULTS

This section presents the results and discussion of results obtained based on the data analysis and model formulation and simulation as well as validation designated for this study (Khang et al., 2022b). This includes the bar graph of the data class, correlation coefficient, and matrix to identify the statistically significant attributes. More so, the performance metrics include the confusion matrix, ROC curve, AUC score, precision, recall, and f1-score.

12.4.1 ANALYSIS OF THE DISTRIBUTION

The data collected is made up of attributes containing hepatocellular carcinoma risk factors including the class (i.e., 0s and 1s) (figures 12.1, 12.2–12.10).

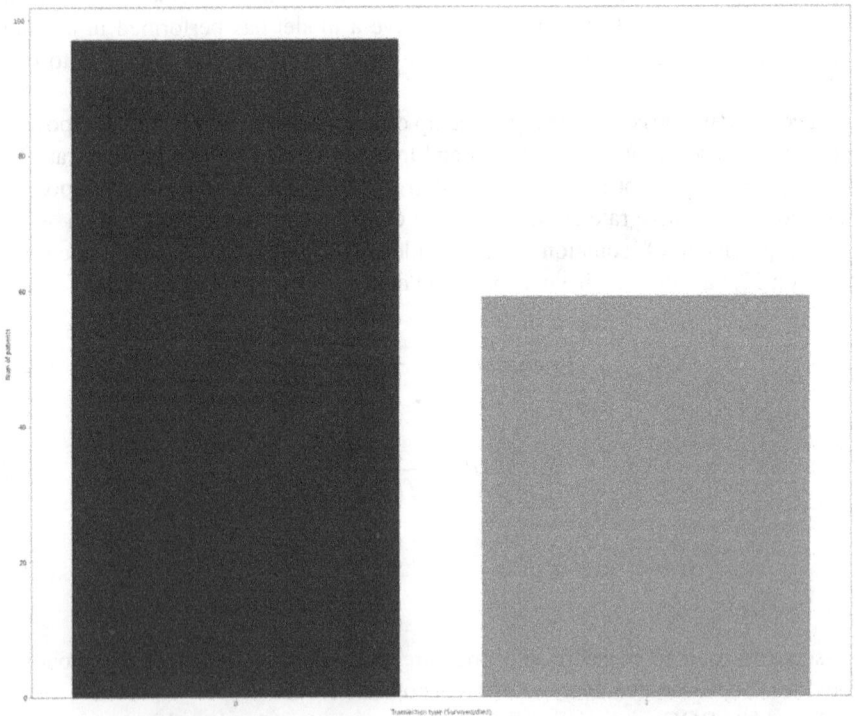

FIGURE 12.1 Bar graph of the class.

Source: Author's owner.

12.4.2   Features Correlation Matrix

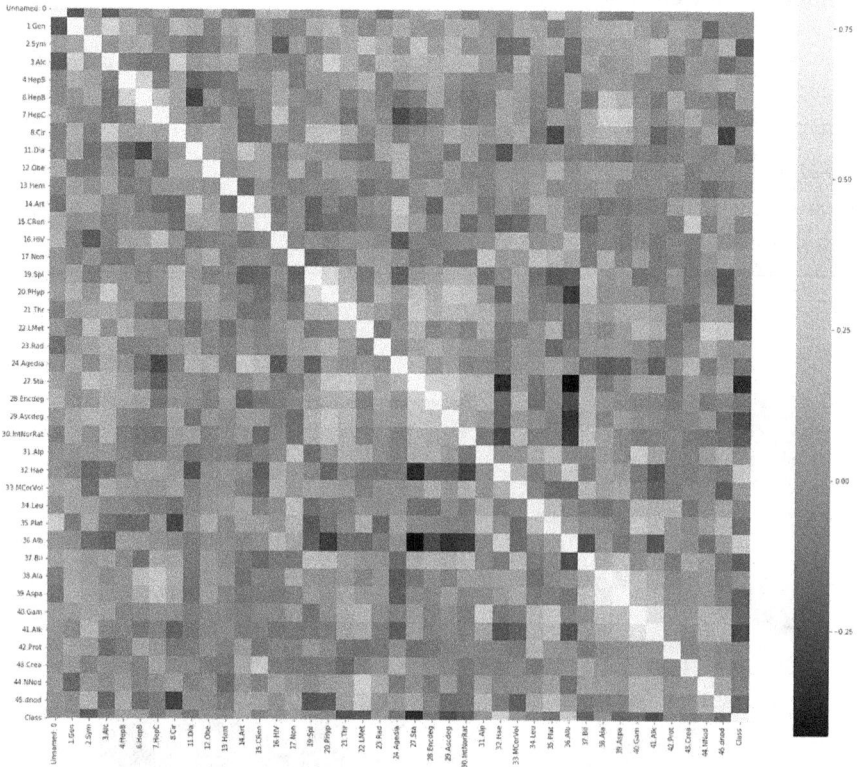

FIGURE 12.2   Features correlation matrix.

Source: Author's owner.

12.4.3   Result of the Models

Outputs of the model are presented below. This includes the performance metric of all fitted models, i.e., random forest algorithm, XGBoost, AdaBoost, and CatBoost (tables 12.1–12.4).

12.4.4   Random Forest Algorithm

TABLE 12.1
Random Forest Output of the Model

	precision	recall	f1-score	support
Died	0.69	0.75	0.72	12
Survived	0.84	0.80	0.82	20

(Continued)

TABLE 12.1 (Continued)
Random Forest Output of the Model

	precision	recall	f1-score	support
accuracy			0.78	32
macro avg	0.77	0.78	0.77	32
weighted avg	0.79	0.78	0.78	32

Accuracy: 0.78125
Source: Author's owner.

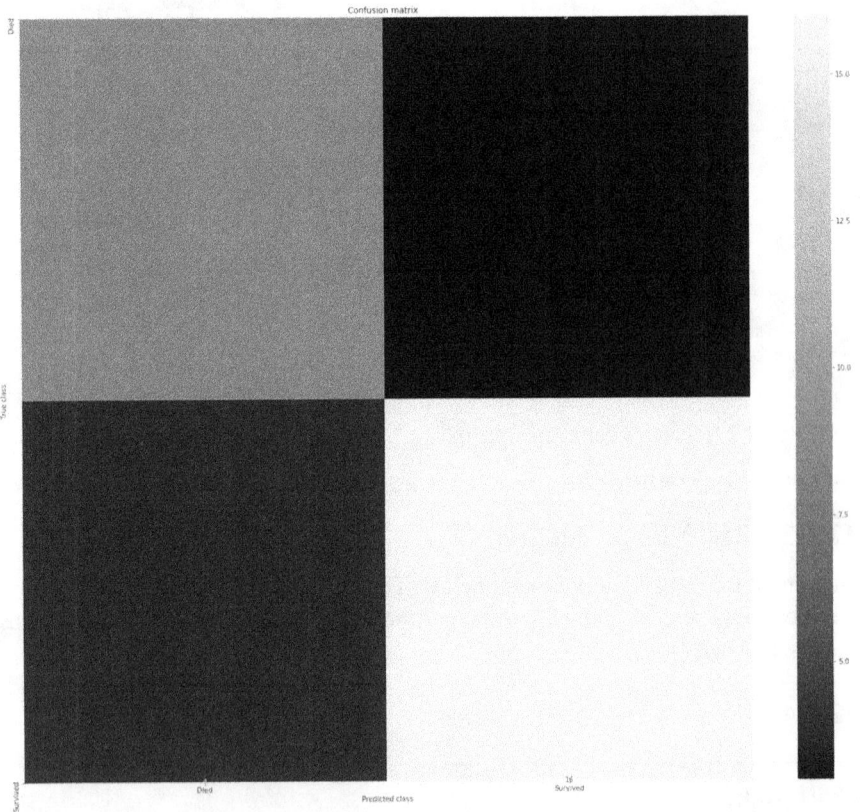

FIGURE 12.3 Confusion matrix for random forest classifier.

Source: Author's owner.

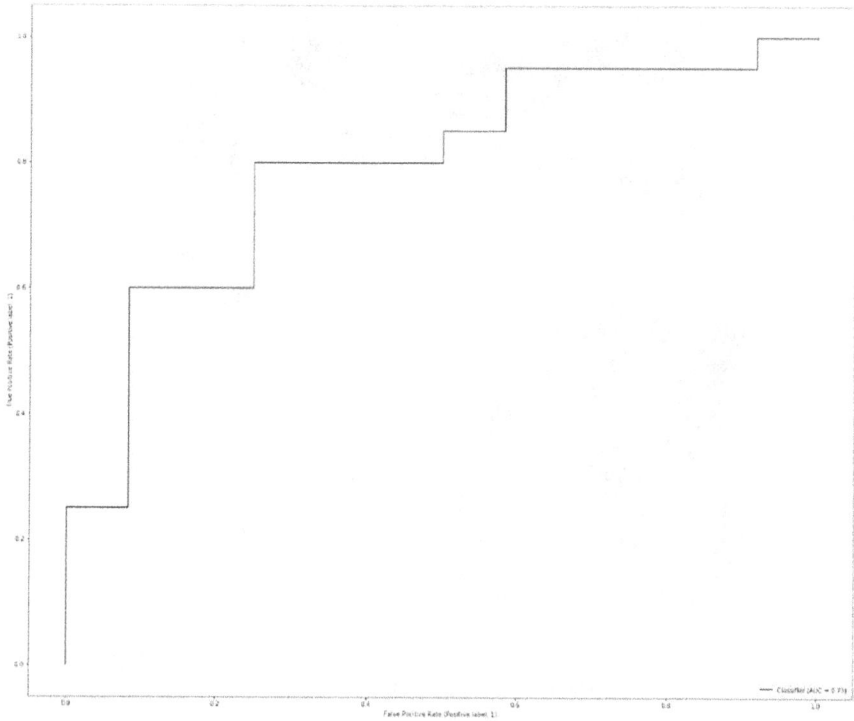

FIGURE 12.4   ROC and AUC score of random forest.

Source: Author's owner.

12.4.5   EXTREME GRADIENT BOOST (XGB) ALGORITHM

TABLE 12.2
Extreme Gradient Boost Output of the Model

	precision	recall	f1-score	support
Died	0.54	0.58	0.56	12
Survived	0.74	0.70	0.72	20
accuracy			0.66	32
macro avg	0.64	0.64	0.64	32
weighted avg	0.66	0.66	0.66	32

Accuracy: 0.65625
Source: Author's owner.

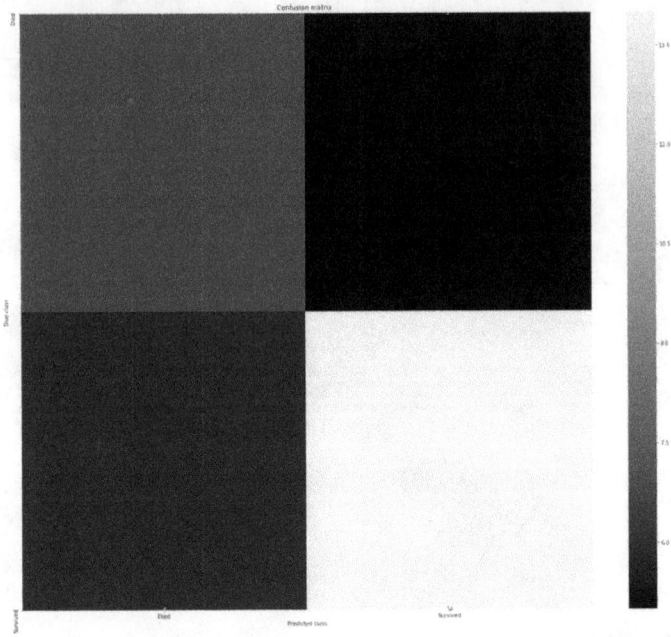

FIGURE 12.5 Extreme gradient boost confusion matrix.

Source: Author's owner.

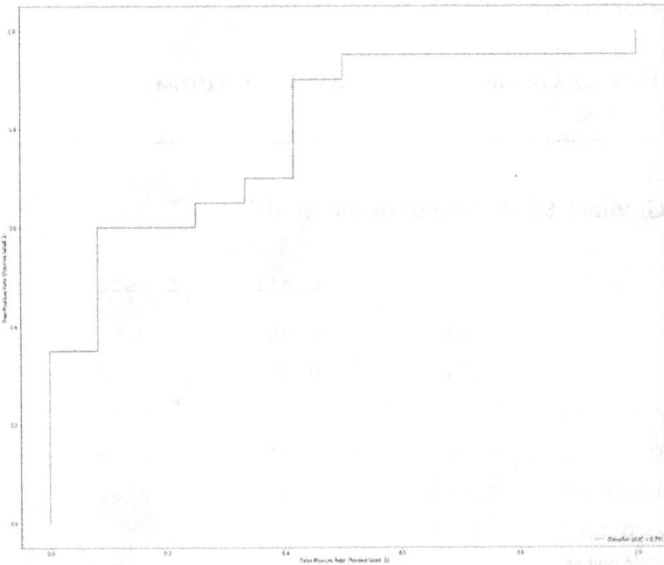

FIGURE 12.6 ROC and AUC score of extreme gradient boost.

Source: Author's owner.

12.4.6   CATBOOST ALGORITHM

TABLE 12.3
CatBoost Output of the Model

	precision	recall	f1-score	support
Died	0.62	0.67	0.64	12
Survived	0.79	0.75	0.77	20
accuracy			0.72	32
macro avg	0.70	0.71	0.70	32
weighted avg	0.72	0.72	0.72	32

Accuracy: 0.71875
Source: Author's owner.

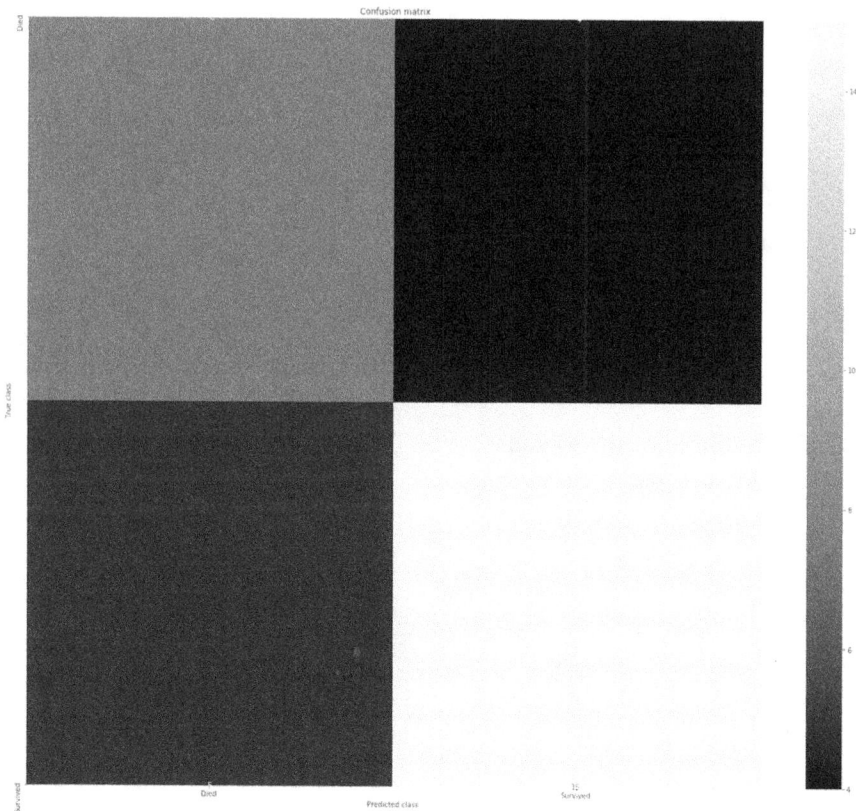

FIGURE 12.7   CatBoost confusion matrix.
Source: Author's owner.

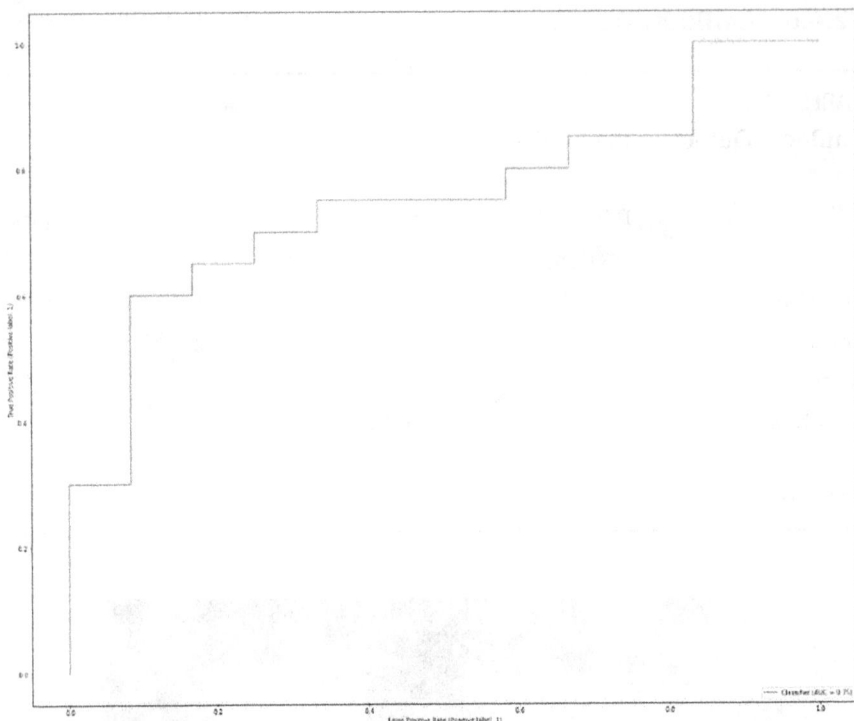

FIGURE 12.8   ROC and AUC score for CatBoost.

Source: Author's owner.

12.4.7   ADABOOST ALGORITHM

TABLE 12.4
AdaBoost Output of the Model

	precision	recall	f1-score	support
Died	0.65	0.92	0.76	12
Survived	0.93	0.70	0.80	20
accuracy			0.78	32
macro avg	0.79	0.81	0.78	32
weighted avg	0.83	0.78	0.78	32

Accuracy 0.78125

Source: Author's owner.

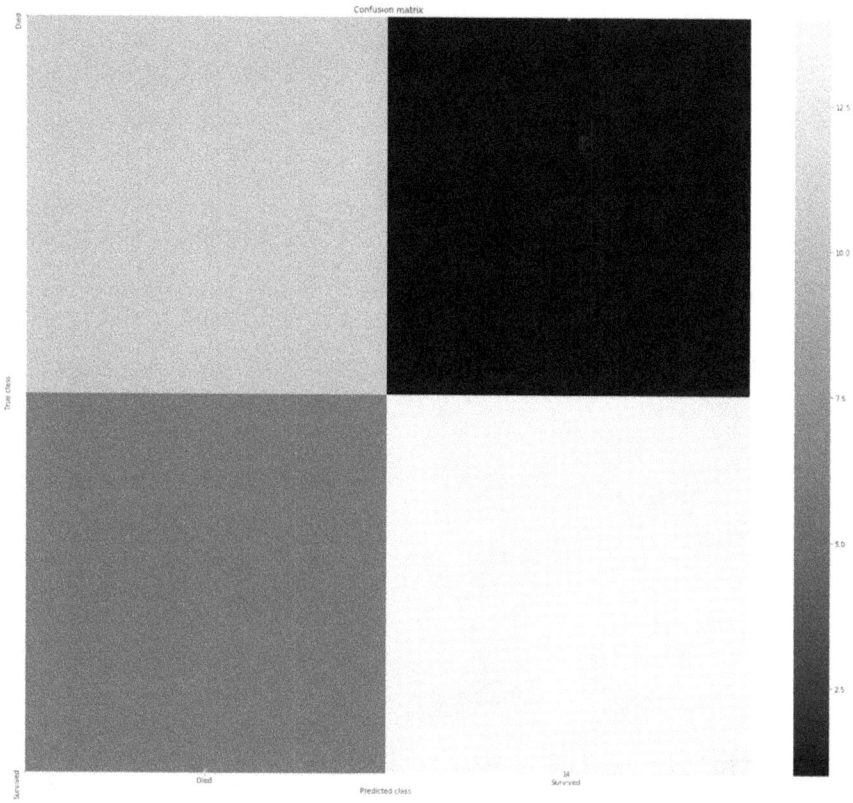

FIGURE 12.9   AdaBoost confusion matrix.

Source: Author's owner.

12.4.8 PERFORMANCE COMPARISON

The performance comparison of the four ensemble machine learning techniques used are presented below.

12.5 DISCUSSION

Figures 12.11 and 12.12 show the summary as well as performance comparison of algorithms used for the hepatocellular carcinoma classification survival model.

According to the results presented in figure 12.11 and figure 12.12, it was identified that AdaBoost is the best performing algorithm, having the highest percentage value in both accuracy and ROC_AUC Score, with 78.125% and 79.58%, respectively.

Although random forest has a joint percentage value with AdaBoost algorithms, it was outshined at the ROC_AUC score, making AdaBoost the best algorithm for the classification survival model for hepatocellular carcinoma. The least performed

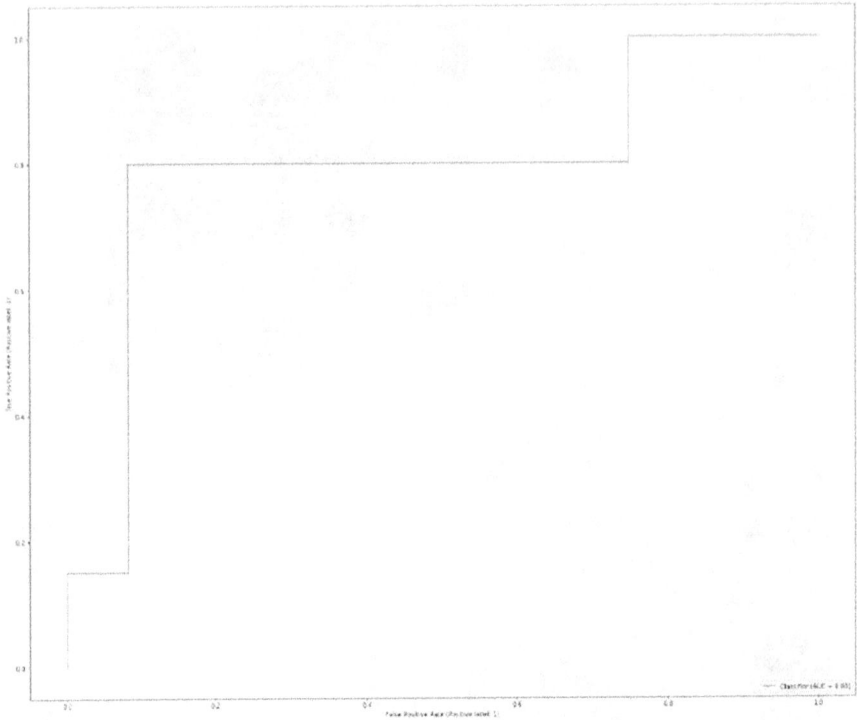

FIGURE 12.10   ROC and AUC score for AdaBoost.

Source: Author's owner.

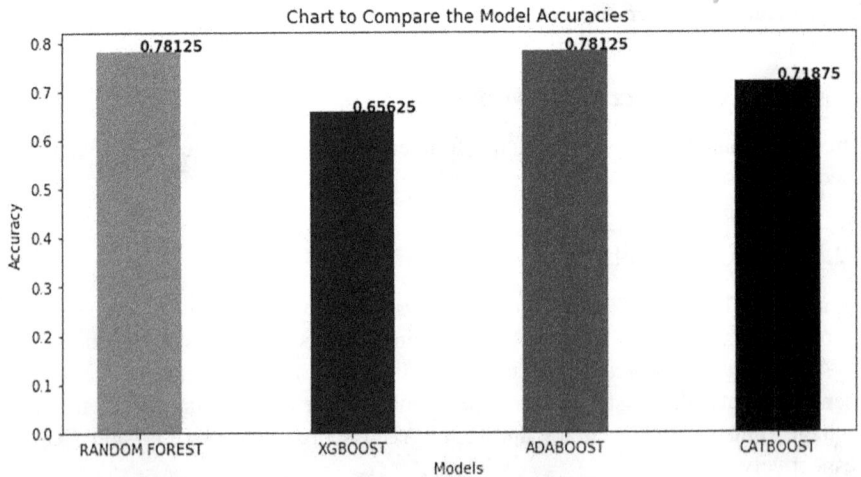

FIGURE 12.11   Accuracies model comparison chart.

Source: Author's owner.

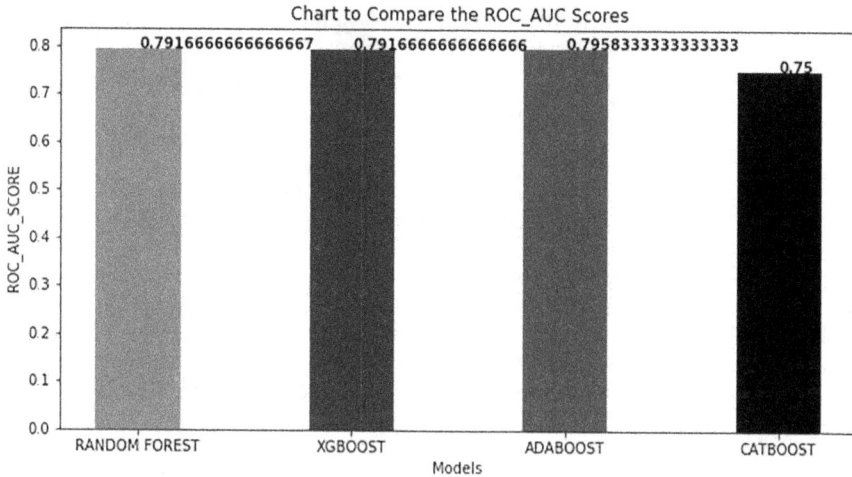

FIGURE 12.12 ROC_AUC score comparison chart.

Source: Author's owner.

algorithm was XGBoost in terms of accuracy and CatBoost was the least performed in terms of ROC_AUC score.

12.6 CONCLUSION

The purpose of this study was to carry out performance comparative analysis using various ensemble learning techniques – adaptive boosting (AdaBoost) and extreme gradient boosting (XGBoost), categorical boosting (CatBoost), and random forest for a hepatocellular carcinoma classification survival model (Khang et al., 2022a).

Taking into consideration the result, it was concluded that ensemble learning algorithms adopted produced a high predicting value suitable enough to correctly classify hepatocellular carcinoma survival. For the classification report (accuracy measure, precision, recall, and F1-score), random forest and AdaBoost ensemble learning output higher values than the other algorithms, as indicated in figure 12.11.

Figure 12.12 shows that AdaBoost performs better than random forest and the rest of algorithms. Thus, based on the overall results, AdaBoost can be considered to be the best ensemble learning algorithm for a hepatocellular carcinoma classification survival model.

Further studies could be involved for more thorough pre-processing and robust hyperparameter tuning to improve the model (Vrushank et al., 2023).

REFERENCES

Anifowose, F. (2020). Ensemble Machine Learning Explained in Simple Terms. *The Way Ahead.* https://www.sciencedirect.com/science/article/pii/S0920410517300712

Azmi, S. S., & Baliga, S. (2020, May 5). An Overview of Boosting Decision Tree Algorithms utilizing AdaBoost and XGBoost Boosting strategies. *International Research Journal of Engineering and Technology (IRJET)*, 7(5), 6866–6870. https://www.academia.edu/download/64615371/IRJET-V7I51293.pdf

Bertuccio, P., Turati, F., Carioli, G., & Rodriguez, T. (2017). Global trends and predictions in hepatocellular carcinoma mortality. https://scholar.google.com/scholar_lookup?title=Global%20trends%20and%20predictions%20in%20hepatocellular%20carcinoma%20mortality&author=P.%20Bertuccio&author=F.%20Turati&author=G.%20Carioli&publication_year=2017

Bhambri, P., Rani, S., Gupta, G., & Khang, A. (2022). *Cloud and Fog Computing Platforms for Internet of Things*. ISBN: 978-1-032-101507, CRC Press. 10.1201/9781003213888

Bobkov, V., Bobkova, A., Porshnev, S., & Zuzin, V. (2016). The application of ensemble learning for delineation of the left ventricle on echocardiographic records. *Dynamics of Systems, Mechanisms and Machines*, pp. 1–5. https://ieeexplore.ieee.org/abstract/document/7818984/

Chen, T., & Guestrin, C. (2016). XGBoost: a scalable tree boosting system. *In Proceedings of the 22nd ACM SIGKDD International Conference on Knowledge Discovery and Data Mining*, (pp. 785–794). https://dl.acm.org/doi/abs/10.1145/2939672.2939785

Cheng, Z., Yang, P., Qu, S., Zhou, J., Yang, J., Yang, X., Xia, Y., Li, J., Wang, K., Yan, Z., Wu, D., Zhang, B., Hüser, N., & Shen, F. (2015). Risk factors and management for early and late intrahepatic recurrence of solitary hepatocellular carcinoma after curative resection. *HPB*, 17(5), 422–427. 10.1111/hpb.12367

Chiu, H.-C., Ho, T.-W., Lee, K.-T., Chen, H.-Y., & Ho, W.-H. (2013). Mortality Predicted Accuracy for Hepatocellular Carcinoma Patients with Hepatic Resection Using Artificial Neural Network. *The Scientific World Journal*, 2013, 10. 10.1155/2013/201976

Dyakonov, A. (2021, March 15). Ensemble in Machine Learning with Examples. https://dasha.ai/en-us/blog/ensemble-in-machine-learning

Freund, Y., & Schapire, R. E. (2012). Foundation and algorithms. *MIT press, Cambridge*. https://www.jmlr.org/papers/volume10/rudin09a/rudin09a.pdf

Gomez-Rios, A., Luengo, J., & Herrera, F. (2017). A Study on the Noise Label Influence in Boosting Algorithms: AdaBoost, GBM and XGBoost. *Hybride Artificial Intelligence System*, 268–280. https://link.springer.com/chapter/10.1007/978-3-319-59650-1_23

He, H., Zhang, W., & Zhang, S. (2018). A novel ensemble method for credit scoring: adaption of different imbalance ratios. *Expert System with Applications*. https://www.sciencedirect.com/science/article/pii/S0957417418300125

Howal, S. (2018, December 15). Ensemble Learning in Machine Learning | Getting Started. *Medium*. https://towardsdatascience.com/ensemble-learning-in-machine-learning-getting-started-4ed85eb38e00

IBM (2022). What is Machine Learning? | *This introduction to machine learning provides an overview of its history, important definitions, applications, and concerns within businesses today.* https://www.ibm.com/cloud/learn/machine-learning

Khang, A., Ragimova, N. A., Hajimahmud, V. A., & Alyar, A. V. (2022a). Advanced Technologies and Data Management in the Smart Healthcare System. *AI-Centric Smart City Ecosystems: Technologies, Design and Implementation* (1st Ed.). CRC Press. 10.1201/9781003252542-16

Khang, A., Chowdhury, S., & Sharma, S. (Eds.). (2022b). *The Data-Driven Blockchain Ecosystem: Fundamentals, Applications, and Emerging Technologies* (1st ed.). CRC Press. 10.1201/9781003269281

Khang A., Rana, G., Tailor, R. K., & Hajimahmud, V. A. (Eds.). (2023a). *Data-Centric AI Solutions and Emerging Technologies in the Healthcare Ecosystem* (1st Ed.). CRC Press. 10.1201/9781003356189

Khang, A., Rani, S., Gujrati, R., Uygun, H., & Gupta, S. K. (Eds.). (2023b). *Designing Workforce Management Systems for Industry 4.0: Data-Centric and AI-Enabled Approaches* (1st Ed.). CRC Press. 10.1201/99781003357070

Khanh, H. H., & Khang, A. (2021). The Role of Artificial Intelligence in Blockchain Applications. *Reinventing Manufacturing and Business Processes through Artificial Intelligence*, 20–40. CRC Press. 10.1201/9781003145011-2

Lee, S. H., Kim, S. U., Jang, J. W., Bae, S. H., Lee, S., Kim, B. K., Park, J. Y., Kim, D. Y., Ahn, S. H., & Han, K.-H. (2015). Use of transient elastography to predict de novo recurrence after radiofrequency ablation for hepatocellular carcinoma. *OncoTargets and Therapy*, 8, 347–356. 10.2147/OTT.S75077

McGlynn, K. A., Petrick, J. L., & El-Serag, H. B. (2021). Epidemiology of Hepatocellular Carcinoma. *Hepatology*, 73(S1), 4–13. 10.1002/hep.31288

Rana, G., Khang, A., Sharma, R., Goel, A. K., & Dubey, A. K.. (2021). *Reinventing Manufacturing and Business Processes through Artificial Intelligence*, (Eds.). CRC Press. 10.1201/9781003145011

Rani, S., Chauhan, M., Kataria, A., & Khang, A. (2021). IoT Equipped Intelligent Distributed Framework for Smart Healthcare Systems. *Networking and Internet Architecture*, (Eds.). CRC Press. 10.48550/arXiv.2110.04997

Rani, S., Bhambri, P., Kataria, A., Khang A., & Sivaraman, A. K. (Eds.). (2023). *Big Data, Cloud Computing and IoT: Tools and Applications* (1st Ed.). Chapman and Hall/CRC. 10.1201/9781003298335

Sato, M., Tateishi, R., Moriyama, M., Fukumoto, T., Yamada, T., Nakagomi, R., Kinoshita, M. N., Nakatsuka, T., Minami, T., Uchino, K., Enooku, K., Nakagawa, H., Shiina, S., Ninomiya, K., Kodera, S., Yatomi, Y., & Koike, K. (2021). Machine Learning–Based Personalized Prediction of Hepatocellular Carcinoma Recurrence After Radiofrequency Ablation. *Gastro Hep Advances*. https://www.ghadvances.org/article/S2772-5723(21)00008-X/abstract

Shiina, S., Tateishi, R., Arano, T., Uchino, K., Enooku, K., Nakagawa, H., Asaoka, Y., Sato, T., Masuzaki, R., Kondo, Y., Goto, T., Yoshida, H., Omata, M., & Koike, K. (2012). Radiofrequency ablation for hepatocellular carcinoma: 10-year outcome and prognostic factors. *The American Journal of Gastroenterology*, 107(4), 569–577; quiz 578. 10.1038/ajg.2011.425

Vrushank, S., Vidhi, T., & Khang, A. (2023). Electronic Health Records Security and Privacy Enhancement using Blockchain Technology. *Data-Centric AI Solutions and Emerging Technologies in the Healthcare Ecosystem*. (1st ed.), (2023), P (1). CRC Press. 10.1201/9781003356189

Zhu, Y., Gu, L.-L., Zhang, F.-B., Zheng, G.-Q., Chen, T., & Jia, W.-D. (2022). Long-Term Survival and Risk Factors in Patients with Hepatitis B-Related Hepatocellular Carcinoma: A Real-World Study. *Canadian Journal of Gastroenterology and Hepatology*, 2022, 9. 10.1155/2022/7750140

13 Heart Disease and Liver Disease Prediction Using Machine Learning

Divvela Vishnu Sai Kumar, Ritik Chaurasia, Anuradha Misra, Praveen Kumar Misra, and Alex Khang

CONTENTS

13.1 INTRODUCTION

Heart disease portrays a scope of conditions that influence your heart. Infections under the umbrella of coronary illness incorporate coronary conduit sickness, like coronary course infection, arrhythmias, and intrinsic heart issues (inborn heart absconds), among others.

Cardiovascular infection which is a kind of coronary illness normally alludes to conditions including little or obstructed corridors that can prompt respiratory failure, chest torment (angina), or stroke. Other heart conditions, for example, those influencing your heart muscle, valves, or cadence, are likewise viewed as sorts of coronary illness (Babu et al., 2017).

Coronary illness is one of the significant reasons for ailment, demise, etc. among individuals on the planet. Anticipating coronary illness is viewed as one of the main subjects in the clinical information examination stage.

The information in the medical care industry is exceptionally gigantic. Information mining deciphers a huge assortment of green medical services information into data that can assist with settling on informed choices and surmises (Khang et al., 2022).

With the expanding pattern of stationary living things and an absence of actual work, liver-related infections have become very normal nowadays (Khang et al., 2023). In country regions, the tension is as yet taken care of, yet in metropolitan regions, particularly in enormous urban communities, liver illness is a typical sight nowadays.

- Liver illness kills a huge number of individuals consistently.
- Hepatitis B alone causes 1.34 million passing every year.

Issues with liver patients not effortlessly analyzed early in light of the fact that they will work ordinarily regardless of whether patients are somewhat harmed.

Early findings of liver issues will expand the endurance pace of patients. Liver disappointment is a significant danger among Indians. It is normal that by 2025 India will turn into the World Capital for Liver Diseases. The predominance of liver illness in India has been credited to a work area way of life, an increment in liquor utilization, and smoking.

13.2   PREDICTION OF DISEASE

Diagnosis and prediction of heart, liver disease is an important issue. Due to this reason, a lot of work has been done in this area. We categorize this process into two steps, they are: The first introduces the steps of selecting the appropriate patient with a selection of features, secondly to test those learning algorithms that provide high accuracy.

13.2.1   FEATURES SELECTION

The feature selection is one of the significant difficulties to prepare the machine learning algorithms with the given information (Cai et al., 2018). So as per a few examinations and explorations in this issue for grouping the heart disease, it utilizes 13 features. They are Age, Sex, cp, trestbps, chol, fbs, restecg, thalach, exang, oldpeak, slope, ca, thal. And for liver disease classification, we are going to use only ten features. They are Age, Gender, Total_Bilirubin, Direct_Bilirubin, Alkaline_ Phosphotase, and Alamine_Aminotransferase. If the number of attributes is 13, then the accuracey will be more; the number of attributes should be ten for better accuracy.

13.2.2   MACHINE LEARNING ALGORITHMS

For good accuracy prediction, an efficient machine learning algorithm is required. Prediction of heart and liver disease is very complex and critical; it is included with so many procedures, and simple mistake in this procedure and can lead to the patient's death also. So, we have to use the highest accuracy algorithm.

In this step, we have evaluated the algorithms of machine learning using an accuracy score method and we have selected the algorithm with high accuracy (Oladeji et al., 2019) (Fang et al., 2018).

13.3   DATASET COLLECTION

In this research paper, we have used the dataset of people who are already tested for the tests related to heart disease in any hospital. This dataset is a data frame that can be represented by a table with rows and columns to represent the features of the dataset, which is helpful to train the ML model (Rani et al., 2021).

13.3.1   MANUAL EXPLORATION

In this step of manual exploration, we have manually checked the data; that is, if the patient has any disease or not by checking the target data column. To give a target data to the algorithm, we have used this process (Khang et al., 2023).

13.3.2   DATA PRE-PROCESSING

Data pre-processing is a very important step because the data we collected had null values; we had to understand in which column the null value was present and how many null values were coming (Rana et al., 2021).

So that if null values are less, then we could remove those data; otherwise, we have to replace those null values with any analysis like mean of the column. So we have to pre-process the data before sending it to the machine learning model (Khanh & Khang, 2021).

13.3.3   SPLITTING DATASET

Prior to preparing the machine learning model, we gave the objective segment in the informational index and then we split the information involving the train test split capacity in the ScikitLearn bundle. We partitioned the information into training and testing datasets; later, that training set was consequently isolated into training and validation as shown in figure 13.1.

13.3.4   MODEL EVALUATION

In this step, we executed the algorithms of machine learning such as logistic regression, KNN, decision tree classifier, and SVM on the prediction of heart disease

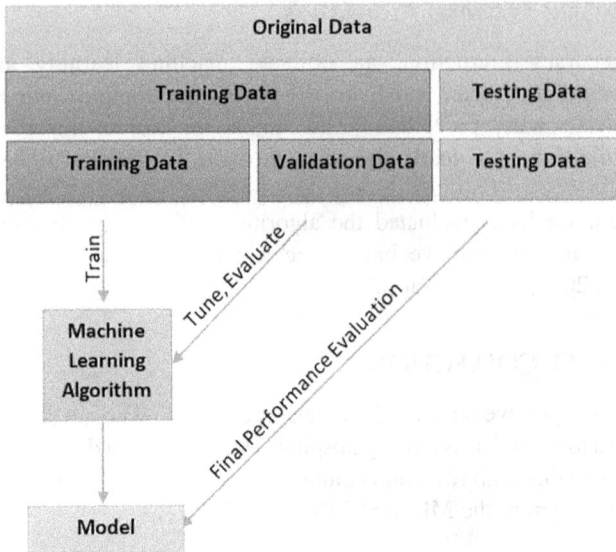

FIGURE 13.1   Training and testing of data.

Source: Author's owner.

and we applied models like logistic regression, random forest classifier, and decision tree classifier on the classification of liver disease.

Here, our methodology was to apply various algorithms on the two heart and liver illness datasets to approve and assess the accuracy of each model. We used this score of accuracy to test the algorithms. Accuracy score is the number of correct predictions to the total number of predictions, as shown in (figure 13.2).

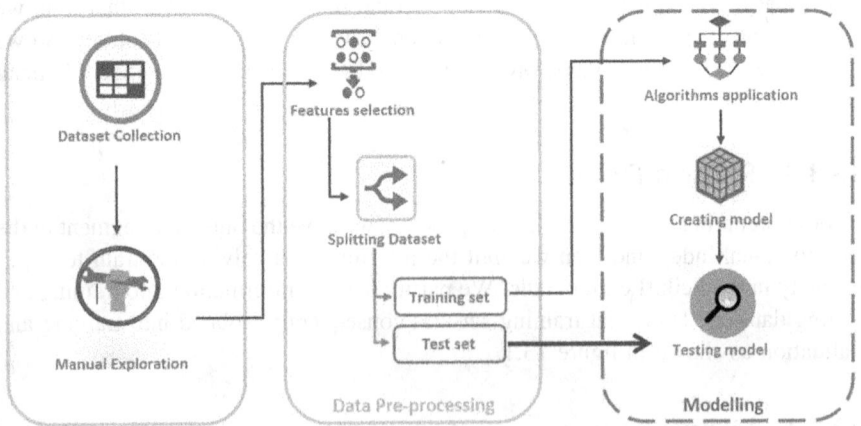

FIGURE 13.2   Model evaluation process of data.

Source: Author's owner.

13.4 RESULTS AND DISCUSSION

We applied different machine learning algorithms, as mentioned above, to achieve the final results. The Process that we followed is discussed next.

13.4.1 Data Collection

Data collection is defined as the method involved with gathering the information and investigating the information for precise experiences for research. The disease dataset of heart problems dates from 1988 and consisted of four databases: Cleveland, Hungary, Switzerland, and Long Beach V.

Four of these databases are Cleveland, Hungary, Switzerland, and Long Beach V. They contain 76 attributes, including the predicted attribute, but all published experiments used a subset of 14 of them. We used the Pandas library to load the datasets (Dhai Eddine Salhi et al., 2021) (figures 13.3 and 13.4).

13.4.2 Manual Exploration

We performed manual exploration to explore a large dataset in an unstructured way to cover all the fields and features of data, like what is the target of the data. Above in the heart disease dataset, the target column decided whether the patient was having the disease or not. In the liver disease dataset, the target column decided whether the patient was having the disease or not.

- In heart illness data, if 1 was there in the target data, then that patient was having the heart disease or if 0 is in target data, then patient was not having the heart disease.

In [73]: heart_dataset.head()

Out[73]:

	age	sex	cp	trestbps	chol	fbs	restecg	thalach	exang	oldpeak	slope	ca	thal	target
0	63	1	3	145	233	1	0	150	0	2.3	0	0	1	1
1	37	1	2	130	250	0	1	187	0	3.5	0	0	2	1
2	41	0	1	130	204	0	0	172	0	1.4	2	0	2	1
3	56	1	1	120	236	0	1	178	0	0.8	2	0	2	1
4	57	0	0	120	354	0	1	163	1	0.6	2	0	2	1

In [4]: heart_dataset.tail()

Out[4]:

	age	sex	cp	trestbps	chol	fbs	restecg	thalach	exang	oldpeak	slope	ca	thal	target
298	57	0	0	140	241	0	1	123	1	0.2	1	0	3	0
299	45	1	3	110	264	0	1	132	0	1.2	1	0	3	0
300	68	1	0	144	193	1	1	141	0	3.4	1	2	3	0
301	57	1	0	130	131	0	1	115	1	1.2	1	1	3	0
302	57	0	1	130	236	0	0	174	0	0.0	1	1	2	0

FIGURE 13.3   Heart disease data.

Source: Author's owner.

```
In [2]:  #load the data set using pandas
         liver_dataset = pd.read_csv('indian_liver_patient.csv')

In [3]:  liver_dataset.head(10)
```

Out[3]:

	Age	Gender	Total_ Bilirubin	Direct_ Bilirubin	Alkaline_ Phosphotase	Alamine_ Aminotransferase	Aspartate_ Aminotransferase	Total_ Protiens	Albumin	Albumin_and_ Globulin_Ratio	Dataset
0	65	Female	0.7	0.1	187	16	18	6.8	3.3	0.90	1
1	62	Male	10.9	5.5	699	64	100	7.5	3.2	0.74	1
2	62	Male	7.3	4.1	490	60	68	7.0	3.3	0.89	1
3	58	Male	1.0	0.4	182	14	20	6.8	3.4	1.00	1
4	72	Male	3.9	2.0	195	27	59	7.3	2.4	0.40	1
5	46	Male	1.8	0.7	208	19	14	7.6	4.4	1.30	1
6	26	Female	0.9	0.2	154	16	12	7.0	3.5	1.00	1
7	29	Female	0.9	0.3	202	14	11	6.7	3.6	1.10	1
8	17	Male	0.9	0.3	202	22	19	7.4	4.1	1.20	2
9	55	Male	0.7	0.2	290	53	58	6.8	3.4	1.00	1

FIGURE 13.4   Liver disease data.

Source: Author's owner.

- In the liver disease dataset, if 1 is there in target data, then patient was having the liver disease or if 2 was there in the target data then the patient was not having the liver disease.

13.4.3   DATA PRE-PROCESSING

In the data pre-processing step we checked if null data was present or not in the dataset (Hajimahmud et al., 2022). In heart disease, data did have any null data but in liver disease data had some null data in the Albumin_and_Globulin_Ratio column so we filled those null values by the mean value of that column.

And after that, in the liver disease data set, we replaced the male and female by 1 and 0 and then only the algorithm was able to predict the data, as in table 13.1.

Table 13.1 presents the details of selected features in heart disease data with attributes of age, sex, cp, trestbps, chol, fbs, restecg, thalach, exang, oldpeak, slope, ca, thal, and target.

13.4.3.1   Feature columns for liver disease dataset
- Age of the patient
- Gender of the patient
- Total bilirubin
- Direct bilirubin
- Alkaline phosphotase
- Alamine aminotransferase
- Aspartate aminotransferase
- Total proteins
- Albumin
- Albumin and globulin ratio

Dataset: field used to split given data into two sets (patient with liver disease, or no disease) as in figure 13.5.

TABLE 13.1

Features of Heart Disease Data

Attribute	Description	Values
Age	Age	29 to 62 years
Sex	Sex	• male • female
CP	Type of chest pain	typical angina pectoris atypical angina 3- non-anginal pain 4- asymptomatic
trestbps	Resting blood pressure in mm/Hg	Numeric value:example: 140 mm/Hg
Chol	Serum cholesterol in mg/dl	Numeric value: example: 289 mg/hg
Fbs	Fasting blood pressure>120 mg/dl	Numeric value: example: 129 mm/Hg
Restecg	Resting electro-cardio-graphic	0-normal, 1- have the ST-T 2- hypertrophy
thalach	Maximum heart rate	Numeric value: Example: 140,173
Exang	Exercise angina	• Yes • No
Oldpeak	ST induced by the exercise relative to taking rest	Numeric Value
Slope	The slope of exercise segment	• on the rise • flat 3- the downhill slope
Ca	Number of vessels that are majorly colored with fluoroscopy	0 to 3 vessels
Thal	Thalassemia	3- normal, defect repaired, reversible defect

Source: Author's owner.

13.4.3.2 Correlation matrix for liver disease data

We divided our dataset into two parts; the first part was having the training data, which was of size 80% and the second part was having test data of size 20% (figure 13.6).

13.4.4 MODEL EVALUATION

We applied ML algorithms such as logistic regression, KNN, decision tree classifier, and SVM for heart illness data and algorithms such as logistic regression, random forest classifier, and decision tree classifier for liver disease data.

13.4.5 TESTING ALGORITHMS

After applying those ML algorithms on the given two datasets, we tested those models using accuracy score. After calculating the accuracy score, we compared those accuracies by pasting in tables, as in figure 13.7 and figure 13.8.

```
fig, ax = plt.subplots(figsize=(8,6))
sns.heatmap(liver_dataset.corr(), annot=True, fmt='.1g', cmap="viridis", cbar=False);
```

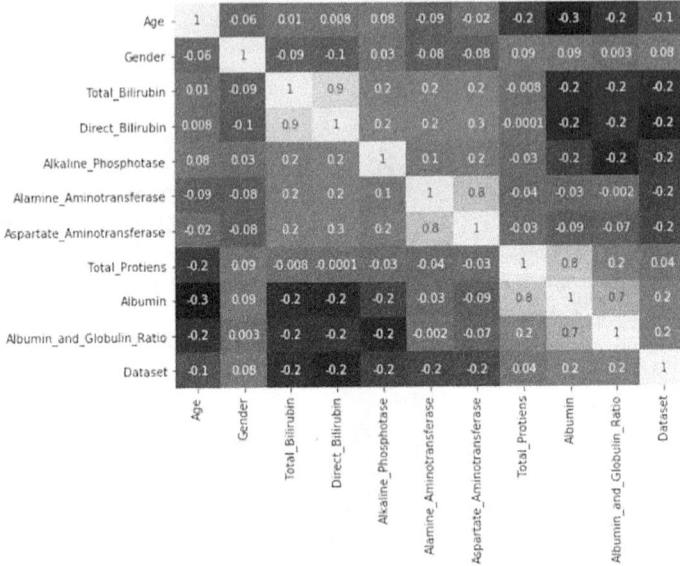

	Age	Gender	Total_Bilirubin	Direct_Bilirubin	Alkaline_Phosphotase	Alamine_Aminotransferase	Aspartate_Aminotransferase	Total_Protiens	Albumin	Albumin_and_Globulin_Ratio	Dataset
Age	1	-0.06	0.01	0.008	0.08	-0.09	-0.02	-0.2	-0.3	-0.2	-0.1
Gender	-0.06	1	-0.09	-0.1	0.03	-0.08	-0.08	0.09	0.09	0.003	0.08
Total_Bilirubin	0.01	-0.09	1	0.9	0.2	0.2	0.2	-0.008	-0.2	-0.2	-0.2
Direct_Bilirubin	0.008	-0.1	0.9	1	0.2	0.2	0.3	-0.0001	-0.2	-0.2	-0.2
Alkaline_Phosphotase	0.08	0.03	0.2	0.2	1	0.1	0.2	-0.03	-0.2	-0.2	-0.2
Alamine_Aminotransferase	-0.09	-0.08	0.2	0.2	0.1	1	0.8	-0.04	-0.03	-0.002	-0.2
Aspartate_Aminotransferase	-0.02	-0.08	0.2	0.3	0.2	0.8	1	-0.03	-0.09	-0.07	-0.2
Total_Protiens	-0.2	0.09	-0.008	-0.0001	-0.03	-0.04	-0.03	1	0.8	0.2	0.04
Albumin	-0.3	0.09	-0.2	-0.2	-0.2	-0.03	-0.09	0.8	1	0.7	0.2
Albumin_and_Globulin_Ratio	-0.2	0.003	-0.2	-0.2	-0.2	-0.002	-0.07	0.2	0.7	1	0.2
Dataset	-0.1	0.08	-0.2	-0.2	-0.2	-0.2	-0.2	0.04	0.2	0.2	1

FIGURE 13.5 Correlation matrix of liver disease data.

Source: Author's owner.

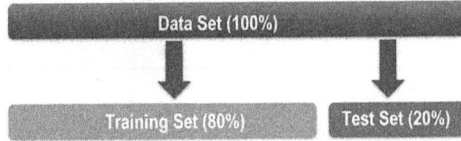

FIGURE 13.6 Train test split of data.

Source: Author's owner.

Out[47]:

	Model	Training Accuracy %	Testing Accuracy %
0	Logistic Regression	86.187845	84.426230
1	K-nearest neighbors	73.480663	63.114754
2	Decision Tree Classifier	100.000000	81.967213
3	Support Vector Machine	100.000000	50.819672

FIGURE 13.7 Accuracy result of heart disease prediction.

Source: Author's owner.

`Out[90]:`

	Model	Training Accuracy %	Testing Accuracy %
0	Logistic Regression	74.498567	65.384615
1	Random Forest Classifier	100.000000	72.222222
2	Decision Tree Classifier	100.000000	68.376068

FIGURE 13.8   Accuracy result for liver disease prediction.

Source: Author's owner.

13.4.6   Choose the Best Algorithm

After analyzing the models using accuracy score, we got the results. By observing the results, we concluded that logistic regression is the highest accuracy algorithm for heart illness prediction and random forest classifier is the best algorithm for liver disease prediction (Khang et al., 2022a).

13.5   CONCLUSION

Heart and liver diseases have become more successive among individuals of such countless nations. So, therefore, predicting the heart and liver disease before getting infected to those diseases can be helpful to decrease the risk of death. This type of prediction of diseases is widely in research areas (Khang et al., 2023).

This is based on the applications of machine learning where we used four algorithms (logistic, KNN, decision tree, SVM) for heart illness prediction and we used three algorithms (logistic, random tree, decision tree) for liver disease prediction and we got very good results: 85% and (100%, 75%) for heart and liver disease detection (Khang et al., 2022a).

We made a study on feature selection also and we used a correlation matrix to know the relation and dependencies among the attributes of the datasets. This method can be implemented in several aspects; for example, we can use deep learning (DL) algorithms and we can increase the size of the dataset to see more accurate results (Jain et al., 2023).

REFERENCES

Babu, S., Vivek, E., Famina, K., Fida, K., Aswathi, P., Shanid, M., Hena, M., "Heart diagnosis of disease using the technique data mining" 2017 (ICECA). vol. 1, pp. 750–753. IEEE (2017). https://ieeexplore.ieee.org/abstract/document/8203643/

Cai, J., Luo, J., Wang, S., Yang, S., "Feature selection in machine learning: A new perspective," *Neurocomputing* 300, 70–79 (2018). https://www.sciencedirect.com/science/article/pii/S0925231218302911

Fang, X., Hodge, B. M., Du, E., Zhang, N., Li, F., "Modelling wind power spatial- temporal correlation in multi-interval optimal power flow: A sparse correlation matrix approach," *Applied Energy* 230, 531–539 (2018). https://www.sciencedirect.com/science/article/pii/S0306261918312972

Hajimahmud, V. A., Khang, A., Hahanov, V., Litvinova, E., Chumachenko, S., Alyar, A. V., "Autonomous Robots for Smart City: Closer to Augmented Humanity," *AI-Centric Smart City Ecosystems: Technologies, Design and Implementation* (1st Ed.) (2022). CRC Press. 10.1201/9781003252542-7

Jain, P., Tripathi, V., Malladi, R., Khang, A., "Data-driven AI Models in the Workforce Development Planning," *Designing Workforce Management Systems for Industry 4.0: Data-Centric and AI-Enabled Approaches*, 179–198, (1st Ed.) (2023). CRC Press. 10.1201/9781003357070-10

Khang, A., Ragimova, N. A., Hajimahmud, V. A., Alyar, A. V., "Advanced Technologies and Data Management in the Smart Healthcare System," *AI-Centric Smart City Ecosystems: Technologies, Design and Implementation* (1st Ed.) (2022a). CRC Press. 10.1201/9781003252542-16

Khang, A., Hahanov, V., Litvinova, E., Chumachenko, S., Hajimahmud, V. A., Alyar, A. V., "The Key Assistant of Smart City - Sensors and Tools," *AI-Centric Smart City Ecosystems: Technologies, Design and Implementation* (1st Ed.) (2022b). CRC Press. 10.1201/9781003252542-17

Khang, A., Rani, S., Gujrati, R., Uygun, H., Gupta, S. K., (Eds.). *Designing Workforce Management Systems for Industry 4.0: Data-Centric and AI-Enabled Approaches* (1st Ed.). (2023). CRC Press. 10.1201/99781003357070

Khang A., Rana, G., Tailor, R. K., Hajimahmud, V. A., (Eds.) *Data-Centric AI Solutions and Emerging Technologies in the Healthcare Ecosystem* (1st Ed.). (2023). CRC Press. 10.1201/9781003356189

Khanh, H. H., Khang, A., "The Role of Artificial Intelligence in Blockchain Applications," *Reinventing Manufacturing and Business Processes through Artificial Intelligence*, 20–40. (2021). CRC Press. 10.1201/9781003145011-2

Oladeji, F. A., Idowu, P. A., Egejuru, N., Faluyi, S. G., Balogun, J. A., "Model for Predicting the Risk of Kidney Stone using Data Mining Techniques," *International Journal of Computer Applications*, (2019), Volume 182 - Number 38. https://lgurjcsit.lgu.edu.pk/index.php/lgurjcsit/article/view/212

Rana, G., Khang, A., Sharma, R., Goel, A. K., Dubey, A. K. *Reinventing Manufacturing and Business Processes through Artificial Intelligence*, (Eds.). (2021). CRC Press. 10.1201/9781003145011

Rani, S., Chauhan, M., Kataria, A., Khang, A., "IoT Equipped Intelligent Distributed Framework for Smart Healthcare Systems," *Networking and Internet Architecture*, (Eds.). (2021). CRC Press. 10.48550/arXiv.2110.04997

Dhai Eddine Salhi, Abdelkamel A Kamel Tari, M-Tahar Kechadi, "Using ML for Heart Disease Prediction," *Advances in Computing Systems and Applications*, (2021), 10.1007/978-3-030-69418-0_7. https://ashpublications.org/bloodadvances/article-abstract/6/5/1525/476859

Tailor, R. K., Pareek, R., Khang, A., (Eds.). "Robot Process Automation in Blockchain," *The Data-Driven Blockchain Ecosystem: Fundamentals, Applications, and Emerging Technologies*, 149–164 (1st Ed.) (2022). CRC Press. 10.1201/9781003269281-8

14 A Novel Improved Logistic Regression Model for Diagnosing Heart Disease

Arkadip Ray, Avijit Kumar Chaudhuri, and Sulekha Das

CONTENTS

14.1   INTRODUCTION

The well-being of the human race is under threat from a number of diseases transmitted by viruses, as well as lifestyle disorders such as cardiovascular diseases (CVDs). In the prior case, intensive research and development are demanding needs, while in the second case, the detection of root causes would sustain humankind (Babasaheb et al., 2023).

A data mining approach can be recommended for gaining insights due to the wide availability of datasets. The extent of CVD has been increasing over time, with the World Health Organization (WHO) reporting 17.9 million deaths in 2016, and CVD is the number one cause of fatality globally.

The situation is particularly serious in emergent nations, where CVD accounts for over three-quarters of deaths. The WHO has earmarked behavioral risk factors as the cause of CVD, and CVD correlates with the existence of other conditions, such as hypertension and diabetes.

To detect CVD, cardiologists typically interpret a patient's present diagnostic test results. However, a problem arises when outcomes of tests conflict with each other, such as when a patient has high blood pressure (hypertension) but low cholesterol levels. In the next diagnostic step, cardiologists assess whether there are behavioral risk factors such as smoking; if there are, then a conclusion can be drawn, but it is problematic if there are no such factors.

Further investigation based on the doctor's acumen yields results, but with varying accuracy levels. The theory of bounded rationality implies that consistency of results among doctors is difficult to achieve (Khang et al., 2023). Researchers also agree that human or manual determination of the risks, or a diagnosis of CVD based on risk factors, is a challenging task (Ray & Chaudhuri, 2021). Hence, the data-mining approach can reveal patterns and insights.

With pathological test data at hand, one can gain insights at a higher level of accuracy. There have been studies that have used data mining in the study of CVD, but these studies have revealed inconsistent predictive accuracy.

Liu et al. (2017), using a rough-set-based technique with various datasets, predicted CVD risk with an accuracy rate as high as 93%. However, any shortfall in prediction can be fatal in cases of CVD, and type II errors may cause adverse results.

Data scientists focus not only on overall accuracy but also on three main issues: consistency, sensitivity, and specificity. There is very little evidence in studies on the application of data mining to the prediction of diseases in general and CVD in particular, nor that do these approaches meet the three criteria (Rani et al., 2023).

To enhance the classification, researchers look forward to bagging and boosting methods. To train a classifier in dealing with individual samples, bagging performs a bootstrap to obtain object samples (Breiman, 1996).

Bootstrap sampling appears to result in low-diversity ensembles compared to other methods of creating an ensemble, although the classifier models used in bagging are sensitive to minor data changes.

Larger sizes of ensembles are suitable for bagging and this issue can be overcome by using the random forest (RF) method (Breiman, 2001). The RF method also utilizes bootstrapping to create samples, but it varies in how it constructs individual decision trees.

RF makes use of an F algorithm that leads to the implementation of higher diversity without reducing the accuracy of every classifier. The individual classifiers are built parallel to each other, rather than being dependent on one another. However, this foundation does not imply that the outputs are nonaligned.

Boosting, conversely, assists to improve the efficiency of a weak classifier. It represents a family of methods, with AdaBoost being the most prevalent member of the family. Typically, AdaBoost works out to be superior when equaled to bagging and RF. A previous study has shown that bagging and RF have their application niches (Li et al., 2011).

All classifiers perform identically when dealing with large group sizes (Banfield et al., 2004). Thus, the challenge remains in the case of small ensemble sizes.

AdaBoost has significant capability to generate diversity, but in unison, it can produce inaccurate classifiers because it compels the classifiers to focus on hard objects and dispense with the data remnants. Research has revealed that it is difficult to get classifiers both to generate high levels of diversity and to attain greater accuracy (Chaudhuri et al., 2021).

The most widely used machine-learning techniques have poor prediction when the dataset is imbalanced (Branco et al., 2016). For example, in this study, the number of patients with CVD constitutes only 32.11% of the whole dataset. Researchers have overcome this problem by identifying and using significant variables through feature selection approaches (Chaudhuri et al., 2021).

However, this leads to a loss of information as variables get left out of the study. In this paper, the author proposes the use of the improved logistic regression (ILR) classifier to address these issues – that is, to ensure both diversity and accuracy (Khang et al., 2022a).

This paper endeavors to fulfill the following research questions: Which is the best data-mining technique (DMT) for the prediction of diseases such as CVD? Which DMT framework can help meet the three criteria? The authors considered the most popular approaches and explored their ensemble to arrive at the highest levels of consistency, sensitivity, and specificity (Khang et al., 2022d).

Previous authors have emphasized the reduction of variables to improve prediction. However, this approach leads to a loss of information. Thus, in this paper, the authors establish a framework (figure 14.1) that proposes the application of data-mining approaches, the measurement of consistency using Kappa, and suggested improvement of the specificity and sensitivity parameters using an ensemble learning approach, without any variable reduction.

In this research, the authors propose an ILR approach (figure 14.2) to construct an ensemble of classifiers. This classifier applies n number of LR classifiers (as an alternative for decision tree (DT) as a default classifier) as well as the adoptive boosting technique by altering its defined base classifier to LR and changing its weight iteratively.

This proposed classifier integrates the n individual decisions and generates a robust classifier with 83% accuracy. Thus, the framework in this paper contributes to the well-being of humankind by enabling higher levels of prediction of diseases.

14.2 RELATED WORK

CVD is one of the most common diseases affecting people in middle or old age, and it leads to severe complications in many cases. Heart ailments are the cause of almost 33% of total deaths worldwide (Uyar & İlhan, 2017). Some authors (Vasighi et al., 2013) also predict the wide spread of CVD in the Asian region.

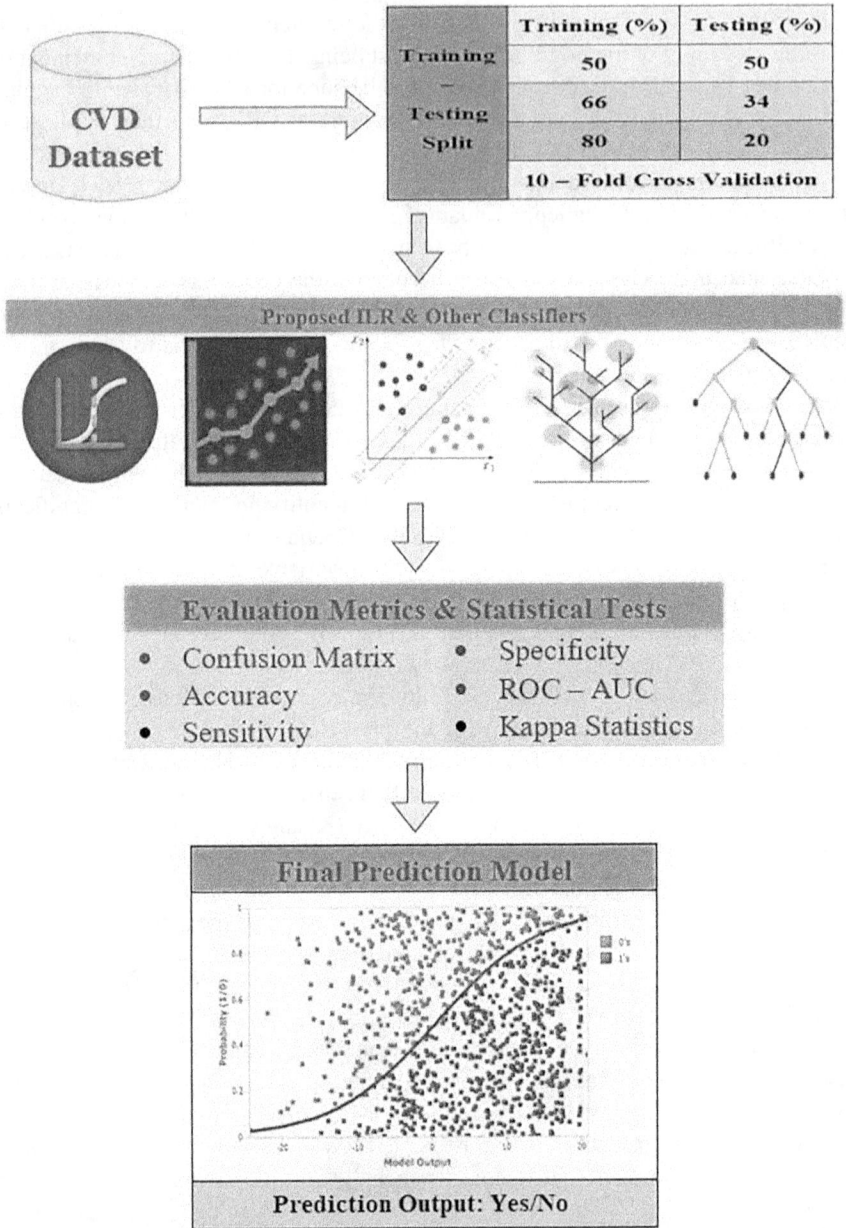

	Training (%)	Testing (%)
Training – Testing Split	50	50
	66	34
	80	20
10 – Fold Cross Validation		

Proposed ILR & Other Classifiers

Evaluation Metrics & Statistical Tests

- Confusion Matrix
- Accuracy
- Sensitivity
- Specificity
- ROC – AUC
- Kappa Statistics

Final Prediction Model

Prediction Output: Yes/No

FIGURE 14.1 CVD prediction model.

Source: Author's owner.

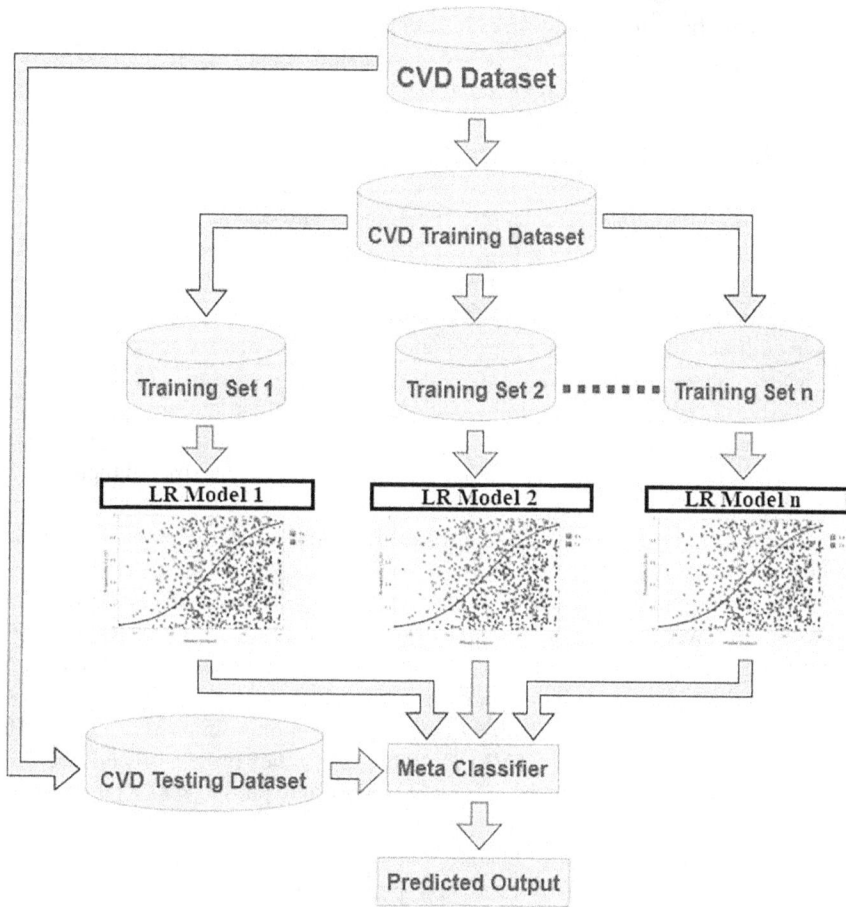

FIGURE 14.2 Workings of the proposed classifier.

Source: Author's owner.

In the case of India, researchers have noted WHO estimations that CVD is responsible for around a quarter of all deaths caused by non-transmissible diseases (Chauhan & Aeri, 2015). Even in developed countries, CVD is listed as one of the primary reasons for death (K. & Singaraju, 2011).

The complication arises because CVD is the outcome of behavioral factors (excess body weight, smoking, poor diet, lack of physical exercise, physical immobility), biological and genetic factors (age, sex, family history), and other deficiencies (high level of glucose in the blood, cholesterol). Several authors have stressed that lifestyle behaviors are the primary cause of CVD (Nahar et al., 2013).

Data-mining or machine-learning techniques help to generate predictive and diagnostic policies automatically. These methods can be beneficial in predicting risk at an early stage of CVD, as shown in figure 14.1.

Researchers have tried and tested different classifiers for predicting the disease, namely support vector machines (SVMs), decision trees (DTs), random forests (RFs), logistic regression (LR), Naive-Bayes (NB), genetic algorithms (GAs), neural networks (NNs), artificial neural networks (ANNs), and K-nearest neighbor (KNN) (Rani et al., 2022).

Srinivas et al. (2010) used rule-based algorithms, DT, NB, and ANN, in healthcare and heart attack prediction. The authors introduced two new classifiers, ODANB and NCC2, and concluded that NB techniques showed greater accuracy than other predictors. However, success was limited to around 84%.

Other researchers (Soni et al., 2011) showed that the results of NB were comparable with other methods, namely, NN and DT. They compared the results of DT, NB, KNN, cluster-based classification, and NN, and concluded that DT and NB were the best predictors among the techniques used in their study.

However, they suggested that the application of GA could enhance prediction. Several authors advocated the use of NN and DT, while some restricted their choice to the application of DT. Yazdani & Ramakrishnan (2015) developed and introduced a clinical decision support system based on ANN to help doctors predict the CVD risk.

This difference in accuracy levels led researchers to use associative classification and to move towards ensemble learning (Fida et al., 2011). Singh & Kaur (2016) showed that an ensemble of GA techniques and NN with fuzzy logic for feature extraction resulted in a significant boost in accuracy of up to 99.97%.

Takci (2018) subsequently highlighted feature selection to improve accuracy. He concluded that the linear kernel SVM algorithm and relief F method were the best feature selection techniques. These two techniques jointly produced 84.81% accuracy in prediction.

Haq et al. (2018) used seven standard machine-learning algorithms, three feature selection algorithms, the cross-validation process, and seven classification performance evaluation metrics, such as execution time, classification specificity, precision, sensitivity, matthews correlation coefficient, etc.

Their proposed system was related to treating healthy people with heart disease. However, these methods led to a loss of information. Thus, the question remains: how can the accuracy level be improved without a reduction in features (Khang et al., 2022b)?

Abdar et al. (2019) achieved 93.08% efficiency of prediction by using N2Genetic-nuSVM and 91.51% with F1-score techniques. Chandra Shekar et al. (2019) described a hybrid technique of ensemble machine-learning classifiers for a comparatively efficient solution for the prediction. Their hybrid model showed good results.

The authors used output features as input in DT analysis. This approach helped to identify the presence of CVD as well as its type. Finally, the authors initialized the factors by DT and used GA to test the fitness.

The varied outcome of the different approaches led to different association rules. Thus, the existing studies lacked consistency, and in most cases, the accuracy was restricted to between 80% and 90%.

There is very little evidence of a framework that ensures the comparison of outcomes; identification of the right factors; measures to ensure consistency, specificity, and sensitivity; and, finally, prediction of the condition at close to 100% accuracy level.

In the present research, the authors proposed a framework to ensure all criteria are met, and they introduce a new ensemble-based classifier, namely, the ILR, to produce an accurate classification. The paper draws on the new approach that shifts from the use of DT as the default classifier to the use of the LR classifier as a learner for training purposes.

14.3 METHODOLOGY

14.3.1 DATASET

This research used the UCI Machine Learning Repository: Heart failure (HF) clinical records dataset (Chicco & Jurman, 2020) to examine medical records of patients with HF that was published in July 2017 by Ahmad and colleagues (Ahmad et al., 2017). They used classic biostatistics time-dependent models (such as Cox regression (Fitrianto & Jiin, 2013) and Kaplan–Meier survival plots (Kleinbaum & Klein, 2011) to predict death and identify critical variables from the health check-up records of 299 Pakistani patients with HF.

Ahmad and co-workers made their dataset publicly available online (the "Dataset" part) along with their analysis description and findings, making it freely accessible to the scientific community. Following that, Zahid & colleagues (2019) used the same dataset to develop two separate sex-based mortality prediction models: one for males and one for females.

Although the results of the two studies (Ahmad et al., 2017) were promising, they used traditional biostatistics methods for prediction, leaving the potential for machine learning (ML) approaches (Khanh & Khang, 2021).

The authors of this study want to close this gap by employing a variety of machine learning approaches to forecast patient survival. As a significant finding, the authors show that machine learning approaches using ensembles may provide the best prediction results without reducing features (Khang et al., 2022c).

The authors explored a dataset containing the clinical records of 299 HF sufferers attained from Faisalabad Institute of Cardiology and the Allied Hospital in Faisalabad (Punjab, Pakistan) between April and December 2015 (Ahmad et al., 2017). The patients ranged from 40 to 95 years in age, with 105 women and 194 men partaking in this study (shown in table 14.1).

All of them suffered from left ventricular systolic dysfunction and were categorized as class III or IV heart failure patients (classification provided by New York Heart Association (NYHA)).

The dataset has 13 attributes that provide clinical, physical, and lifestyle data (described in table 14.1), which the authors discussed briefly in the following section.

Anemia, high blood pressure, diabetes, sex, and smoking are examples of binary features (described in table 14.1). The hospital physician diagnosed anemia if a patient's hematocrit readings were less than 36%. Unfortunately, high blood pressure is not defined in the original dataset study.

TABLE 14.1

Meaning, Measurement Unit, and Intervals of Each Feature of the Dataset

Sl. no.	Feature	Explanation	Measurement	Statistical trait
1	Age	Age of Patient	Years	Range: 40–95 Mean: 60.83
2	Anemia	Red Blood Cell/ Hemoglobin Deficiency	Boolean	0, 1
3	High Blood Pressure	Patient with High Blood Pressure	Boolean	0, 1
4	Creatinine Phosphokinase (CPK)	CPK Enzyme Level in Blood	mcg/L	Range: 23–7861 Mean: 581.84
5	Diabetes	Patient with Diabetes	Boolean	0, 1
6	Ejection Fraction	Percentage of Blood Discharge from Heart at Each Contraction	Percentage	Range: 14–80 Mean: 38.08
7	Sex	Man/Woman	Binary	0, 1
8	Platelets	Platelets Found in Blood	kiloplatelets/mL	Range: 25.01–850.00 Mean: 263.36
9	Serum Creatinine	Level of Creatinine in Blood	mg/dL	Range: 0.50–9.40 Mean: 1.39
10	Serum Sodium	Level of Sodium in Blood	mEq/L	Range: 114–148 Mean: 136.63
11	Smoking	Patient Smokes or Not	Boolean	0, 1
12	Time	Period of Follow-up	Days	Range: 4–285 Mean: 130.30
13	(Target) Death Event	Demise of Patient during Follow-up Period	Boolean	0, 1

Source: Author's owner.
mcg/L: micrograms per litre; mL: microliter; mEq/L: milliequivalents per litre

The creatinine phosphokinase (CPK) enzyme level in blood is the release of CPK into the bloodstream when muscle tissue is injured. As a result, elevated levels of CPK in a patient's blood may suggest cardiac failure or damage (Chicco & Jurman, 2020).

The ejection fraction is the proportion of blood pushed out by the left ventricle during each contraction. When a muscle breaks down, creatinine produces a waste product called serum creatinine. Doctors pay special attention to serum creatinine levels in the blood to assess renal function. Serum creatinine levels that are high in a patient may suggest renal impairment (Chicco & Jurman, 2020).

Sodium is a mineral indispensable for the opposite functioning of muscles and nerves. The serum sodium test is a common blood test that determines if a patient's sodium level in the blood is normal. Heart failure may be the cause of an unusually low sodium level in the blood (Chicco & Jurman, 2020).

The authors employed the death event feature as the target in this binary classification analysis, which denotes whether the patient perished or stayed alive before the completion of the average follow-up time of 130 days.

Unfortunately, the original dataset report does not specify whether any patient had primary renal disease and does not offer any more information regarding the sort of follow-up that was performed. In terms of the dataset imbalance, there are 32.11% alive patients or 203 individuals (death event = 0) and 67.89% deceased patients or 96 individuals (death event = 1).

The authors of the present study arranged the dataset with 299 rows (patients) and 13 attributes (features), keeping in line with the original data curators. Table 14.2 provides the quantitative properties of the dataset.

14.3.2 Choice of Models

This paper compares data-mining models, namely RF, DT, LR, NB, and SVM, for analysis of the cause of heart disease and accurate prediction of the disease. It recommends the use of ILR. The following sections discuss the criteria for the choice of the DMT.

14.3.3 Proposed Classifier: Improved Logistic Regression

The proposed improved logistic regression (ILR) utilizes an ensemble approach of classifiers to generate accurate classification output. Ensemble-based boosting techniques are classification methods that turn the power of a weak classifier into a robust classifier by improving the accuracy.

ILR performs the stage-wise estimation of variable weights for fitting an additive LR model. In this process, the LR classifiers of an ensemble get added one at a time, enabling the training of the subsequent LR classifiers on data that could not be classified by the previous ensembles.

The method assigns weights in such a way that higher weights are assigned to objects that are difficult to classify. In the process, it signals the subsequent classifiers to focus on these objects (Hajimahmud et al., 2022).

The method uses an iterative approach, and the selected LR classifier reduces the mean training error in each iteration. By utilizing this mechanism, the ILR classifier combines many LR classifiers.

The AdaBoost technique, by default, uses the weak learner, DT classifier as its base estimator or base classifier to train the model. In this proposed model, the authors have changed the default classifier to LR classifier as a learner for training purposes.

The ILR works according to the following steps.

- **Step 1:** ILR randomly selects a partition of data, which is called a training subset.
- **Step 2:** The ILR model is trained by the subset iteratively and it will calibrate the next training data subset determined by the correct predictions from the prior training.

TABLE 14.2
Statistical Quantitative Description of Category Features

Number of Records in Dataset: 299 Individuals

Number of Dead Patients: 96 Individuals

Number of Survived Patients: 203 Individuals

Dataset Features	Complete Dataset		Dead Patients		Survived Patients	
	Number of Records	Percentage of Records	Number of Records	Percentage of Records	Number of Records	Percentage of Records
Anemia (value - false)	170	56.86	50	52.08	120	59.11
Anemia (value - true)	129	43.14	46	47.92	3	40.89
High blood pressure (value - false)	194	64.88	57	59.38	137	67.49
High blood pressure (value - true)	105	35.12	39	40.62	66	32.51
Diabetes (value - false)	174	58.19	56	58.33	118	58.13
Diabetes (value - true)	125	41.81	40	41.67	85	41.87
Sex (woman - false)	105	35.12	34	35.42	71	34.98
Sex (man - true)	194	64.88	62	64.58	132	65.02
Smoking (value - false)	203	67.89	66	68.75	137	67.49
Smoking (value - true)	96	32.11	30	31.25	66	32.51

Source: Author's owner.

- **Step 3:** Some higher values are assigned to incorrectly classified interpretations by the ILR so that these interpretations will have higher possibilities for classification in the subsequent iteration.
- **Step 4:** Some weight values are allocated to the trained classifier depending on the accuracy value of that particular classifier by the ILR model in each iterative step (for higher accuracy, the weight value should be high).
- **Step 5:** The preceding steps should resume iteratively until the total training data subset fits without producing any error or the number of estimators accomplishes the maximum allocated value.

14.3.4 ALGORITHM FOR THE ILR

Suppose we are considering a set of training data, $\{(a_i, b_i)\}_{i=1}^{N}$, where $a_i \in R^Q$ and $b_i \in \{-1, 1\}$ and suppose we are given a potentially large number of logistic regression classifiers as weak classifiers, denoted by $f_m(a) \in \{-1, 1\}$ and a 0–1 loss function I, defined as

$$I(f_m(a), b) = \begin{cases} 0 \text{ if } f_m(a_i) = b_i \\ 0 \text{ if } f_m(a_i) \neq b_i \end{cases}$$

Then, the algorithm of the AdaBoost can be illustrated as follows:

end for

end for end for

After learning, the final classifier is based on a linear combination of the logistic regressions:

$$g(a) = \text{sign}\left(\sum_{x=1}^{X} \alpha_x f_x(a)\right)$$

Essentially, AdaBoost is a greedy algorithm that builds up a "strong classifier," i.e., g (a), incrementally, by optimizing the weights for, and adding, one weak (logistic regression) classifier at a time (figure 14.2).

14.3.5 DECISION TREE (DT)

DT enables supervised classification and allows the processing of erroneous datasets and missing values. This method calculates the value of the dependent aspect (attribute) given the values of independent (input) attributes (Shouman et al., 2012).

A DT classification method such as J48 employs the C4.5 algorithm. This algorithm develops a DT on the significant informative feature. The features are based on the concept of entropy. A feature forms a node in the tree when an information gain is enhanced owing to a split in this feature. It is an iterative process where all features are tested to qualify as a node.

This method does not require any form of normalization or scaling of variables to set the relationship between dependent and independent attributes. The results attained from DTs are not influenced by outliers, as the classification is constructed on the proportion of samples with split ranges and not on absolute values.

This method does not demand linearity in relationships between the dependent and independent attributes. DT explains the results well and is very intuitive. A DT method works well in medical or healthcare databases as it enables patients to be classified according to different labels, such as with or without the disease. This approach becomes difficult when the database is enormous, leading to the use of the RF technique or the SVM model.

14.3.6 Random Forest (RF)

RF, a supervised machine-learning algorithm, is a blended arrangement technique that is based on the statistical learning hypothesis (Breiman, 2001). RF creates multiple DTs and combines the results to give the best classification.

To generate the individual classifiers, it uses either a bagging method or a random selection of features (Chaudhuri et al., 2021). It is a classifier strategy, called the unweight majority of class votes, to minimize errors. A large number of trees makes an RF from the selected samples.

Technically, RF uses a divide-and-conquer-based ensemble model to randomly generate several DTs in a split dataset. Votes from every tree are considered and the most prevalent class gets selected as the result of a classification problem.

The introduction of the right kind of randomness impacts the accuracy of RF. The formation of the tree with minimal depth has an advantage as it is unrelated with the measurement of prediction error (Chen et al., 2012).

14.3.7 Logistic Regression (LR)

LR allows the effect of several explanatory variables on a response variable to be analyzed simultaneously. The LR equation gives the probability of an event, such as the occurrence of CVD or no CVD. The use of LR for categorical factors in the field of medical research has increased since the 1990s.

LR is a classification technique for estimating the contribution of a set of features to a binary outcome; for example, a person with or without CVD. This method gives the linear combination variables that predict the occurrence (or otherwise) of the disease (Tailor et al., 2022).

LR is one of the most popular models, especially in clinical practice, since it enables the regression of dependent variables over broad types of variables. Its rationalization is upfront, and it helps in quick decision making. However, the problem with LR is its tendency to generate over-fit models (Babyak, 2004).

14.3.8 Naive-Bayes (NB)

The NB algorithm calculates a series of probabilities by counting the frequency and value combinations of a given dataset. It is known as a simple probabilistic classifier. It uses the Bayes theorem as its base algorithm and assumes that all features are self-sufficient.

The Bayes algorithm employs conditional probability to find out the probability of a randomly selected feature to be chosen as a classifier in a particular category. NB assumes that any two randomly chosen features are statistically independent of each other, which avoids the problem arising from a large number of vectors in the Bayesian classifier. This conditional presumption of independence seldom holds in real-world applications; hence, the characterization of this algorithm is "naive."

However, the algorithmic rule continues to perform well and learn quickly in numerous supervised classification problems (Dimitoglou et al., 2012). Simplicity, robustness, and prediction accuracy of the Bayes theorem make it one of the most frequent classification techniques to be applied to comparatively small and simple datasets.

However, a NB classifier performs poorly with sizeable datasets and datasets with complex attribute dependencies. Chaudhuri et al. (2021) showed that the Bayesian classifier performs better in comparison to NB on a dataset with 375 features.

14.3.9 SUPPORT VECTOR MACHINE (SVM)

Cortes and Vapnik created the SVM algorithm as a regulatory algorithm in 1995 (Cortes et al., 1995). The basis of this technique is to use exactness to generalize errors. This technique generates one "hyperplane" and divides the data into classes to categorize the samples.

In some cases, SVM might not find a hyperplane to segregate the most appropriate hyperplane, which then requires the introduction of a soft margin that accepts some myocardial infraction classifications.

SVM shows good results for multi-domain or binomial applications in a big data environment. It performs faster after training is done. However, this method is statistically complex and computationally expensive. A large dataset is likely to contain noise, and SVM yields poor results in such cases (Rani et al., 2021).

This low performance is because SVM makes use of hyperplanes and support vectors that classify in higher-dimensional space. This drawback can be overcome by combining SVM with other machine-learning techniques. The efficiency of SVM lies in its use of the appropriate kernel function and it's fine-tuning (Chaudhuri et al., 2021).

14.3.10 ASSESSMENT OF PERFORMANCE OF MACHINE LEARNING ALGORITHMS

In this paper, statistical metrics are applied to evaluate the classification performance of machine learning algorithms. The metrics include accuracy, sensitivity, specificity, and F1-Score, Kappa statistic for each model, receiver operating characteristic (ROC) curve, and area under the curve (AUC) values.

14.3.10.1 Accuracy

For the binary classification, assessment metrics consist of accuracy, sensitivity, and specificity. To review performance, the F1 score, which is the harmonic mean of recall and precision, weighs up both metrics. The metrics are defined as shown in equations 14.1, 14.2, 14.3, 14.4.

$$Accuracy = \frac{TP + TN}{TP + TN + FP + FN} \qquad (14.1)$$

$$Sensitivity = \frac{TP}{TP + FN} \qquad (14.2)$$

$$Specificity = \frac{TN}{TN + FP} \qquad (14.3)$$

$$F1\text{-}Score = \frac{2TP}{2TP + FP + FN} \qquad (14.4)$$

where TP, TN, FP, and FN indicate true positive, true negative, false positive, and false negative, respectively.

In other words, the term *accuracy* measures the rate of correctly classified cases, sensitivity determines the rate of incorrectly classified cases with CVD, and specificity quantifies the rate of correctly classified cases without CVD.

14.3.10.2 Kappa Statistic for Each Model

Cohen's Kappa statistic or k-coefficient assesses the degree of concurrence between a pair of variables, commonly used as a metric of interrater concurrence, i.e., Kappa most often contends with data that are the result of a judgment, not a measurement (Bhambri et al., 2022). Kappa compares the probability of concurrence to that of expected if the ratings are nonpartisan. The values range in [−1, 1] with 1 presenting complete concurrence and 0 meaning no concurrence or independence. A negative statistic implies that the concurrence is worse than random. The criterion for a "good" or "acceptable" Kappa value is subjective.

14.3.10.3 ROC Curve and AUC Values

AUC is a performance statistic for binary classifiers. It compares the ROC curve to the region below the curve to determine how much of the curve is up in the northwest corner. A score of 0.5 is thought to be superior to a random guess.

A rating close to 0.9 suggests a decent model, whereas a score of 1 indicates an exceptional model. When comparing models and offering clarity, the composite statistic, ROC-AUC score is often more useful than accuracy, sensitivity, and specificity (Vandewiele et al., 2021).

14.3.11 Training-Testing Partition

Obtaining different (independent) samples from an initial dataset is a typical method in machine learning for building and modifying prediction (supervised) models. The most common strategy is "train and test."

The basic approach is to use an independent test specimen to create a predictive model with a preparatory test and then approve the model. This strategy reduces the

TABLE 14.3
Training and Testing Set Partition

Training-Testing Partition	Total Training Records	Positive Records in Training Set	Negative Records in Training Set
50–50	149	41 (27.51%)	108 (72.49%)
66–34	197	52 (26.40%)	145(73.60%)
80–20	239	71 (29.70%)	168(70.60%)
10-fold cross-validation	299	96 (32.10%)	203(67.90%)

Source: Author's owner.

likelihood of model over-fitting, offers an acceptable estimate of model correctness, and enhances generalization when applying the model to fresh data.

The authors used this concept in this study by separating the heart disease dataset into two disjointed subsets (as shown in table 14.3).

14.4   RESULTS AND DISCUSSION

Using the Python programming language, the authors created and simulated a proposed model (shown in figure 14.1). The authors carried out a comparison study in this model between five advanced machine learning algorithms, namely NB, LR, RF, DT, and SVM, and the suggested model.

Among these five common machine learning approaches, some perform better than others in terms of accuracy. The authors applied advanced ensemble machine learning and suggested an ensemble meta-algorithmic approach to improving the accuracy and overall performance of the weak classifier.

The machine learning approaches used on the UCI Machine Learning Repository: Heart failure clinical records dataset yielded an accuracy of 83%.

As shown in table 14.4 and figure 14.3, different approaches yielded different levels of accuracy, with DT recording an accuracy of 63%, while the proposed ILR exhibited the highest (83%) accuracy.

TABLE 14.4
Comparison of accuracies

Training-testing partition	Accuracies					
	LR	NB	SVM	DT	RF	ILR
50–50	0.79	0.79	0.81	0.67	0.76	0.83
66–34	0.77	0.78	0.77	0.73	0.75	0.81
80–20	0.78	0.73	0.75	0.63	0.68	0.77
10-fold cross-validation	0.79	0.78	0.77	0.70	0.74	0.80

Source: Author's owner.

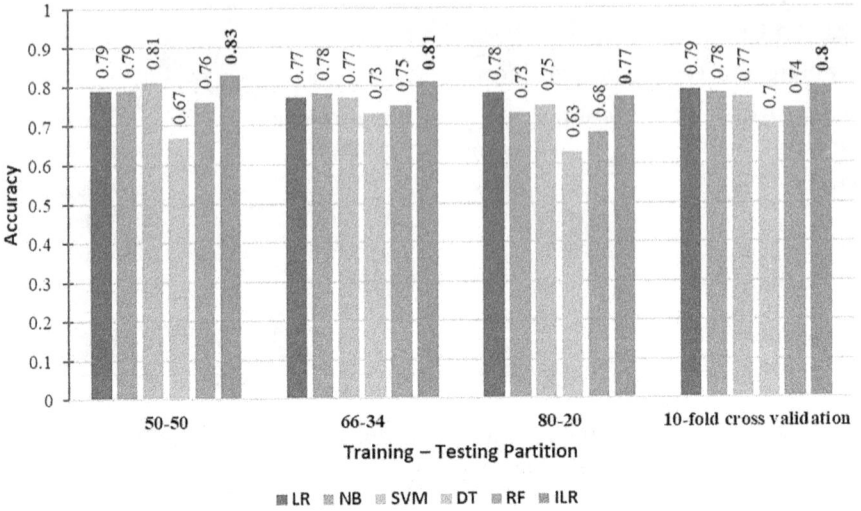

FIGURE 14.3 Comparison of accuracies.

Source: Author's owner.

The statistics of real and predicted classifications derived from the examination of several classification methods are shown in a confusion matrix. The data collected in this matrix is used to measure the performance of all such systems.

Table 14.5 demonstrates the outcomes of utilizing several machine learning techniques to build confusion matrices.

The sensitivity, specificity, and accuracy of our suggested model, as well as the performances of other techniques, were assessed using true positive (TP), true negative (TN), false negative (FN), and false positive (FP) terms, as shown in figure 14.4.

Table 14.5 compares this suggested model to other frequently used independent classification algorithms. The comparison findings show that the suggested classification approach has the greatest accuracy and specificity values (83% accuracy, 83% specificity) for the heart disease dataset (figure 14.5).

According to the authors' findings from several studies in this research, the LR's classification accuracy was 79%, with 92% sensitivity and 77% specificity. The RF attained a classification accuracy of 76%, with a sensitivity of 88% and a specificity of 76%. The SVM's classification accuracy was 81%, with 88% sensitivity and 78% specificity.

However, of the six classifiers tested, our suggested classifier performed the best, achieving 83% classification accuracy, 88% sensitivity, and 83% specificity. Table 14.4 and Table 14.5 display the entire set of results.

The analytical results of our suggested classifier are also promising. The enhanced specificity to predict CVD using this suggested classifier is a noteworthy outcome. The LR and NB classifiers yielded 92% and 96% sensitivity, respectively, although their specificities were relatively low.

ILR overcomes that limitation, yielding sensitivity and specificity results of 88% and 83%, respectively, implying that fewer individuals would need to be tested for

TABLE 14.5
Comparison of Sensitivity and Specificity

Training-Testing Partition	LR		NB		SVM		DT		RF		ILR	
	Sensitivity	Specificity	Sensitivity	Specificity	Sensitivity	Specificity	Sensitivity	Specificity	Sensitivity	Specificity	Sensitivity	Specificity
50–50	0.88	0.77	0.90	0.77	0.88	0.78	0.56	0.71	0.76	0.76	0.84	0.83
66–34	0.92	0.73	0.96	0.72	0.86	0.73	0.72	0.73	0.88	0.71	0.88	0.78
80–20	0.88	0.75	0.91	0.69	0.81	0.73	0.58	0.66	0.71	0.67	0.82	0.75
10-fold cross-validation	0.79	0.69	0.78	0.73	0.77	0.70	0.70	0.52	0.74	0.61	0.80	0.71

Source: Author's owner.

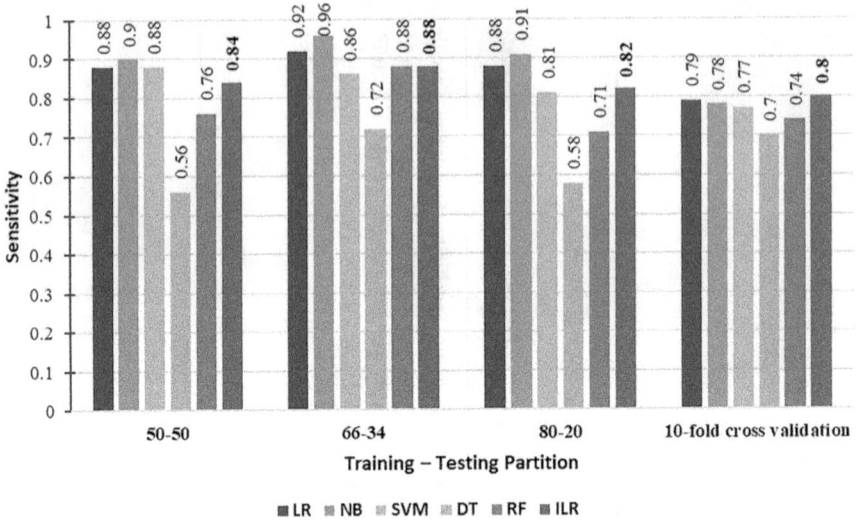

FIGURE 14.4   Comparison of sensitivity.

Source: Author's owner.

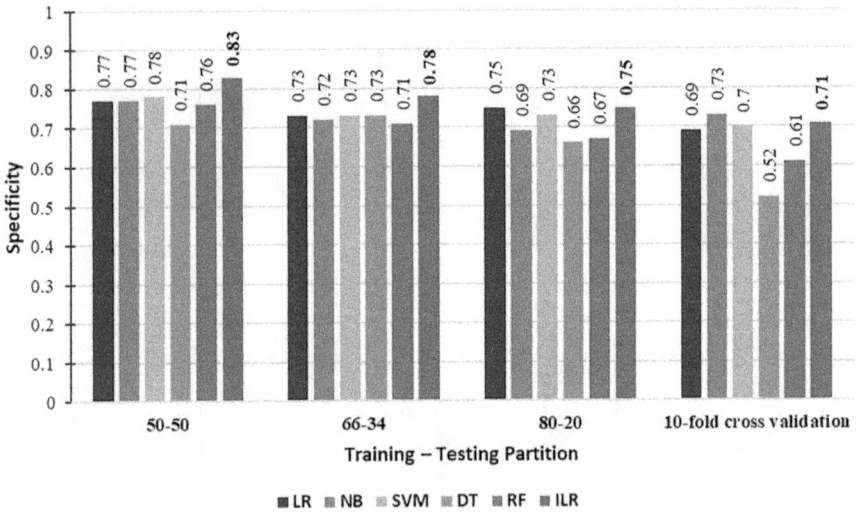

FIGURE 14.5   Comparison of specificity.

Source: Author's owner.

CVD due to improved specificity. Simultaneously, a high sensitivity value would save money and reduce the waiting periods of seriously ill patients, both of which would be crucial to saving lives.

Table 14.6 and figure 14.6 show the F-Score analysis findings for the five most prevalent machine learning approaches and the suggested model. These findings

TABLE 14.6

Comparison of F-Score

Training-Testing Partition	LR	NB	SVM	DT	RF	ILR
50–50	0.64	0.64	0.67	0.48	0.61	0.75
66–34	0.67	0.66	0.67	0.65	0.62	0.75
80–20	0.68	0.56	0.63	0.50	0.51	0.68
10-fold cross-validation	0.80	0.77	0.76	0.76	0.76	0.81

Source: Author's owner.

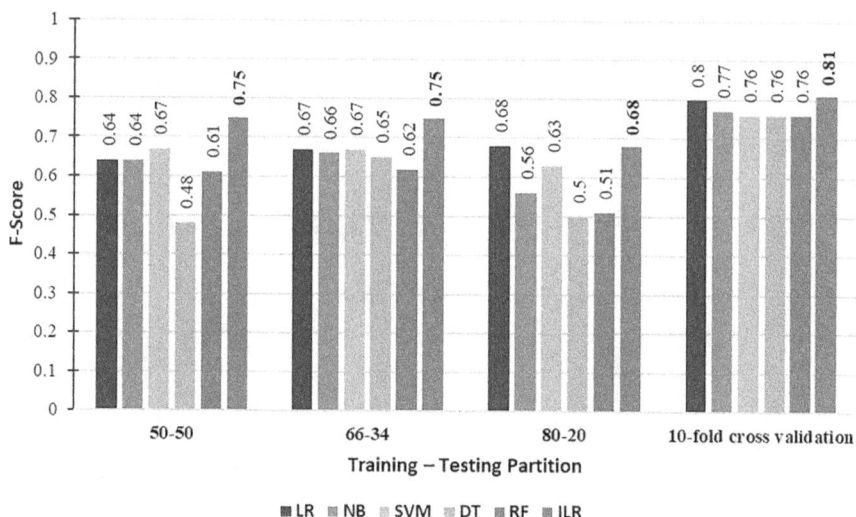

FIGURE 14.6 Comparison of F-score.

Source: Author's owner.

clearly show that the proposed model outperformed other classifiers consistently (value = 0.81).

Table 14.7 and figure 14.7 show the ROC values for these experiments using distinct machine learning algorithms. ROC values obtained by several classifiers are displayed in different areas of this table for various train-test partitions and 10-fold cross-validation.

The experimental findings reveal that our suggested classifier outperformed most of the other previously used approaches stated in the literature review. The computed AUC value for the suggested model is 0.95.

Comparing the performances of different machine learning classifiers might generate an ambiguous result if the comparison has been based only on accuracy-based

TABLE 14.7

Comparison of ROC and AUC

Training-Testing Partition	LR	NB	SVM	DT	RF	ILR
50–50	0.73	0.73	0.75	0.61	0.71	0.80
66–34	0.74	0.74	0.74	0.71	0.71	0.80
80–20	0.75	0.69	0.72	0.61	0.64	0.75
10-fold cross-validation	0.99	0.95	0.97	0.67	0.84	0.95

Source: Author's owner.

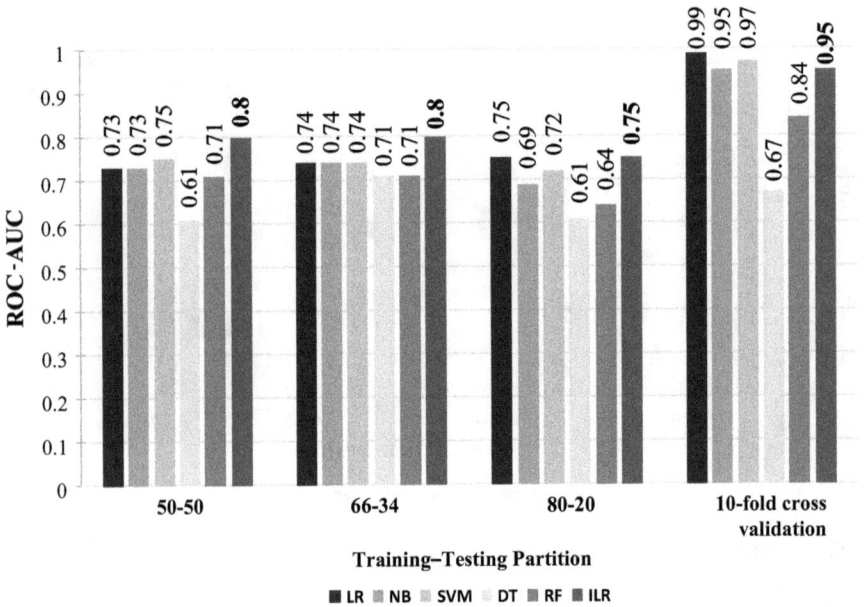

FIGURE 14.7 Comparison of ROC and AUC.

Source: Author's owner.

metrics. The Cohen's Kappa Statistic (CKS) value is utilized to assist in producing error-free relative efficiency of various classifiers considering the cost of error.

In this respect, the CKS is an exceptional measure taking values between −1 and +1, for reviewing classifications that may be due to chance.

As the classifier's calculated Kappa value approaches 1, its performance is believed to be more accurate than "by chance." Therefore, the CKS value is a recommended metric for measurement objectives in the performance analysis of classifiers. This Kappa value is calculated by using equation 14.5:

$$CKS = (pa - pac)/(1 - pac) \qquad (14.5)$$

where pa represents total agreement probability and pac represents probability "by chance." The results of the CKS analysis of the five popular machine learning techniques and our proposed model are shown in table 14.8 and figure 14.8.

These results demonstrate that the proposed model performed much better than other classifiers (value = 0.63).

A comparison of performance of our proposed classifier with previous studies has been stated in table 14.9. Improved logistic regression (ILR) clearly outperformed the previous works in terms of accuracy, sensitivity, specificity, and ROC-AUC measure. Despite the imbalanced nature of the heart failure dataset, ILR produced remarkable scores without applying feature selection.

TABLE 14.8

Kappa Statistic for Each Model

Training-Testing Partition	LR	NB	SVM	DT	RF	ILR
50–50	0.51	0.51	0.55	0.24	0.45	0.63
66–34	0.52	0.51	0.50	0.43	0.45	0.61
80–20	0.53	0.40	0.46	0.22	0.30	0.50
10-fold cross-validation	0.51	0.43	0.41	0.30	0.38	0.52

Source: Author's owner.

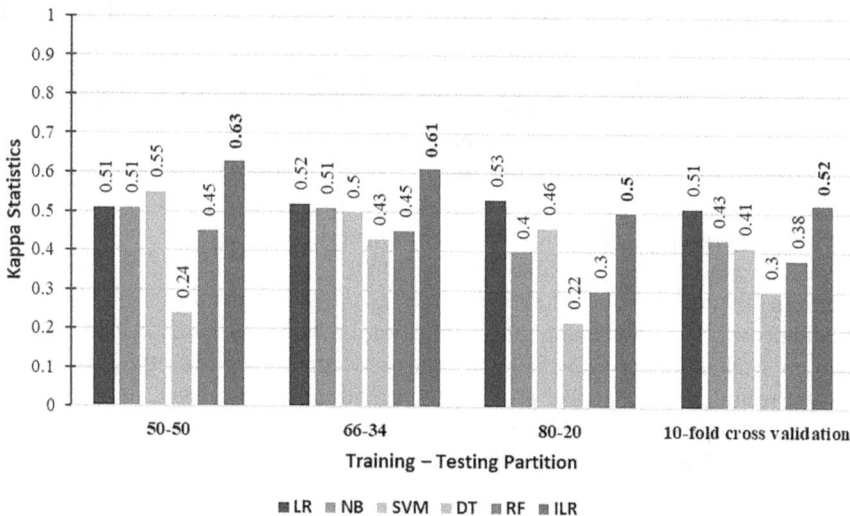

FIGURE 14.8   Comparison of Kappa values.

Source: Author's owner.

TABLE 14.9

Performance Comparison of Different Studies on Heart Failure Dataset

Literature Reference	Method	Accuracy (%)	Sensitivity/ Specificity (%)	F1-Score	Kappa	ROC or AUC
Chicco & Jurman, 2020	RF with univariate feature selection	58.5	54.1/85.5	×	×	69.8
Kim et al., 2020	RF + SMOTE	×	71.23/75.11	×	×	×
Al Mehedi Hasan et al., 2021	DT + MRMR + RFE	80	51.72/93.44			72.58
Newaz et al., 2021	BRF + Chi2	76.25	80.21/74.45	×	×	77.33
This Study	**ILR**	**83**	**88/83**	**0.81**	**0.63**	**95**

Source: Author's owner.

14.5 CONCLUSION

Benchmarking is required to compare the performance of common machine learning models with our suggested model. The suggested classifier is examined to see whether it is the best model and whether it increases performance and classification accuracy.

In most research publications, accuracy is determined by the number of feature selection strategies used and the outcomes provided by the other models. The suggested classifier has no constraints when it comes to picking the characteristics to employ.

In this model, the best results are obtained by taking into account all of the characteristics present in the dataset. The findings produced by employing this suggested classifier with all characteristics from the dataset demonstrate that it is effective in properly predicting heart disease in patients when compared to other known existing machine learning techniques.

So, the main contribution of this research paper is not only the development of an ensemble learning model but also the restructuring of the default structure of the boosting algorithm by changing the base estimator.

This proposed classifier also has important features, such as its ability to determine the best possible ratio on the training dataset versus the testing dataset to simultaneously find the optimum combination of both sets based on the defined ratio, as well as its experimentation to find an accurate rule using the ILR.

Test results show that this proposed ensemble learning classification model is effective in improving performance metrics and classification accuracy compared to its foundation learner and other independent learners specified in the literature. The following are some of the potential implications of the present research work and the proposed classifier.

CVD detection is frequently accompanied by several tiresome and expensive processes like regular medical tests in laboratories in the presence of experts or doctors or in the course of hospital admission. This proposed model makes use of some features extracted from conventional lifestyles and a few medical test reports from laboratories in textual or numeral format to predict the sickness with greater accuracy.

For medical service providers or doctors, this proposed model is intended to provide an accurate classification of CVD based on fewer precise and explanatory test data from patients. As a result, with the aid of this model, the primary consumer (i.e., medical practitioners or doctors) can predict heart disease more quickly and accurately (including in cases of clinical assumption) and they can indicate the risk level of the disease efficiently. So, it can help to save lives and significantly minimize medical costs (Vrushank et al., 2023).

For research scholars/academics, this proposed model for classification provides a wide scope for future research on improving the prediction accuracy not only of heart disease but of other medical conditions, too.

In summary, concerning other healthcare datasets, our proposed model is capable of successfully performing medical decision support tasks for various diseases; however, it may produce better classification accuracy with real-world datasets. Researchers can restructure different boosting algorithms by using different weak classifiers as the base classifier to enhance the classification accuracy for clinical and non-clinical datasets.

14.6 FUTURE SCOPE

The machine learning methods used in this proposed classifier to predict the early diagnosis of heart disease are shown to be highly effective. The proposed model in this study is tested with a small dataset containing a limited number of features.

However, the same model needs testing on more divergent real-life CVD datasets, on data from various other disease and nonmedical datasets, and on data that can be obtained from specific electronic health record repositories. Data collected from patient surveys, observational cohort studies, and clinical trials can also help understand the success, safety, and cost of the model.

AI-based systems are classified into four types of machines: reactive AI machines, limited memory AI machines, theory of mind AI machines, and self-aware AI machines (Rana et al., 2021).

REFERENCES

Abdar, M., Książek, W., Acharya, U. R., Tan, R.-S., Makarenkov, V., Pławiak, P.: A new machine learning technique for an accurate diagnosis of coronary artery disease. *Computer Methods and Programs in Biomedicine*, 179, 104992 (2019). 10.1016/j.cmpb.2019.104992

Ahmad, T., Munir, A., Bhatti, S. H., Aftab, M., Raza, M. A.: Survival analysis of heart failure patients: A case study. *PLOS ONE*, 12 (2017). 10.1371/journal.pone.0181001

Al Mehedi Hasan, M., Shin, J., Das, U., Yakin Srizon, A.: Identifying prognostic features for predicting heart failure by using machine learning algorithm. *2021 11th International Conference on Biomedical Engineering and Technology*. (2021). 10.1145/3460238.3460245

Babasaheb, J., Sphurti, B., Khang, A.: Industry Revolution 4.0: Workforce Competency Models and Designs. *Designing Workforce Management Systems for Industry 4.0: Data-Centric and AI-Enabled Approaches*, (1st ed.), 14–31, (2023). CRC Press. 10.1201/9781003357070-2

Babyak, M. A.: What you see may not be what you get: A brief, nontechnical introduction to overfitting in regression-type models. *Psychosomatic Medicine*, 66, 411–421 (2004). 10.1097/00006842-200405000-00021

Banfield, R. E., Hall, L. O., Bowyer, K. W., Bhadoria, D., Kegelmeyer, W. P., Eschrich, S.: A comparison of ensemble creation techniques. *Multiple Classifier Systems*, 223–232 (2004). 10.1007/978-3-540-25966-4_22

Bhambri, P., Rani, S., Gupta, G., Khang, A.: *Cloud and Fog Computing Platforms for Internet of Things*. ISBN: 978-1-032-101507, (2022). CRC Press. 10.1201/9781003213888

Branco, P., Torgo, L., Ribeiro, R. P.: A survey of predictive modeling on imbalanced domains. *ACM Computing Surveys*, 49, 1–50 (2016). 10.1145/2907070

Breiman, L.: Bagging predictors. *Machine Learning*, 24, 123–140 (1996). 10.1007/bf00058655

Breiman, L.: Random forests. *Machine Learning*, 45, 5–32 (2001). 10.1023/a:1010933404324

Chandra Shekar, K., Chandra, P., Venugopala Rao, K.: An ensemble classifier characterized by genetic algorithm with decision tree for the prophecy of heart disease. *Innovations in Computer Science and Engineering*, 9–15 (2019). 10.1007/978981-13-7082-3_2

Chaudhuri, A. K., Banerjee, D. K., Das, A.: A dataset centric feature selection and stacked model to detect breast cancer. *International Journal of Intelligent Systems and Applications*, 13, 24–37 (2021). 10.5815/ijisa.2021.04.03

Chaudhuri, A. K., Banerjee, D. K., Das, A., Ray, A.: A multi-stage approach combining feature selection with machine learning techniques for higher prediction reliability and accuracy in heart disease diagnosis. *International Journal of Engineering Research & Technology* (IJERT), 10, 73–85 (2021). 10.17577/IJERTV10IS070057

Chaudhuri, A. K., Ray, A., Banerjee, D. K., Das, A.: A multi-stage approach combining feature selection with machine learning techniques for higher prediction reliability and accuracy in cervical cancer diagnosis. *International Journal of Intelligent Systems and Applications*, 13, 46–63 (2021). 10.5815/ijisa.2021.05.05

Chaudhuri, A. K., Sinha, D., Banerjee, D. K., Das, A.: A novel enhanced decision tree model for detecting chronic kidney disease. *Network Modeling Analysis in Health Informatics and Bioinformatics*, 10 (2021). 10.1007/s13721-021-00302-w

Chauhan, S., Aeri, B. T.: The rising incidence of cardiovascular diseases in India: Assessing its economic impact. *Journal of Preventive Cardiology*, 4, 735–740 (2015).

Chen, X., Ishwaran, H.: Random forests for genomic data analysis. Genomics, 99, 323–329 (2012). 10.1016/j.ygeno.2012.04.003

Chicco, D., Jurman, G.: Machine learning can predict survival of patients with heart failure from serum creatinine and ejection fraction alone. *BMC Medical Informatics and Decision Making*, 20 (2020). 10.1186/s12911-020-1023-5

Cortes, C., Vapnik, V.: Support-vector networks. *Machine Learning*, 20, 273–297 (1995). 10.1007/bf00994018

Dimitoglou, G., Adams, J. A., Jim, C. M.: Comparison of the C4.5 and a naive bayes classifier for the prediction of lung cancer survivability. *Journal of Computing*, 4, 1–9 (2012). 10.48550/arXiv.1206.1121

Fida, B., Nazir, M., Naveed, N., Akram, S.: Heart disease classification ensemble optimization using genetic algorithm. *2011 IEEE 14th International Multitopic Conference.* (2011). 10.1109/inmic.2011.6151471

Fitrianto, A., Jiin, R. L., Several types of residuals in cox regression model: An empirical study. *International Journal of Mathematical Analysis*, 7, 2645–2654 (2013). 10.12988/ijma.2013.38193

Hajimahmud, V. A., Khang, A., Hahanov, V., Litvinova, E., Chumachenko, S., Alyar, A. V.: Autonomous Robots for Smart City: Closer to Augmented Humanity. *AI-Centric Smart City Ecosystems: Technologies, Design and Implementation*, (1st ed.), (2022). CRC Press. 10.1201/9781003252542-7

Haq, A. U., Li, J. P., Memon, M. H., Nazir, S., Sun, R.: A hybrid intelligent system framework for the prediction of heart disease using machine learning algorithms. *Mobile Information Systems*, 1–21 (2018). 10.1155/2018/3860146

K, V., Singaraju, J.: Decision support system for congenital heart disease diagnosis based on signs and symptoms using neural networks. *International Journal of Computer Applications*, 19, 6–12 (2011). 10.5120/2368-3115

Khang A., Hahanov, V., Abbas, G. L., Hajimahmud, V. A.: Cyber-Physical-Social System and İncident Management. *AI-Centric Smart City Ecosystems: Technologies, Design and Implementation*, (1st ed.), (2022a). CRC Press. 10.1201/9781003252542-2

Khang A., Hahanov, V., Litvinova, E., Chumachenko, S., Hajimahmud, V. A., Alyar, A. V.: The Key Assistant of Smart City - Sensors and Tools. *AI-Centric Smart City Ecosystems: Technologies, Design and Implementation*, (1st ed.), (2022b). CRC Press. 10.1201/9781003252542-17

Khang, A., Ragimova, N. A., Hajimahmud, V. A., Alyar, A. V.: Advanced Technologies and Data Management in the Smart Healthcare System. *AI-Centric Smart City Ecosystems: Technologies, Design and Implementation*, (1st ed.), (2022c). CRC Press. 10.1201/9781003252542-16

Khang A., Chowdhury, S., & Sharma, S. (Eds.): *The Data-Driven Blockchain Ecosystem: Fundamentals, Applications, and Emerging Technologies*, (1st ed.), (2022d). CRC Press. 10.1201/9781003269281

Khang, A., Rani, S., Gujrati, R., Uygun, H., Gupta, S. K., (Eds.): *Designing Workforce Management Systems for Industry 4.0: Data-Centric and AI-Enabled Approaches*, (1st ed.), (2023). CRC Press. 10.1201/99781003357070

Khanh, H. H., Khang, A.: The Role of Artificial Intelligence in Blockchain Applications. *Reinventing Manufacturing and Business Processes through Artificial Intelligence*, 20–40, (2021). CRC Press. 10.1201/9781003145011-2

Kim, Y.-T., Kim, D.-K., Kim, H., Kim, D.-J.: A comparison of oversampling methods for constructing a prognostic model in the patient with heart failure. *2020 International Conference on Information and Communication Technology Convergence* (ICTC). (2020). 10.1109/ictc49870.2020.9289522

Kleinbaum, D. G., Klein, M.: Kaplan-Meier survival curves and the log-rank test. *Statistics for Biology and Health.* 55–96 (2011). 10.1007/978-1-4419-66469_2

Li, J., Heap, A. D., Potter, A., Daniell, J. J.: Application of machine learning methods to spatial interpolation of environmental variables. *Environmental Modelling & Software*, 26, 1647–1659 (2011). 10.1016/j.envsoft.2011.07.004

Liu, X., Wang, X., Su, Q., Zhang, M., Zhu, Y., Wang, Q., Wang, Q.: A hybrid classification system for heart disease diagnosis based on the RFRS method. *Computational and Mathematical Methods in Medicine*, 2017, 1–11 (2017). 10.1155/2017/8272091

Nahar, J., Imam, T., Tickle, K. S., Chen, Y.-P.P.: Computational intelligence for heart disease diagnosis: A medical knowledge driven approach. *Expert Systems with Applications*, 40, 96–104 (2013). 10.1016/j.eswa.2012.07.032

Newaz, A., Ahmed, N., Shahriyar Haq, F.: Survival prediction of heart failure patients using machine learning techniques. *Informatics in Medicine Unlocked*, 26, 100772 (2021). 10.1016/j.imu.2021.100772

Rana, G., Khang, A., Sharma, R., Goel, A. K., Dubey, A. K.: *Reinventing Manufacturing and Business Processes through Artificial Intelligence*, (2021). CRC Press. 10.1201/9781003145011

Rani, S., Bhambri, P., Kataria, A., Khang, A.: Smart City Ecosystem: Concept, Sustainability, Design Principles and Technologies. *AI-Centric Smart City Ecosystems: Technologies, Design and Implementation*, (1st ed.), (2022). CRC Press. 10.1201/9781003252542-1

Rani, S., Bhambri, P., Kataria, A., Khang A., & Sivaraman, A. K. (Eds.): *Big Data, Cloud Computing and IoT: Tools and Applications*, (1st ed.), (2023). Chapman and Hall/CRC. 10.1201/9781003298335

Rani, S., Chauhan, M., Kataria, A., Khang, A.: IoT Equipped Intelligent Distributed Framework for Smart Healthcare Systems. *Networking and Internet Architecture*, (2021). CRC Press. 10.48550/arXiv.2110.04997

Ray, A., Chaudhuri, A. K.: Smart healthcare disease diagnosis and patient management: Innovation, improvement and skill development. *Machine Learning with Applications*, 3, 100011 (2021). 10.1016/j.mlwa.2020.100011

Shouman, M., Turner, T., Stocker, R.: Applying K-nearest neighbour in diagnosing heart disease patients. *International Journal of Information and Education Technology*. 220–223 (2012). 10.7763/ijiet.2012.v2.114

Singh, J., Kaur, R.: Cardio vascular disease classification ensemble optimization using genetic algorithm and neural network. *Indian Journal of Science and Technology*, 9 (2016). 10.17485/ijst/2016/v9is1/98900

Soni, J., Ansari, U., Sharma, D., Soni, S.: Predictive data mining for medical diagnosis: An overview of heart disease prediction. *International Journal of Computer Applications*, 17, 43–48 (2011). 10.5120/2237-2860

Srinivas, K., Rani, B. K., Govrdhan, A.: Applications of data mining techniques in healthcare and prediction of heart attacks. *International Journal on Computer Science and Engineering (IJCSE)*, 2, 250–255 (2010).

Tailor, R. K., Pareek, R., Khang, A., (Eds.): Robot Process Automation in Blockchain. *The Data-Driven Blockchain Ecosystem: Fundamentals, Applications, and Emerging Technologies*, (1st ed.), 149–164. (2022). CRC Press. 10.1201/9781003269281-8

Takci, H.: Improvement of heart attack prediction by the feature selection methods. *Turkish Journal of Electrical Engineering & Computer Sciences*, 26, 1–10 (2018). 10.3906/elk-1611-235

Uyar, K., İlhan, A.: Diagnosis of heart disease using genetic algorithm based trained recurrent fuzzy neural networks. *Procedia Computer Science*, 120, 588–593 (2017). 10.1016/j.procs.2017.11.283

Vandewiele, G., Dehaene, I., Kovács, G., Sterckx, L., Janssens, O., Ongenae, F., De Backere, F., De Turck, F., Roelens, K., Decruyenaere, J., Van Hoecke, S., Demeester, T.: Overly optimistic prediction results on imbalanced data: *A case study of flaws and benefits when applying over-sampling. Artificial Intelligence in Medicine*, 111, 101987 (2021). 10.1016/j.artmed.2020.101987

Vasighi, M., Zahraei, A., Bagheri, S., Vafaeimanesh, J.: Diagnosis of coronary heart disease based on1H NMR spectra of human blood plasma using genetic algorithm-based feature selection. *Journal of Chemometrics*, 27, 318–322 (2013). 10.1002/cem.2517

Vrushank S., Vidhi T., Khang, A., 2023: Electronic Health Records Security and Privacy Enhancement Using Blockchain Technology. *Data-Centric AI Solutions and Emerging Technologies in the Healthcare Ecosystem*, (1st ed.), (2023), P(1). CRC Press. 10.1201/9781003356189

Yazdani, A., Ramakrishnan, K.: Performance evaluation of artificial neural network models for the prediction of the risk of heart disease. *IFMBE Proceedings*, 179–182 (2015). 10.1007/978-981-10-0266-3_37

Zahid, F. M., Ramzan, S., Faisal, S., Hussain, I.: Gender based survival prediction models for heart failure patients: A case study in Pakistan. *PLOS ONE*, 14 (2019). 10.1371/journal.pone.0210602

15 Systematic Review

An Early Detection of Skin Disease Using Machine Learning

Punam Rattan and Anchal Kumari

CONTENTS

15.1 INTRODUCTION

Today, skin disease or skin lesion considered as one of the most dangerous forms of cancer for humans. There are many causes of skin disease, such as fungal infections, bacteria, allergies or virus3es, air pollution, UV rays, and unhealthy lifestyles, etc. To identify these skin diseases machine learning techniques used and help to prevent ourselves from cancer at an early stage (Prasad and Nadu, 2020).

The Skin Cancer Foundation (SCF) has currently established that melanoma has a predominant form of skin lesion. Melanoma is likely to spread to other parts of the body. When it is spreads to other parts of the body, it becomes difficult for treatment. Studies show that when it is detected in the early stage, it completely cures.

According to the Indian Cancer Society 2015, India has a higher incidence of skin cancer than other countries such as the United States, Canada, and the United

DOI: 10.1201/9781003356189-15

Kingdom. Approximately 125,693 new cancer cases have reported, but more than 45,395 cases expected to die from cancer (Poornima and Shailaja, 2017). It is very crucial part of early detection of skin cancer. Skin cancer can be serious if it is not detected in the primary stage (Koklu and Ozkan, 2017). It acts as part of the excretory system for removing sweat from the body.

The exposed skin area is called the epidermis and the hidden skin area called the dermis (Bakheet, 2017). The skin is composed of three different cells: squamous epithelial cells, basal cells, and melanocytes. Skin cancer caused by exposure to ultraviolet light (UV) (Arif et al., 2022).

The color and texture of the skin may change, it may be chronic and contagious, and it may progress to skin cancer. Therefore, skin diseases must be diagnosed early to reduce their growth and also minimize the spreading rate (Journal, 2017).

Treatment and diagnosis of skin diseases is very time consuming and costly to the patient's financial and physical costs (Alquran et al., 2017).

In general, most people are unaware of the type and stage of skin condition. Some skin diseases show symptoms after a few months and allowing the disease to progress and spread further (Gound and Gaikwad, 2018).

This is due to the lack of medical knowledge among the peoples. It can be difficult for a dermatologist to diagnose the condition of the skin and required expensive clinical examination of the condition of the skin (Soliman and Alenezi, 2019).

Skin cancer typically classified into three types: basal cell carcinoma (BCC), melanoma, and squamous cell carcinoma (SCC). Diagnosis of melanoma can be improved with ABCD rules based on a computerized system, as shown in figure 15.1.

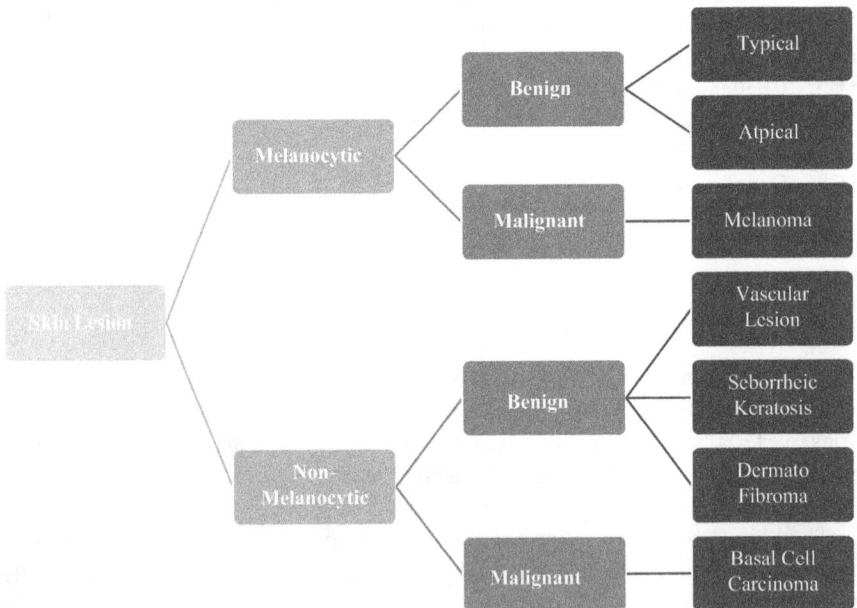

FIGURE 15.1   Diagnosis structure for skin lesion (Arif et al., 2022).

Source: Author's owner.

These systems usually consist of separate units for image segmentation, feature extraction, or classification (Koklu and Ozkan, 2017).

15.2 RELATED WORK

15.2.1 Types of Skin Lesions

15.2.1.1 Melanocytic

15.2.1.1.1 Benign
Benign are non-cancerous growths in the human body. Unlike cancerous tumors, they do not spread to other parts of the body. Benign can form anywhere in the body. Benign has further two types i.e., typical benign and atypical benign.

15.2.1.1.2 Malignant
A malignant lesion is invasive, which implies it can invade the surrounding tissues. Malignant tumors contain malignant cells that are out of control and capable of metastasizing, or spreading to other parts of the body.

15.2.1.1.3 Melanoma
Melanoma said to be the deadliest disease and an emerging skin cancer form in the world. The most important source of melanoma is DNA impairment due to the ultra-radiation exposures like sunlight and tanning beds. The occurrence of malignant melanoma also happens in the area of legs for women and chest in men.

15.2.1.2 Non-Melanocytic
Non-melanoma skin cancers develop most frequently on sun-exposed skin. To detect skin cancer early, it is helpful to understand how your skin naturally appears.

15.2.1.2.1 Benign
Vascular Lesion: Vascular lesions, often known as birthmarks, are relatively common anomalies of the skin and underlying tissues. Vascular lesions are classified into three types: pyogenic granulomas, hemangiomas, and vascular malformations.
Seborrheic Keratosis: Seborrheic keratosis is a frequent benign (non-cancerous) skin lesion. Seborrheic keratosis is typically dark, black, or light tan in color.
Dermato Fibroma: Dermatofibromas are non-cancerous (benign) skin lesions that can form anywhere on the body but most commonly on the lower legs, upper arms, or upper back.

15.2.1.2.2 Malignant: Basal Cell Carcinoma
The numerous kinds of non-cancerous tumors developed from varieties of skin cells. The medical term for mole is considered *nevus* from which the benign tumor can be developed. They also affect children and young adults.

15.2.2 Types of Skin Disease

After checking the symptoms of skin disease, it is necessary to classify the skin classes and also check if the input image is cancerous or not. The following types of skin diseases are given in figure 15.2.

1. **Atomic Dermatitis:** This is a form of eczema, which is the most common type of skin inflammation produced by itchy rash and an overactive immune system.
2. **Psoriasis:** An autoimmune disorder characterized by a range of skin eruptions.
3. **Cellulitis:** A red, warm, painful rash results from inflammation of the dermal and subcutaneous layers.
4. **Rosacea:** A poorly understood skin illness that develops a red rash on the face and seems to be acne.
5. **Urticaria:** it is commonly known as hives, is a skin reaction induced by allergy or stress that is characterized by swelling, lumps, itching, and burning that arise and disappear anywhere on the body.
6. **Fungal Infection:** Mycosis refers to a fungal infection. Although most fungi are harmless to humans, some can cause diseases under certain situations. Athlete's foot, ringworm, yeast infection, and other common fungal infections
7. **Acne:** Acne is the most prevalent skin disorder, affecting about 85% of people at some point in their lives.

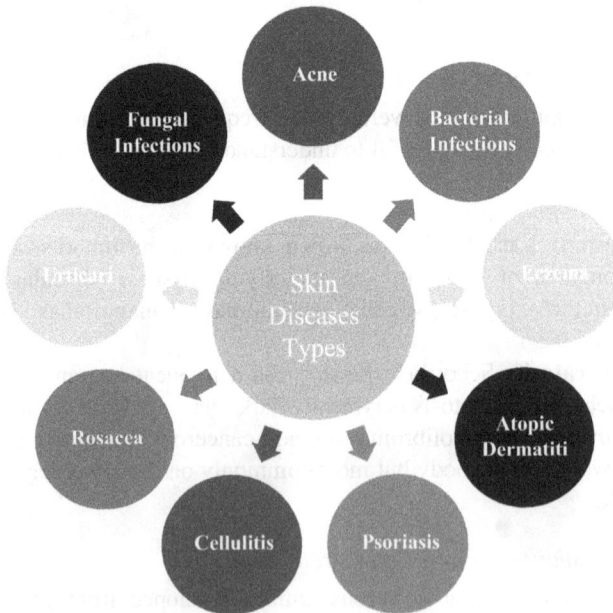

FIGURE 15.2 Types of skin disease.

Source: Author's owner.

8. **Bacterial infection:** Bacterial infection occurs when harmful bacteria enter a person's body or wound and multiply, resulting in illness, organ damage, tissue damage, or disease. Bacteria have the ability to infect any part of the body.
9. **Eczema:** Eczema is a condition in which patches of skin become inflamed, itch, and crack. Some types can also cause blisters.

15.2.3 ARTICLE STRUCTURE

According to a literature review, this chapter provides a comprehensive review of research articles published between 2015 and mid-2022 that used machine learning to diagnose different skin disorders with varied accuracies. This chapter is organized as follows:

- Section 15.2: Discuss the comparative analysis.
- Section 15.3: Present the details of dataset used in studies.
- Section 15.4: Discuss the existing studied methodologies.
- Section 15.5: Describe the challenges in skin lesion area.
- After that, conclusions of the chapter are followed by the references in Section 15.6.

15.3 MACHINE LEARNING ALGORITHMS

Comparative analysis on various machine learning algorithms (ANN, SVM, KNN, CNN, and Hybrid Classifier) are shown in table 15.1.

15.4 DATASET USED

From the literature review, it analyzed that different datasets from different online dataset library i.e., PH2 dataset, Dermnetnz, UCI repository, ISIC-Archive, HAM10000, ISIC 2016, ISIC 2017, ISIC 2018, etc. are taken to classify the skin cancer, in table 15.2.

15.5 CHALLENGES FACED IN THIS AREA

A systematic review of the existing method gives us a clear picture about different problems in detection of skin lesions. Diagnosis of skin disease from an image is a challenging problem as there are different skin lesion classes. Misclassification of skin diseases can cause major problems for people (Vrushank et al., 2023). Researchers have reported the following issues in the classification of skin diseases:

- There are many types of lesions in the disease.
- Many illnesses can share similar visual features, which often confuses dermatologists to identify the illness by visual inspection.
- Detecting images of light-skinned people in standard datasets is another challenge. As a result, a dataset comprising enough lesion photos of dark-skinned and light-skinned persons is required to improve the detection accuracy.

TABLE 15.1

Comparative Analysis of Machine Learning Techniques

Reference	Skin Disease Name	Techniques Used	Evaluation Matrix	Feature Extraction	Classification Method Used	Accuracy
Poornima and Shailaja, 2017	Melanoma	SVM	Accuracy	Contour segmentation Local Binary Pattern	SVM	Good accuracy
Bakheet, 2017	Melanoma	SVM	Accuracy	HOG feature	SVM	97.32%
Arif et al., 2022	Melanoma	Hybrid CNN	Accuracy	GLCM and Histogram based features	Hybrid CNN	97.3%
Journal, 2017	skin cancer images	Machine Learning	Accuracy	NA	SVM	95%
Alquran et al., 2017	Melanoma	SVM	Accuracy	GLCM and ABCD feature	SVM	92.10%
Gound and Gaikwad, 2018	Eczema, Fungal infection, Urticarial	Image Processing and Data Mining	Accuracy	ABCD & GLCM Features	SVM,C4.5	Good accuracy
Soliman and Alenezi, 2019; Hajimahmud et al., 2022	3 different skin disease	Image Processing and Machine Learning	Accuracy	pre-trained CNN	SVM with MATLAB 2018b	100%
Vijayalakshmi, 2019	Melanoma	Image Processing and Machine Learning	Accuracy	NA	SVM, BPAN and CNN	SVM has accurate result than other
Mahbod et al., 2019	Melanoma and Seborrheic keratosis	HYBRID DEEP NEURAL NETWORKS	Accuracy	AlexNet, VGG16 and ResNet-18	SVM	83.83% for melanoma classification and 97.55% for seborrheic keratosis
Elngar et al., 2021	Eczema, Melanoma, Psoriasis, Onychosis, Acne, Corn	Machine Learning (CNN-SVM MAA)	Accuracy	CNN	SVM	SVM provide good accuracy
Parikh and Shah, 2016	bacterial infections, fungal infections, eczema and Scabies	SVM	Accuracy	NA	SVM, MATLAB	95.39%

Reference	Disease/Subject	Method	Metric	Technique	Tool/Algorithm	Accuracy
Bakheet, 2017	Melanoma	Shrikrishna Hospital, Karmasad, Gujarat, India, Department of Skin and V.D	Accuracy	SVM	NA	97.32%
Kumar et al., 2019	melanoma	Image processing and SVM	Accuracy	NA	SVM	Good Accuracy
Shoieb et al., 2016	Melanoma, Basal Cell Carcinoma, Eczema, and Impetigo	deep learning	Accuracy	CNN	SVM, MATLAB 9.0	94%
Kumar et al., 2019	Dermatitis, Herpes, and psoriasis	Image Color and Texture Features	Recognition rate	GLCM	SVM	80%-Herpes 90%-Dermatitis 95%-Psoriasis
Shoieb et al., 2016	Melanoma	Artificial Neural Network (ANN)	Accuracy	2DWavelet transform	MATLAB	84%
Wei et al., 2018	Skin Disease Analysis of normal and abnormal skin	Artificial Neural Network (ANN)	Accuracy	NA	MLP algorithm (feedforward neural network)	97%
Aswin et al., 2013	9 different diseases. (Eczema, Acne, Leprosy, Psoriasis, Tinea Corporis, Pityriasis Rosea Scabies, Foot Ulcer, Vitiligo)	Image Processing and Artificial Neural Network (ANN)	Accuracy	YCbCr algorithm	Feed-Forward back-propagation neural network with tenfold cross validation process	90%
Bourouis et al., 2013	bacterial infections, fungal infections, eczema and Scabies	bacterial infections, fungal infections, eczema and Scabies	bacterial infections, fungal infections, eczema and Scabies	bacterial infections, fungal infections, eczema and Scabies	bacterial infections, fungal infections, eczema and Scabies	bacterial infections, fungal infections, eczema and Scabies
Ahmed et al., 2014	Eczema Disease	GENETIC ALGORITHM	Accuracy	Canny Edge Detector	BPNN, ANN	Good accuracy
Parikh et al., 2015	Skin Diseases Diagnosis	Artificial Neural Network (ANN)	Accuracy	NA	MATLAB	94%
Abdulbaki et al., 2017	10 common skin diseases (Atopic Dermatitis, Folliculitis, Pityriasis Versicolor, Seborrheic Dermatitis, Vitiligo, Leprosy Lichen Planus, Warts, Herpes Zoster, Pediculosis Captis)	ANN	Accuracy	NA	ANN & Rf	90%

(Continued)

TABLE 15.1 (Continued)
Comparative Analysis of Machine Learning Techniques

Reference	Skin Disease Name	Techniques Used	Evaluation Matrix	Feature Extraction	Classification Method Used	Accuracy
Filimon and Albu, 2014	Melanoma	Color and Texture based Feature Extraction	Accuracy	HSV and statistical method for texture-based feature extraction	SVM (Support Vector Machine) and Neural Network (CNN)	CNN gives better accuracy then SVM
Kolkur et al., 2018	Melanoma	Deep Learning	Accuracy	NA	CNN (Inception –V3)	83%
Agrahari et al., 2022; Bhambri et al., 2022	Eczema, Melanoma and Impetigo	Image Processing with Data Mining and Deep Learning	Accuracy	NA	SVM and CNN	CNN gives accurate and efficient result as compared to SVM Classifier
Ruthra and Sumathy, 2019	Psoriasis, Lichen Planus, Pityriasis	Image Processing and Machine Learning	Accuracy	Computer Vision algorithm	CNN	Good accuracy
Mirunalini et al., 2017	Atopic dermatitis, Acne vulgaries & scabies	CNN Algorithms	Accuracy	NA	CNN classifier with TensorFlow	88%-dermatitis, 85%-arcane vulgaris and 84.7%-scabies
Hajgude et al., 2019	Benign Nevus and melanoma	Deep Learning	Accuracy	NA	CNN	98%
Kamble et al., 2019	Melanoma	Deep neural networks	Accuracy, Sensitivity, Specificity	NA	ResNet50 CNN	CNN achieves high sensitivity- 82.3 and specificity-77.9%.
Akyeramfo-Sam et al., 2019	Acne, Lichen planus and sjs ten	Machine Learning Algorithms	Accuracy and Error rate	NA	logistic regression kernal SVM, Naïve Bayes, Random Forest and CNN	CNN provide best result with accuracy 96% and error rate 0.04%

Mohamed et al., 2019	Benign or Malignant [BCC: basal cell carcinoma, MM: malignant melanoma; SK: seborrheic keratosis; H/H: hematoma/ hemangioma; SL: senile lentigo]	Deep Learning	Accuracy, Sensitivity, Specificity	CNN	NA	For six-class FRCNN, it was 86.2%; for BCDs and TRNs, it was 79.5% and 75.1%, respectively; and for two-class accuracy, sensitivity, and specificity, it was 91.5%, 83.3%, and 94.5% for FRCNN; 86.6%, 86.3%, and 86.6% for BCD; and 85.3%, 83.5%, and 85.9% for TRN, respectively
Brinker et al., 2019	6 diseases (Acne, Actinic, psoriasis, tina ringworm, eczema and seborrhoea	CNN	Accuracy	NA	CNN (MobileNet Model)	81%
Bhadula et al., 2019	Nevus and Melanoma	CNN	Accuracy	NA	ResNet 50, Densenet121, VGG16	Good Accuracy
Jinnai et al., 2020	Melanoma	Convolutional Neural Network	Accuracy	open CV method	CNN with LeNet architecture	Good Accuracy
Divya and Dsouza, 2019	MelanocyticNevi, Melanoma, Benign keratosis-like lesions,Basal cell Carcinoma, ActinicKeratoses, Vascular lesion and Dermatofibroma	Deep Learning	Accuracy	NA	CNN with Keras application API	93%
Maron et al., 2021	7 classes of skin lesion i.e., Benign keratosis, dermatofibroma melanocytic nevus and actinic keratosis. basal cell carcinoma, melanoma vascular	CNN	Accuracy	NA	DenseNet-20 and ResNet-101	Good Accuracy
Sharma and Bhave, 2019	Skin lesion	Deep Learning	Accuracy	NA	deep CNN and SVM	CNN+SVM-91%
Rao, 2021	Benign and Malignant	Deep Learning	Accuracy	BP-CNN, BN-CNN	NA	CNN provides good accuracy

(Continued)

TABLE 15.1 (Continued)

Comparative Analysis of Machine Learning Techniques

Reference	Skin Disease Name	Techniques Used	Evaluation Matrix	Feature Extraction	Classification Method Used	Accuracy
Harangi et al., 2020	Skin disease	Deep Learning	Accuracy	ResNet	NA	Good accuracy
Gupta et al., 2018	Glaucoma diagnosis, Alzheimer's disease, bacterial sepsis diagnosis	Machine Learning	Accuracy	NA	ANN, SVM and CNN algorithm	CNN has provided good evaluation performance and accurate result
Kumar et al., 2019	Benign Nevus, Melanoma or Seborrheic Keratosis,	CNN	Accuracy, Sensitivity, Specificity	NA	CSARM-CNN	sensitivity-80.22%, specificity-99.40% and accuracy-95.0%
Journal, 2017	Skin images	Deep Learning	Accuracy	ResNet152v2	NA	Good Accuracy
Rayan et al., 2018	Seborrhea keratosis, Actinic keratosis, Rosacea, lupus erythematous, Basal cell carcinoma, and Squamous cell carcinoma	CNN Algorithms	Accuracy and Performance rate	NA	ImageNet, ResNet-50, Inception-v3 Densenet121 Xception and Inception ResNet V2	Inception ResNet-V2 achieved highest accuracy with Performance rate-77.0%
Jiang et al., 2020	Melanoma, bullae, seborrheic keratosis, shingles, and squamous cell carcinoma	Color attributes include a color space with a color moment and an RGB histogram. Texture features: GLCM with Haralick features	Accuracy and F-measure	Gray Level co-occurrence matrix	SVM, k-NN and combined SVM and k-NN classifiers	F-measures of 46.71% and 34% for SVM and k-NN classifiers, respectively, and 61% for SVM and k-NN fusion
Pawale et al., 2021	Melanoma	Combining Deep Learning	Accuracy, Sensitivity, Specificity	Rsurf features and LBP	AlexNet combined with SVM	Accuracy-0.826, Sensitivity-0.533, Specificity- 0.898 and AOC-0.780
Wu et al., 2019; Rani et al., 2023	skin disease caused by bacterium, fungi, and virus	Data Mining	Accuracy, Sensitivity, Specificity	Nearest Neighbor using HSV	Nearest Neighbor using HSV	80%
Sumithra et al., 2015	Melanoma	various classifier	Accuracy	GLCM, wavelet & Tamura	SVM, KNN, DT & ensemble	

Author/Year	Disease	Approach	Metric	Features	Algorithm	Result
Majtner et al., 2021 Khang et al., 2022b	psoriasis, seborrheic dermatitis, lichen planus, pityriasis rosea,mchronic dermatitis	Ensemble Data Mining Techniques	Accuracy	NA	CART, SVM, DT, RF and GBDT	SVM 100%, KNN 87.5%, ensemble 87.5% & DT 75 % / 99%
Density et al., 2018	Melanoma	PSO-SVM hybrid system	Accuracy, Sensitivity, Specificity	Image Histogram, Confusion Matrix, Wavelet Packet Transform	Particle Swarm optimization & SVM (PSO-SVM).	WPT-SFS- SVM - 77.4 % & WPT-PSO-SVM accuracy - 87.1%, sensitivity- 94.1% & specificity- 80.2%
Shahi et al., 2018	Melanoma	Deep neural networks	Accuracy	ABCD rule	Matrix MNN and BpNN	80%
Verma et al., 2019	Melanoma	Artificial Intelligence Algorithm	AUROC, Accuracy, Sensitivity, Specificity	NA	Artificial Intelligence Algorithm	AUROC 95.8% and 100% sensitivity with specificity of 64.8%,
Takruri et al., 2019	Melanocytic nevi, Melanoma, Benign keratosis, BCC, Actinic keratosis, Vascular lesions, Dermatofibroma	DCNN	Accuracy	NA	Inceptionv3 and DenseNet-201	Good Accuracy with Fine tuning method
Sanghavi, 2019	Melanoma	machine learning and the deep learning	Accuracy	Image Quality Assessment,	Discrete Cosine transform and Discrete Wavelet Transform	80%
Phillips et al., 2019	Melanoma	Deep Learning	Accuracy	Local Binary Pattern, Edge Histogram, Histogram of Oriented Gradients and Gabor method	SVM Random Forest, K Nearest Neighbor & Naïve Bayes (NB)	85%
Ray et al., 2020	Melanoma	Hybrid convolutional neural network	Accuracy	NA	Hybrid Convolutional Neural Network	Good Accuracy

(Continued)

TABLE 15.1 (Continued)
Comparative Analysis of Machine Learning Techniques

Reference	Skin Disease Name	Techniques Used	Evaluation Matrix	Feature Extraction	Classification Method Used	Accuracy
Namitha et al., 2020 Khang et al., 2022a	Heart disease	Deep Learning	Accuracy	NA	Fuzzy information system and Bi-LSTM	accuracy of 98.86%, precision of 98.9%, sensitivity of 98.8%, specificity of 98.89%, and F-measure of 98.86%
Seeja and Suresh, 2019	Melanoma	DCNN	Accuracy	NA	DenseNet201, MobileNetV2, Res50V2, ResNet152V2, Xception, VGG16, VGG19, and GoogleNet	GoogleNet had the highest accuracy

Source: Author's owner.

TABLE 15.2

List of Dataset Used

Reference	Datasets used	Sampled images	Accuracy
Arif et al., 2022	ISIC 2017 AND Atlas of dermoscopy (EDRA),	From ISIC dataset, for testing phase used 514 images i.e., 129 melanoma and 385 non-melanoma and 590 images for EDRA, 231 melanoma and 359 non-melanoma images used	Highest Accuracy (SVM)
Alquran et al., 2017	Kwait Incp, International Skin Cancer Collaboration: Melanoma (ISIC 2016) and Skin Vision BV	NA	92.1% (SVM)
Vijayalakshmi, 2019; Mahbod et al., 2019; Ruthra and Sumathy, 2019; Mirunalini et al., 2017; Mohamed et al., 2019; Brinker et al., 2019; Harangi et al., 2020; Majtner et al., 2021; Seeja et al., 2019	International Skin Imaging Collaboration (ISIC) archive, ISIC-2016, ISIC 2017, ISIC 2018	2037 color dermoscopic skin image (411-MM, 254-SK, 1372-BM) (Mahbod et al., 2019) 1800 picture (360-benign, 300-meligent) (Ruthra and Sumathy, 2019), 2000 dermoscopic image (150 for validation, 600 for testing) (Mirunalini et al., 2017), 1300 skin images(50% of benign & 50% of melanoma) (Mohamed et al., 2019), 1512 image (Harangi et al., 2020), 4204 biospy (Brinker et al., 2019), 900 image (727-benign, 173 melanoma) (Majtner et al., 2021), 900 dermoscopic images (Seeja et al., 2019)	SVM has accurate result than other (Vijayalakshmi, 2019) 83.83% for melanoma classification and of 97.55% for seborrheic keratosis (Mahbod et al., 2019) CNN gives better accuracy then SVM (Ruthra and Sumathy, 2019) 82.50% (Mirunalini et al., 2017) Good Accuracy (Harangi et al., 2020) CNN achieves high sensitivity- 82.3 and specificity-77.9%. (Brinker et al., 2019) 85.19% (Seeja et al., 2019)
Elngar et al., 2021	Beni-Suef University Hospital, Cairo University Hospital and various websites	NA	92.1% (CNN)

(Continued)

TABLE 15.2 (Continued)
List of Dataset Used

Reference	Datasets used	Sampled images	Accuracy
Parikh et al., 2016; Parikh et al., 2015	Department of Skin & V.D., Shrikrishna Hospital,Karamsad, Gujarat, India	470 instance (Parikh et al., 2016), 470 image (Parikh et al., 2015)	95.39% (SVM) (Parikh et al., 2016), Good accuracy (SVM+ANN) (Parikh et al., 2016)
Kumar et al., 2019	https://www.kaggle.com/drscarlat/melanoma	600 images	Good accuracy (SVM)
Shoieb et al., 2016	Online databases Dermatology Information System and dermis dataset	337 images (43-melanoma, 26- non-melanoma) and in DermQuest 134 image (76-melanoma,58-Non melanoma)	94% (SVM)
Ahmed et al., 2014	Department of Dermatology, Sir Salimullah Medical College and Mitford Hospital, Dhaka, Bangladesh	775 images of 178 patient	90% (ANN)
Abdulbaki et al., 2017	Dermnetnz		Good accuracy (BpNN,ANN)
Filimon and Albu, 2014	Machine Learning Repository Dermatology Data Set	366 patient images	93.70% (ANN)
Kolkur et al., 2018	G. S. M. C. KEM Hospital, Parel Mumbai, Department of Skin and VD	NA	90% (ANN & RF)
Hajgude et al., 2019	From surveys and websites	From Internet	CNN gives accurate and efficient result as compared to SVM Classifier
Kamble et al., 2019; Phillips et al., 2019	From Clinic images	NA (Kamble et al., 2019), 1500 skin images (Phillips et al., 2019)	Good accuracy (CNN) (Kamble et al., 2019), AUROC 95.8% and 100% sensitivity with specificity of 64.8% (ANN) (Phillips et al., 2019)

Author/Year	Source	Images	Results
Akyeramfo-Sam et al., 2019 Wu et al., 2019	four (4) medical centres in the Sunyani Municipality, Ghana, Xiangya Derm	2656 face images	88%-dermatitis, 85%-arcane vulgaris and 84.7%-scabies (CNN) Inception ResNet-V2 achieved highest accuracy with Performance rate-77.0% (CNN)
		576 images (Wu et al., 2019) (Pawale et al., 2021) (Wu et al., 2019) (Wu et al., 2019) (Wu et al., 2019)	
Divya and Dsouza, 2019; Gupta et al., 2018; Sanghavi, 2019	Dermoscopic images were collected from Internet	1000 images of six types of diseases (Divya and Dsouza, 2019), 996 images (Gupta et al., 2018), 400 images (Sanghavi, 2019)	81% (CNN) (Divya and Dsouza, 2019), CNN+SVM-91% (Gupta et al., 2018), 80% (BpNN) (Sanghavi, 2019)
Maron et al., 2021; Jiang et al., 2020	ISIC 2017, PH2	NA (Maron et al., 2021), 200 image of PH2 i.e., 160 of Nevus & 40 of Melanoma (Jiang et al., 2020)	Good accuracy (CNN) (Maron et al., 2021), sensitivity-80.22%, specificity-99.40% and accuracy-95.0% (CSARM-CNN) (Jiang et al., 2020)
Sharma and Bhave, 2019	Two data sets used: the Pedro Hispano Hospital PH2 dermoscopy picture database and the ISBI 2016 challenge dataset	For PH2 total images 5706, for ISBI 3968 images	Good Accuracy (CNN)
Rao, 2021; Ray et al., 2020; Namitha et al., 2020	ViDIR Group, Department of Dermatology, Medical University of Vienna, obtained the HAM10000 data set	10010 images (Rao, 2021), 7210 images (Ray et al., 2020), 10015 dermoscopic images (Namitha et al., 2020)	93% (CNN) (Rao, 2021), Good Accuracy with Fine tuning method (Ray et al., 2020), 83% (Namitha et al., 2020)
Verma et al., 2019	UCI machine repository	366 instances	98.64% (SVM)
Takruri et al., 2019	Southern Pathology Laboratory in Wollongong NSW, Australia	79 histo-pathological images	WPT-SFS-SVM-77.4% & WPT-PSO-SVM accuracy-87.1%, sensitivity-94.1% & specificity-80.2%. (PSO-SVM)

Source: Author's owner.

- The datasets used to diagnose skin cancer in the real world are extremely imbalanced. Each type of skin cancer has a highly variable quantity of images in the unbalanced collection.
- For software to extract unique features from skin images for better detection, powerful hardware resources with high graphics processing unit (GPU) power are necessary.
- Computer-aided diagnosis is difficult because the skin color and skin type (age) are different. Therefore, feature selection associated with such diseases in computer-aided diagnosis is very important for correctly identifying them (Khang et al., 2023a).

15.6 RESULTS AND DISCUSSION

We first retrieved the paper from Science Direct, Scopus, PubMed, and Web of Sciences and then categorized them into applied classification techniques of machine learning that is SVM, ANN, CNN, and other classifiers. From the review, it analyzed that 27% researcher used support vector machine (SVM), 13% used artificial neural network (ANN), 38% used CNN, and 22% of researchers used other classifiers for detection (Rani et al., 2021).

This graph demonstrates the previous researchers' use of SVM, ANN, and other techniques. As a result, even though numerous new algorithms have been developed, they still do not produce more accurate results.

The methods used to identify and categorize skin cancer became the subject of this study, which also examined the various steps involved, such as image pre-processing, image segmentation, feature extraction, and classification. There are several proposed algorithms and there is a comparison between them based on different performance measures, such as accuracy, sensitivity, and specificity, as shown in figure 15.2 (figure 15.3).

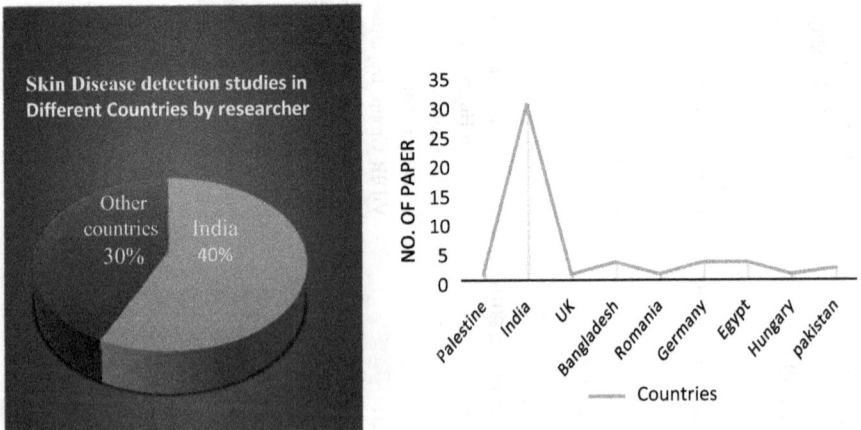

FIGURE 15.3 Detection of skin diseases in different countries.

TABLE 15.3
The list of Used Frameworks

Frame	Major Function	References
MATLAB	Useful results are displayed, statistics, and visualizations	Alquran et al., 2017; Mahbod et al., 2019; Bakheet, 2017; Kumar et al., 2019; Wei et al., 2018; Abdulbaki et al., 2017; Rao, 2021; Wu et al., 2019; Shahi et al., 2018
Keras	Applied to programming implementations, quickly transform ideas into results	Divya and Dsouza, 2019; Maron et al., 2021
Python	GPU acceleration and automatic derivation of robust deep neural networks	Jinnai et al., 2020; Rayan et al., 2018; Density et al., 2018; Namitha et al., 2020
TensorFlow	Applied to programming various machine learning algorithms	Hajgude et al., 2019; Bhadula et al., 2019; Gupta et al., 2018

Source: Author's owner.

Moreover, the rest of the 30% research done by other researchers from other countries like China, Egypt, USA, Pakistan, Hungry, Japan, and Germany, etc.

15.7 SOFTWARE TECHNIQUES USED

From collected literature, only ten papers have been published with MATLAB (Mahbod et al., 2019), a deep learning framework that includes tensors flow (Akyeramfo-Sam et al., 2019), Keras (Divya and Dsouza, 2019), and Python (Rayan et al., 2018). The details shown are in table 15.3.

15.8 CONCLUSION

This research analyzed a number of methods, including ANN, KNN, CNN, and approaches based on image processing (Tailor et al., 2022). These methods demonstrate the tremendous evolution in accuracy, duration, and complexity over time.

This study has demonstrated a literature review on skin disease classification and detection, which provided an important reference for dermatologist and cancer patient in early detection of skin disease.

This study was founded on about 60 related publication and journal articles that find the lesion and cause of skin lesion. It analyzed different machine learning methods that provide different accuracy for detection of skin lesions.

This chapter explained the proposed research methodology for detection skin lesion. From the comparative analysis of ML techniques, it shows the different method of feature extraction and classification method with their accuracy rate. Therefore, it analyzes that a neural network provide highest accuracy, specificity, and sensitivity values for detection skin lesion or reduce the error rate.

15.9 LIMITATIONS

There are some limitations of this study that lie in the coverage of the literature. This study does not work with a real-time dataset and study limited to an online dataset that miss some findings. In addition, we also excluded reports and unpublished works excluded from this study (Khang et al., 2023b).

Meanwhile, this study provides the result based on patient skin type or disease; it does not provide history of patient. This study not provide any result of patient history that is affected by other illnesses.

Various machine learning (ML) strategies for skin cancer detection and classification have been covered in this comprehensive review research (Khang et al., 2023c). It includes a variety of steps, including pre-processing, image segmentation, feature extraction, and classification.

The classification of lesion images using SVM, ANN, KNN, and CNN algorithms remained the primary focus of this work (Khanh and Khang, 2021).

In the future, we can work on improving the accuracy of detection and also reduce the error rate with the help of artificial intelligence (AI) and hybrid techniques (Rana et al., 2021).

Deep learning is also the most powerful techniques that provide promising features for accurate skin disease detection and classification than machine learning (ML).

REFERENCES

A. S. Abdulbaki, S. A. M. Najim, and S. A. Khadim, "Eczema Disease Detection and Recognition in Cloud Computing," vol. 12, no. 24, pp. 14396–14402, 2017. http://www.ripublication.com/ijaer17/ijaerv12n24_56.pdf

P. Agrahari, A. Agrawal, and N. Subhashini "Skin Cancer Detection Using Deep Learning," *Lecture Notes in Electrical Engineering*, vol. 792, pp. 179–190, 2022. doi: 10.1007/978-981-16-4625-6_18.

N. Ahmed, R. Yasir, A. Rahman, and N. Ahmed, "Dermatological Disease Detection Using Image Processing and Artificial Neural Network." *on Electrical and Computer …*, 2014. https://ieeexplore.ieee.org/abstract/document/7026918/

S. Akyeramfo-Sam, A. Addo Philip, D. Yeboah, N. C. Nartey, and I. Kofi Nti, "A Web-Based Skin Disease Diagnosis Using Convolutional Neural Networks," *Int. J. Inf. Technol. Comput. Sci.*, vol. 11, no. 11, pp. 54–60, 2019, doi: 10.5815/ijitcs.2019.11.06.

H. Alquran et al., "The melanoma skin cancer detection and classification using support vector machine," IEEE Jordan Conf. Appl. Electr. Eng. Comput. Technol., 2017, pp. 1–5, doi: 10.1109/AEECT.2017.8257738

M. Arif, F. M. Philip, F. Ajesh, D. Izdrui, M. D. Craciun, and O. Geman, "Automated Detection of Nonmelanoma Skin Cancer Based on Deep Convolutional Neural Network," *J. Healthc. Eng.*, vol. 2022, 2022, doi: 10.1155/2022/6952304

R. B. Aswin, J. A. Jaleel, and S. Salim "Implementation of ANN Classifier using MATLAB for Skin Cancer Detection," pp. 87–94, 2013. https://www.academia.edu/download/32722571/ICMIC13S8.pdf

S. Bakheet, "An SVM Framework for Malignant Melanoma Detection Based on Optimized HOG Features," *Computation*, vol. 5, no. 1, pp. 1–13, 2017, doi: 10.3390/computation5010004

S. Bhadula, S. Sharma, P. Juyal, and C. Kulshrestha, "Machine Learning Algorithms Based Skin Disease Detection," no. 2, pp. 4044–4049, 2019, doi: 10.35940/ijitee.B7686.129219

P. Bhambri, S. Rani, G. Gupta, and Khang, A. *Cloud and Fog Computing Platforms for Internet of Things*, ISBN: 978-1-032-101507, 2022. CRC Press. 10.1201/9781003213888

A. Bourouis, A. Zerdazi, M. Feham, and A. Bouchachia "M-Health: Skin Disease Analysis System Using Smartphone's Camera," *Procedia Computer Science*, vol. 19, pp. 1116–1120, 2013, doi: 10.1016/j.procs.2013.06.157.

T. J. Brinker et al., "Deep Neural Networks Are Superior to Dermatologists in Melanoma Image Classification," *Eur. J. Cancer*, vol. 119, pp. 11–17, 2019, doi: 10.1016/j.ejca.2019.05.023

C. Density, J. T. Davis, and D. E. Brown, "Implementation of Nearest Neighbor Using HSV to Identify Skin Disease Implementation of Nearest Neighbor Using HSV to Identify Skin Disease," 2018, doi: 10.1088/1757-899X/288/1/012153

Conf. Vis. Towar. Emerg. Trends Commun. Networking, *ViTECoN 2019*, no. March, pp. 1–5, 2019, doi: 10.1109/ViTECoN.2019.8899449

N. Divya, and D. P. Dsouza, "Cureskin – Skin Disease Prediction Using MobileNet Model," vol. 3307, pp. 32–37, 2019. http://journals.resaim.com/ijresm/article/view/998

A. A. Elngar, R. Kumar, A. Hayat, and P. Churi, "Intelligent System for Skin Disease Prediction Using Machine Learning," 2021, doi: 10.1088/1742-6596/1998/1/012037

D. Filimon, and A. Albu, "Skin Diseases Diagnosis Using Artificial Neural Networks," pp. 189–194, 2014. https://ieeexplore.ieee.org/abstract/document/6840059/

R. S. Gound, and J. B. Gaikwad, "Skin Disease Diagnosis System Using Image Processing and Data Mining," vol. 179, no. 16, pp. 38–40, 2018. https://scholar.google.com/scholar?hl=en&as_sdt=0%2C5&q=Skin+Disease+Diagnosis+System+using+Image+Processing+and+Data+Mining&btnG=

T. Gupta, S. Saini, A. Saini, S. Aggarwal, and A. Mittal, "A Deep Learning Framework for Recognition of Various Skin Lesions Due to Diabetes," *2018 Int. Conf. Adv. Comput. Commun. Informatics*, ICACCI 2018, no. February 2019, pp. 92–98, 2018, doi: 10.1109/ICACCI.2018.8554897

J. Hajgude, A. Bhavsar, H. Achara, and N. Khubchandani, "Skin Disease Detection Using Image Processing with Data Mining and Deep Learning," pp. 4363–4366, 2019. https://www.academia.edu/download/59879000/IRJET-V6I495420190627-15642-ilfuyg.pdf

V. A. Hajimahmud, Khang, A. V. Hahanov, E. Litvinova, S. Chumachenko, and A. V. Alyar, "Autonomous Robots for Smart City: Closer to Augmented Humanity," *AI-Centric Smart City Ecosystems: Technologies, Design and Implementation* (1st ed.), 2022. CRC Press. 10.1201/9781003252542-7

B. Harangi, A. Baran, and A. Hajdu, "Assisted Deep Learning Framework for Multi-Class Skin Lesion Classification Considering a Binary Classification Support," *Biomed. Signal Process. Control*, vol. 62, p. 102041, 2020, doi: 10.1016/j.bspc.2020.102041

Y. Jiang, S. Cao, S. Tao, and H. Zhang, "Skin Lesion Segmentation Based on Multi-Scale Attention Convolutional Neural Network," *IEEE Access*, vol. 8, pp. 122811–122825, 2020, doi: 10.1109/ACCESS.2020.3007512

S. Jinnai, N. Yamazaki, Y. Hirano, Y. Sugawara, Y. Ohe, and R. Hamamoto, "The Development of a Skin Cancer Classification System for Pigmented Skin Lesions Using Deep Learning," *Biomolecules*, vol. 10, no. 8, pp. 1–13, 2020, doi: 10.3390/biom10081123

I. Journal, "Irjet-Skin Disease Detection Using Neural Network," 47, 777–780. https://academia.edu/download/59879000/IRJET-V6I495420190627-15642-ilfuyg.pdf

I. Journal, "Skin Cancer Detection Using Image Processing," *Int Res J Eng Technol*, 2017. https://www.academia.edu/download/53555135/IRJET-V4I4702.pdf

M. Kamble, N. Kandalkar, and G. Khandagale, "Skin Disease Detection Using Image Processing and Machine Learning," vol. 8, no. 4, pp. 293–297, 2019, doi: 10.17148/IJARCCE.2019.8448

A. Khang, N. A. Ragimova, V. A. Hajimahmud, and A. V. Alyar, "Advanced Technologies and Data Management in the Smart Healthcare System," *AI-Centric Smart City Ecosystems: Technologies, Design and Implementation* (1st ed.), 2022a. CRC Press. 10.1201/9781003252542-16

A. Khang, S., Chowdhury, and S., Sharma (Eds.). *The Data-Driven Blockchain Ecosystem: Fundamentals, Applications, and Emerging Technologies* (1st ed.), 2022b. CRC Press. 10.1201/9781003269281

A. Khang, S. K. Gupta, V. A. Hajimahmud, J. Babasaheb, and G. Morris, *AI-Centric Modelling and Analytics: Concepts, Designs, Technologies, and Applications* (1st ed.), 2023a. CRC Press. 10.1201/9781003400110

A. Khang, S. K. Gupta, V. Shah, and A. Misra, (Eds.). *AI-Aided IoT Technologies and Applications in the Smart Business and Production* (1st ed.), 2023b. CRC Press. 10.1201/9781003392224

H. H. Khanh, and Khang, A. "The Role of Artificial Intelligence in Blockchain Applications," *Reinventing Manufacturing and Business Processes through Artificial Intelligence* pp. 20–40, 2021. CRC Press. 10.1201/9781003145011-2

M. Koklu, and I. A. Ozkan, "Skin Lesion Classification Using Machine Learning Algorithms," *Int. J. Intell. Syst. Appl. Eng.*, vol. 4, no. 5, pp. 285–289, 2017, doi: 10.18201/ijisae.2017534420

M. S. Kolkur, D. R. Kalbande, and V. Kharkar, "Machine Learning Approaches to Multi-Class Human Skin Disease Detection," vol. 14, no. 1, pp. 29–39, 2018. https://www.ripublication.com/ijcir18/ijcirv14n1_03.pdf

V. S. Kumar, and G. S. Jayalakshmi, "Performance Analysis of Convolutional Neural Network (CNN) Based Cancerous Skin Lesion Detection System," *Phys. Rev.*, vol. 47, pp. 777–780, 2019. https://ieeexplore.ieee.org/abstract/document/8862143/

N. V. Kumar, P. V. Kumar, K. Pramodh, and Y. Karuna, "Classification of Skin diseases Using Image Processing and SVM," *Proc. - Int. Conference on Vision ...*, 2019 https://ieeexplore.ieee.org/abstract/document/8899449/

A. Mahbod, G. Schaefer, C. Wang, R. Ecker, and I. Ellinge, "Skin lesion classification using hybrid deep neural networks," IEEE Int. Conf. Acoust. Speech Signal Process., 2019, pp. 1229–1233, doi: 10.1109/ICASSP.2019.8683352.

T. Majtner, S. Yildirim-Yayilgan, and J. Y. Hardeberg, "Combining Deep Learning and Hand-Crafted Features for Skin Lesion Classification," *2016 6th Int. Conf. Image Process. Theory, Tools Appl. IPTA 2016*, no. April 2021, doi: 10.1109/IPTA.2016.7821017

R. C. Maron et al., "Robustness of Convolutional Neural Networks in Recognition of Pigmented Skin Lesions," *Eur. J. Cancer*, vol. 145, pp. 81–91, 2021, doi: 10.1016/j.ejca.2020.11.020

P. Mirunalini, A. Chandrabose, V. Gokul, and S. M. Jaisakthi, "Deep Learning for Skin Lesion Classification," 2017, [Online]. Available: http://arxiv.org/abs/1703.04364

A. Mohamed, W. Mohamed, and A. H. Zekry, "Deep Learning Can Improve Early Skin Cancer Detection," *Int. J. Electron. Telecommun*, vol. 65, no. 3, pp. 507–513, 2019, doi: 10.24425/ijet.2019.129806

S. J. Namitha, N. Nikhilesha, S. S. Bellur, S. S. Sinha, and M. S. Ojus, "Survey on Skin Disease Classification Models," pp. 6013–6015, 2020. https://ieeexplore.ieee.org/abstract/document/9971993/

K. S. Parikh, and T. P. Shah, "Support Vector Machine – A Large Margin Classifier to Diagnose Skin Illnesses," vol. 23, pp. 369–375, 2016, doi: 10.1016/j.protcy.2016.03.039

K. S. Parikh, T. P. Shah, R. Kota, and R. Vora, "Diagnosing Common Skin Diseases Using Soft Computing Techniques," vol. 7, no. 6, pp. 275–286, 2015. https://gvpress.com/journals/IJBSBT/vol7_no6/28.pdf

P. Pawale, G. Ghadage, and M. Sahani, "Skin Disease Prediction," 2021. https://www.ingentaconnect.com/content/wk/ane/2021/00000133/00000004/art00032

M. Phillips et al., "Assessment of Accuracy of an Artificial Intelligence Algorithm to Detect Melanoma in Images of Skin Lesions," *JAMA Netw. Open*, vol. 2, no. 10, pp. 1–12, 2019, doi: 10.1001/jamanetworkopen.2019.13436

M. S. Poornima, and K. Shailaja, "Detection of Skin Cancer Using SVM," *Int. Res. J. Eng. Technol*, 2017. https://scholar.google.com/scholar?hl=en&as_sdt=0%2C5&q=Poornima++Detection+of+Skin+Cancer+Using+SVM&btnG=

S. S. Prasad, and T. Nadu, "Skin Disease Detection Using Computer Vision and Machine," *European Journal of Molecular & Clinical Medicine*, vol. 7, no. 4, pp. 2999–3003, 2020. https://scholar.google.com/scholar?hl=en&as_sdt=0%2C5&q=Prasad+Skin+Disease+Detection+Using+Computer+Vision+And+Machine+Learning+Technique&btnG=

G. Rana, Khang, A. R. Sharma, A. K. Goel, and A. K. Dubey. *Reinventing Manufacturing and Business Processes through Artificial Intelligence* 2021. CRC Press. 10.1201/9781003145011

S. Rani, P. Bhambri, A. Kataria, Khang, A. and A. K. Sivaraman (Eds.). *Big Data, Cloud Computing and IoT: Tools and Applications* (1st ed.), 2023. Chapman and Hall/CRC. 10.1201/9781003298335

S. Rani, M. Chauhan, A. Kataria, and Khang, A. "IoT Equipped Intelligent Distributed Framework for Smart Healthcare Systems," *Networking and Internet Architecture* 2021. CRC Press. 10.48550/arXiv.2110.04997

K. S. Rao, "Skin Disease Detection Using Machine Learning," *International Journal Of*. vol. 9, no. 3, pp. 64–68, 2021. https://scholar.google.com/scholar?hl=en&as_sdt=0%2C5&q=Skin+Disease+Detection+using+Machine+Learning&btnG=

A. Ray, A. Gupta, and A. Al, "Skin Lesion Classification with Deep Convolutional Neural Network: Process Development and Validation," *JMIR Dermatology*, vol. 3, no. 1, pp. 1–7, 2020, doi: 10.2196/18438

Z. Rayan, M. Alfonse, and A. B. M. Salem, "Machine Learning Approaches in Smart Health," *Procedia Comput. Sci.*, vol. 154, no. 1985, pp. 361–368, 2018, doi: 10.1016/j.procs.2019.06.052

V. Ruthra, and P. Sumathy, "Color and Texture Based Feature Extraction for Classifying Skin Cancer Using Support Vector Machine & Convolutional Neural Network," pp. 502–507, 2019. https://www.academia.edu/download/60792159/IRJET-V6I971120191003-9892-10xpo6p.pdf

J. Sanghavi, "A Novel Approach for Detection of Skin Cancer Using Back Propagation Neural Network Jignyasa Sanghavi," *Helix*, vol. 9, no. 6, pp. 5847–5851, 2019, doi: 10.29042/2019-5847-5851

R. D. Seeja, and A. Suresh, "Deep Learning Based Skin Lesion Segmentation and Classification of Melanoma Using Support Vector Machine (SVM)," *Asian Pacific J. Cancer Prev.*, vol. 20, no. 5, pp. 1555–1561, 2019, doi: 10.31557/APJCP.2019.20.5.1555

P. Shahi, S. Yadav, N. Singh, and N. P. Singh, "Melanoma Skin Cancer Detection Using Various Classifiers," *2018 5th IEEE Uttar Pradesh Sect. Int. Conf. Electr. Electron. Comput. Eng. UPCON 2018*, no. November, pp. 1–5, 2018, doi: 10.1109/UPCON.2018.8597093

M. Sharma, and A. Bhave, "Lesion Classification Using Convolutional Neural Network," *Adv. Intell. Syst. Comput.*, vol. 898, no. October, pp. 357–365, 2019, doi: 10.1007/978-981-13-3393-4_37

D. A. Shoieb, S. M. Youssef, and W. M. Aly, "Computer-Aided Model for Skin Diagnosis Using Deep Learning," vol. 4, no. 2, pp. 122–129, 2016, doi: 10.18178/joig.4.2.122-129

N. Soliman, and A. Alenezi, "A Method of Skin Disease Detection Using Image Processing and Machine Learning," *Procedia Comput. Sci.*, vol. 163, pp. 85–92, 2019, doi: 10.1016/j.procs.2019.12.090

R. Sumithra, M. Suhil, and D. S. Guru, "Segmentation and Classification of Skin Lesions for Disease Diagnosis," *Procedia - Procedia Comput. Sci.*, vol. 45, no. March, pp. 76–85, 2015, doi: 10.1016/j.procs.2015.03.090

R. K. Tailor, R. Pareek, and Khang, A. (Eds.). "Robot Process Automation in Blockchain," *The Data-Driven Blockchain Ecosystem: Fundamentals, Applications, and Emerging Technologies* (1st ed.), pp. 149–164, 2022. CRC Press. 10.1201/9781003269281-8

M. Takruri, M. K. A. Mahmoud, and A. Al-Jumaily, "PSO-SVM Hybrid System for Melanoma Detection from Histo-Pathological Images," *Int. J. Electr. Comput. Eng.*, vol. 9, no. 4, pp. 2941–2949, 2019, doi: 10.11591/ijece.v9i4.pp2941-2949

A. K. Verma, S. Pal, and S. Kumar, "Classification of Skin Disease Using Ensemble Data Mining Techniques," 2019, doi: 10.31557/APJCP.2019.20.6.1887

M. M. Vijayalakshmi, "Melanoma Skin Cancer Detection Using Image Processing and Machine Learning." *International Journal of Trend in Scientific ...*, 2019. https://www.academia.edu/download/59920968/169_Melanoma_Skin_Cancer_Detection_using_Image_Processing_and_Machine_Learning20190703-23098-1o8hr8x.pdf

S. Vrushank, T. Vidhi, and Khang, A. "Electronic Health Records Security and Privacy Enhancement Using Blockchain Technology," *Data-Centric AI Solutions and Emerging Technologies in the Healthcare Ecosystem* (1st ed.), 2023, P (1). CRC Press. 10.1201/9781003356189

L. Wei, Q. Gan, and T. Ji, "Skin Disease Recognition Method Based on Image Color and Texture Features," vol. 2018, 2018. https://www.hindawi.com/journals/CMMM/2018/8145713/

Z. Wu et al., "Studies on Different CNN Algorithms for Face Skin Disease Classification Based on Clinical Images," *IEEE Access*, vol. 7, pp. 66505–66511, 2019, doi: 10.1109/ACCESS.2019.2918221

16 Hospital Performance Management

Implementation of Real-Time Monitoring System for Clinical Sector

Babasaheb Jadhav and Biranchi Jena

CONTENTS

16.1 INTRODUCTION

Performance management deals with the outcome of certain functions or activities defined for an individual or organization or a particular system. Performance management at the individual level is the measure of alignment between employees and the organization's goals (Armstrong, 2015). However, it needs great clarity on the aspects of organization goals and targets which can easily connect to the activities done at the associate level (Vrushank et al., 2023).

DOI: 10.1201/9781003356189-16

Performance management on a few occasions is defined as identifying, measuring, and developing the performance of individuals and teams and aligning performance with the strategic goals of the organization (Aguinis, 2013). It is critical to understand the performance management system from the organizational prospect to set up the system in a service industry including hospitals.

Although performance at a micro level revolves around the performance of an employee or group of employees, it would be difficult to measure and manage until the output and outcome of the organization are defined well for a specific period. Thus, performance management system is made up of two important components, one being the performance acceleration and the other one being the performance measurement system (Fried, 2002).

Most organizations are far away from using the performance management models available for the healthcare system (Beyan & Baykal, 2012) and researchers are trying to build a better comparable performance model for the benefit of the system.

Healthcare organizations including hospitals are consciously trying to achieve service standards at a higher level. Achieving higher service standards will ensure high quality of service and so also higher pricing for the services being offered (Khang et al., 2023c).

Tracking indicators for achieving a higher level of performance is becoming a regular business activity in hospital organizations. Recent studies have shown that business performance in terms of efficiency, effectiveness, and patient-centeredness is gaining importance, and more than 70% focus is on maintaining the efficiency of the hospital operation (Carini et al., 2020).

Few organizations have defined more indicators as quality indicators over process and outcome indicators (Gandjour et al., 2002). Thus, indicators are important in the process of performance management.

Although the majority of the international projects on performance management of hospitals followed a common methodology for designing, there is a difference in approach for philosophy, scope, and coverage of these projects (Groene et al., 2008). Thus, understanding the performance issues in the hospital from the philosophy of management is of utmost importance and that would help in driving the performance management projects in a better way.

Process adherence is considered one of the important aspects of the performance management activities in a hospital setup followed by the outcome (Hajimahmud et al., 2022). In a study of a wide range of indicators, more than half of the indicators were created for measuring the adherence to processes of care while little more than one-third of the indicators were related to the outcome of care (Cornell et al., 2009).

Considering the inconsistency in maintaining a good review system for clinical and efficiency-related outcomes in the hospitals, the current research has defined a structured tool for building and implementing a real-time or near real-time tracking of indicators for better operational achievements (Rana et al., 2021).

16.2 METHODOLOGY

A structured review of literature was done for listing out the clinical and operational indicators in a hospital setup. Based on the same, the researchers had taken up a consultancy project for establishing the performance management system in a corporate hospital (Khang et al., 2022a). The following methods have been adopted in the current research:

1. Heads of the department (HoD) were invited for a brainstorming session.
2. A list of operational and clinical indicators was presented to them to ascertain their level of understanding and scope of application in the hospital.
3. All the HoDs were asked to list all the indicators based on the importance of the hospital and their concern for the business and clinical excellence.
4. Based on the feedback from the HoDs, a list of functionalities in the hospital was shortlisted and included in the study.
5. A list of eight performance parameters has been enlisted. These parameters include both clinical and operational and contribute significantly to the performance of patient outcomes.
6. The parameters finalized for analysis are patient grievances management, Medical Record Department (MRD) update management, average length of stay (ALOS) optimization, Out Patient Department (OPD) performance, and planned discharge performance, Operation Theatre (OT) scheduling performance, tracking of critical patients and patient referral tracking (Rani et al., 2021).
7. Appropriate indicators were defined to track the performance on a real-time basis.
8. All the indicators were scrutinized through the "TRUE" indicator test.
9. TRUE indicator is a functional-based test for the development indicators designed by researchers and the tool being adopted in leading organizations and management of social and developmental projects.
10. TRUE is a test for the selection and establishment of appropriate indicators for performance management. It has got four components and each component provides necessary checks for sustaining the indicator and supports the performance management functions of the organization.

16.2.1 COMPONENT 1 (T) – TALLIED

All the indicators must have defined through a formula. If an indicator does have a defined numerator and denominator, it would be difficult to measure them through the right data points. If it is not TALLIED, it may have a lot of subjectivity in it and tracking and action was taken on it would be difficult.

16.2.2 COMPONENT 2 (R) – RELEVANT

All the indicators must be relevant to the clinical or operational outcome. When the indicators are formed, they must have a specific purpose to support and achieve. If it does not connect to those specific needs, the indicator may lose its importance and it will not be sustained for longer. The indicator must be checked for its relevance through the approval of the top management.

16.2.3   Component 3 (U) – Universally Accepted

An indicator is not only developed to achieve a particular operational or clinical outcome, but it also requires all departments' and stakeholders' consent and support in terms of the provision of data and works towards the same. Once accepted by all the stakeholders, it becomes easy and swift to create and track the indicator until the desired result is achieved.

16.2.4   Component 4 (E) – Ease of Data Collection and Compiling

Since an indicator requires a lot of information regularly and consistently, the "ease of data collection and compilation" is one of the most important parameters for the development of indicators in the process of performance management.

If the data needed for the calculation of the indicator is well defined and captured automatically through process automation, the indicators can also be automated and tracking and review would also be easy and effective.

On the other hand, if the data collection is cumbersome and the data capturing is not automated, the sustaining of the performance management through the particular indicator is doubtful.

So, all the indicators designed for performance management have been toughly evaluated through the "TRUE" test for indicator and all those indicators included that have cleared the "TRUE" test.

All the indicators were then placed in a specifically designed template as a master list for managing the performance of the particular department or operational area as in table 16.1.

The following concepts for performance management are used in the above indicator listing template.

16.2.4.1   Type of Indicator

Indicators can be input indicators or activity indicators (process indicators) or output indicators or outcome indicators or impact indicators (Khang et al., 2023a). For the current research and operational understanding, the types of indicators are defined as follows:

a. **Input Indicator:** For every activity, inputs are needed. Inputs could be manpower or machine or functionality status of a machine etc. Any kind of activity would be not optimal if there is a shortfall in the input.
b. **Activity Indicators/Process Indicators:** Activity or process indicators are built for ensuring that a particular activity defined in a process is done with 100% adherence. The absence of a process indicator will not guarantee the right output.
c. **Output Indicators:** Outputs are the final products or services that can be used for the satisfaction of a particular need of a patient or customer. The output indicators could be directed toward volume or quality or efficiency. The output efficiency mostly is measured through the output-to-input ratio.

TABLE 16.1
Designed Template as a Master List for Managing the Performance of the Particular Department or Operational Area

INPUT/ACTIVITY/ OUTPUT/ OUTCOME/ IMPACT (describe it)	Name of the Indicator (the measure which would indicate whether the INPUT/ACTIVITY/ OUTPUT/ OUTCOMES are achieved)	Periodicity of calculating and tracking the Indicator (Frequency) (also note down if this can be automated)	Source of Information (The source which would provide the data/information for calculation of the indicator)	Formula For Calculation (Please write down the formula for the calculation of Indicator(s)	Remarks (Any deviation in the calculation and source of the information expected during the project duration)

Source: Author's owner.

d. **Outcome Indicators:** Outcome indicators are the measurement of the extent to which a particular need of the customer is fulfilled through a particular output. The outcome indicators measure the effectiveness of a particular product or service offering.

e. **Impact Indicators:** Impact indicators are the measurement of the long-term impact on the patient or customers. A positive impact creates a better brand value for the service offering or the organization.

16.2.4.2   Name of the Indicator
The name of the indicator is to be defined with the well-versed terminology being used in the organization.

16.2.4.3   Periodicity of Calculation of the Indicator
For performance management, a particular indicator needs to be measured in a specific period. This information may also include if the indicator needs to be measured on a real-time basis for tracking and taking action on the same immediately.

16.2.4.4   Source of Information
The source of information needs to be specified very clearly as the sharing of information from other departments or secondary sources will be managed accordingly. Such information will help communicate with the concerned department and the IT team for the integration of the same. This document can be a reference document for data privacy for the department and organization.

16.2.4.5   Formula for Calculation of the Indicator
Since the TRUE indicator test is ensuring the formula for calculating the indicator, documentation of the same would bring clarity among all the stakeholders connected in the performance management. The formula will also be used by the IT department for the automation of the indicator development of the daily real-time tracking tool as a part of performance management (Bhambri et al., 2022).

16.2.4.6   Remarks
If any deviation in the indicator management is expected, the same can be documented.

1. Once all the indicators were tested and finalized through the "TRUE" indicator test, "standards" for each indicator were defined so that the current status of the indicator in the organization can be compared with the standards. These standards were taken from the National Accredited Board for Hospitals (NABH), 4th Edition. Where the standards are not available in the NABH, 4th Edition, the national standards are taken from the existing literature. And if the national level standards are not available, the management consensus was taken and the target is frozen for the project period.

2. The data requirements for the list of indicators were informed to the Information Technology (IT) department of the hospital and a necessary

data warehouse was formed to ensure that the indicators are tracked on a "near real-time basis" (Hajimahmud et al., 2022).

3. The IT department was requested to build an intra-web application for the stakeholders to access and track the indicators. A role-based access functionality was created in the system for integrating the performance management model with the operation.

4. Few decision-making facilities were also designed so that actions can be taken instantly to ensure the improvement in the status of the indicator.

5. For the scope of the current article, four operational areas or processes have been covered in terms of the preparation of indicators and daily tracking procedures. Other processes were not included in the scope of the article. However, readers may reach out to the authors if any information related to those processes is needed.

16.3   OUTCOMES

The outcome of the performance management was designed in form of an intranet web-based application. The application had all the defined indicators and real-time tracking of these indicators was facilitated through the necessary IT-based support system and services, as shown in figure 16.1.

- Patient grievance management
- Medical record update management
- Average length of stay (ALOS) of the patients
- Patient discharge management
- Scheduled Operation Theatre (OT) time management

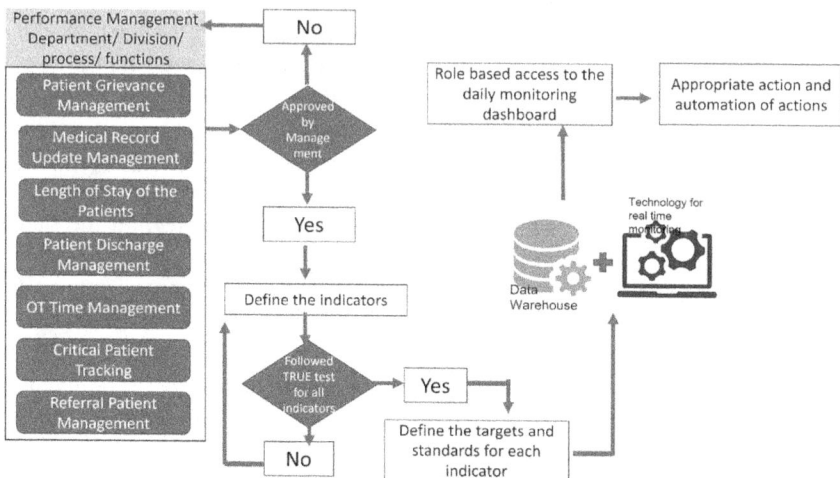

FIGURE 16.1   Real-time monitoring of hospital performance.

Source: Author's owner.

- Critical patient tracking management
- Referral patient management
- Out Patient Department (OPD) management

16.3.1 Patient Grievance Management

Better patient satisfaction along with continual Improvement in the patient experience can help a hospital improve its financial performance by strengthening customer loyalty, building reputation and brand, and boosting utilization of hospital services through increased referrals to family and friends (Delloite, 2018).

To improve the patient experience, patient grievances need immediate attention and resolution. Patient complaints and grievances are commonly related to treatment and communication which accounts for more than one-third of the total complaints (Reader et al., 2014). It was found that after complaining, most of the patients are dissatisfied with the action taken and the response of the hospital staff to their complaints (Friele et al., 2008).

It is therefore important to handle the complaints and grievances effectively and communicate the same back to the patients. Improving the complaint-handling process will reduce financial claims and other disputes between patients and the hospital (Feijter et al., 2012).

Developing a structured tracking system for patient complaints and grievances and actions taken on them will help the management to review systematically and improve its performance accordingly. The current research has designed a set of indicators for the same and implemented the same. The details of the indicators are given in table 16.2.

Four indicators were designed and implemented in the hospital. The complete system was done on a manual basis with the entry of the complaints manually in an Excel-based spreadsheet in the patient grievance cell and there were no indicators in place for tracking the grievances except for the total number of grievances received.

With the system in place, grievance management was automated with the help of the IT team. The implementation team along with the IT team defined the process of managing the grievances and the process was automated. Patients were given an application to lodge their complaints and the hospital customer service team entered the grievance into the system when the patient preferred to complain orally.

For confirmation of the lodge of the complaint, an automated short messaging service (SMS) was also introduced. This not only ensured that all the grievances are accepted in the system but also an acknowledgment is sent immediately to the patient. This improved the patient experience as the patient was aware that their grievances were taken care of.

The newly designed process also grouped all the grievances into seven categories and mapped them to different departments or professionals who would be primarily responsible for the resolution of the same.

The system improved the grievance management system in the hospital to a greater extent with 100% automation of the system. Tracking of the performance by the senior management helped to prioritize the grievances and the capacity building to handle these effectively. The grievance resolution rate has clocked at 93% and

TABLE 16.2

List of Indicators Designed for Improving the Performance of Patient Grievances

INPUT /ACTIVITY (Process) /OUTPUT / OUTCOME /IMPACT	Name of the Indicator	Periodicity of Calculating and Tracking the Indicator (Frequency)	Source of Information/ Data Ownership	Formula for Calculation	Remarks (Other Information Needed for the Project Team)
Output Indicator	grievances reported rate	Daily on a real-time basis	• Patient grievance cell (online+ offline)	**IPD** Total grievance received/ Total admitted patients * 100 **OPD** Total grievance received/ Total OPD footfall * 100	• Can be designed for daily tracking • Can be done for a given period • Can be done for different departments
Process Indicator	% of grievances forwarded to the respective dept.	Daily on a real-time basis	1. Patient grievance cell (online + offline) 2. Information received at respective dept. for action	Total grievance forwarded to the concerned dept. or person/Total grievances received * 100	Department or professional wise allotment of grievances was also tracked
Output Indicator	% of grievances resolved	Daily on a real-time basis	Patient grievance cell (online + offline)	Total grievances resolved/ Total grievances received * 100	Department or professional wise resolution of grievances was also tracked
Output Indicator	% of grievances resolved within 12 hours	Daily on a real-time basis	Patient grievance cell (online + offline)	Total grievance resolved within 12 hours/Total grievances received * 100	Department or professional wise resolution of grievances was also tracked

Source: Author's owner.

the resolution within 12 hours was done for 76% of cases within three months of the implementation.

16.3.2   Medical Record Department (MRD) Update Management

The Medical Record Department (MRD) helps in documenting of patient's medical history, current treatment, and care given. This needs to be done timely and systematically as the records are crucial in future treatment and also for any medico-legal cases. Archiving the records electrically is one of the major functions of the MRD and timely updating patient records improves the operational efficiency of the hospital organizations.

The initial assessment by the implementation team witnessed more than 50% of the patient's treatment documents reach the MRD after 48 hours of patient discharge. This increases the risk of misplacement of the patient record. Again, there is no proof of the patient's record reaching MRD on time. There was evidence of misplaced patient records. Thus, tracking the records helps in providing the exact status.

Updating records is important and there is a delay in updating and archiving the records at MRD. Such a delay was due to multiple reasons, including the absence of clinical notes, and the signature of the consultants among others. The current implementation of the tracking system at MRD introduced the following indicators, as shown in table 16.3.

The introduction of the indicators was done only for the improvement of operational efficiency. After the finalization of indicators, there is an improvement in the process flow and better coordination between the nursing administration and MRD. The misplacement of patient records was reduced from around 5% to 0.1%.

The tracking improves confidence among the senior management as far as the follow-up clinical intervention and management of medico-legal cases are concerned.

16.3.3   Average Length of Stay (ALOS) of the Patients

Longer hospital stay is neither good for the patients nor good for the hospital organizations. Reduction in the number of inpatient days helps in reducing the risk of infection and medication side effects, improvement in the quality of treatment, and increased hospital profit with more efficient bed management (Baek et al., 2018).

Although many studies and strategies have been done across the industry, tracking of the information on an operational level for the understanding of the breadth and width of the issue was not very evident. Although project-based studies are common for studying the length of stay in hospitals, integrating it with regular operational tracking and management review is rare (Babasaheb et al., 2023).

The consulting and implementation team has introduced the following indicators for regular and real-time tracking for the performance review of the length of stay of patients in the hospital is shown in table 16.4.

The above indicators allowed the hospital management to define the standards for the maximum number of days of stay for every procedure for which the patient was admitted. Therefore, clinical attention was improved and care protocols were adhered to more stringently.

TABLE 16.3

List of Indicators Designed for Improving the Performance of the Medical Record Department (MRD)

INPUT /ACTIVITY (Process) /OUTPUT / OUTCOME /IMPACT	Name of the Indicator	Periodicity of Calculating and Tracking the Indicator (Frequency)	Source of Information/ Data Ownership	Formula for Calculation	Remarks (Other Information Needed for the Project Team)
Process Indicator	Total Discharges	Daily on a real-time basis	• HIMS and IPD	Total patients completed all the formalities for discharge	Can be designed for daily tracking of different specialties in the hospital Can be designed for a specific day or set of days with a starting date and ending date specialty wise tracking can be done for any given period
Process Indicator	% of patient records reaching MRD within 24 hours of discharge	Daily on a real-time basis	IPD nursing cell + MRD (online or/and offline records)	Total records received at MRD within 24 hrs of discharge (receive time- discharge time= < 24 hrs)/ Total discharges in a given period *100	
Process Indicator	% of patient records updated and archived at MRD within 48 hours of receiving	Daily on a real-time basis	MRD cell	Total records archived at MRD within 48 hrs of receipt (archived-time– receipt time= < 48 hrs)/ Total receipt of records at MRD in a given period * 100	specialty wise tracking can be done for any given period

Source: Author's owner.

TABLE 16.4

List of Indicators Designed for Improving Performance Related to the Length of Stay (LOS) of the Patients

INPUT /ACTIVITY (Process) /OUTPUT/ OUTCOME /IMPACT	Name of the Indicator	Periodicity of Calculating and Tracking the Indicator (Frequency)	Source of Information/Data Ownership	Formula for Calculation	Remarks (other Information Needed for the Project Team)
Process Indicator	Total inpatients (at the tracking time)	Daily on a real-time basis	• HIMS and IPD	Total patients currently admitted and remain as an inpatient	Can be designed for daily tracking of different specialties in the hospital
Process Indicator	% of in-patients with stay less than 4 days	Daily on a real-time basis	IPD nursing cell + HMIS	Total in-patients in hospital with stay up to 4 days (current time- admitted time = < 96 hrs)/Total in-patients in a given period *100	specialty wise tracking can be done for any given period
Process Indicator	% of in-patients stay between 4-8 days	Daily on a real-time basis	IPD nursing cell + HMIS	Total in-patients in hospital with a stay between 4–8 days (current time – admitted time = < 192 hrs and >96 hrs)/Total in-patients in a given period *100	specialty wise tracking can be done for any given period
Process Indicator	% of in-patients with stay more than 8 days	Daily on a real-time basis	IPD nursing cell + HMIS	Total in-patients in hospital with stay more than 8 days (current time- admitted time > 192 hrs)/Total in-patients in a given period * 100	specialty wise tracking can be done for any given period
Process Indicator	Average Length of Stay	Daily/Weekly/ Monthly or any given period	IPD nursing cell + HMIS	Sum of days stay of all the patients who are already discharged in a given period/ total patients discharged * 100	specialty wise tracking can be done for any given period

Source: Author's owner.

The tracking of the indicators provided easy and valuable information to the hospital administrator (both medical administrators, nursing administrators, and operational team) about the proportion of patients who are in the bracket of 4 to 8 days and more than 8 days. This information prompted them to prioritize the patients in terms of optimizing the treatment including financial counseling.

The regular flashing of numbers for the administrator prompted them to take necessary and immediate action. The implementation of the tracking system reduced the proportion of patients staying more than 8 days from 37% to less than 20% within a span of three months. The average length of stay during this period was also positively affected by the reduction of 1.98 days.

16.3.4 PATIENT DISCHARGE MANAGEMENT

Patient discharge from the hospital is an important event in healthcare management. The discharge process not only makes the patient leave the hospital, but it also ensures a bed is vacated in a planned way so that the next patient planning can be done quite well.

The discharge process although crucial for the operational efficiency of the hospital, preparing the patient for the continuum of care also defines the clinical effectiveness of the overall hospital service delivery model.

Preparation of discharge information for the effective self-management of post-hospitalization tasks during the transition of patients from hospital to home is less explored (Flink & Ekstedt, 2017). Discharge planning also varies from patient to patient based on the criticality and post-hospitalization care needs.

Discharge of older patients is particularly challenging as these patients need the continuum of care in the primary care setup or home healthcare setup (Bauer et al., 2009). Therefore, it is important to plan all the discharges well in advance so that enough time is available for the clinical and care team to define a continuum of care in the discharge documentation and ensure complete information for patient management at home (Khang et al., 2022a).

While management of the challenges related to the discharge processes, a well-structured tracking of critical information on a real-time basis related to the discharge process carries the most important consideration for the operation team. This will create better synchronization between the operation team and the clinical team (Khang et al., 2022b).

The following indicators were designed for the discharge process optimization in the implementation hospital, as shown in table 16.5.

The implementation of the indicators for improving the discharge process has resulted in better coordination with the clinical team and the administration team. When the main motive of the operational team is to adhere to the timelines for discharge, the clinical team may miss out on the mandatory information flow and other important processes, which will enhance the continuum of care at home or primary care units.

The implementation of the daily tracking system improved the discharge within the cut-off time from 57% to 72% within a period of three months. Document adherence was also improved from 45% to 65% during the same period.

TABLE 16.5

List of Indicators Designed for Improving Performance Related to the Discharge of Patients

INPUT /ACTIVITY (Process)/ OUTPUT / OUTCOME /IMPACT	Name of the Indicator	Periodicity of Calculating and Tracking the Indicator (Frequency)	Source of Information/Data Ownership	Formula for Calculation	Remarks (other Information Needed for the Project Team)
Process Indicator	Total inpatients (at the tracking time/day)	Daily on a real-time basis	• HIMS and IPD	Total patients currently admitted and remain as an inpatient	Can be designed for daily tracking of different specialties in the hospital
Process Indicator	% of in-patients planned for discharge at least 24 hours in advance	Daily on a real-time basis	IPD nursing cell + HMIS	Total in-patients in hospital with discharge approval (planned discharge time – discharge decision time = < 24 hrs)/ Total in-patients in a given period *100	specialty wise tracking can be done for any given period The hospital may have a specific time for discharge (just to accommodate the admission time)-the same time can be used for clarity in the calculation of indicators and tracking
Output Indicator	% of in-patients discharged within the cut-off time	Daily on a real-time basis	IPD nursing cell + HMIS	Total in-patients discharged from the hospital within the defined cut-off time/Total in-patients planned for discharge * 100	specialty wise tracking can be done for any given period The Standard to achieve is >95%
Output Indicator	% of in-patients discharged with 100% process adherence	Monthly Audit	IPD nursing cell + HMIS	Total patients discharged from hospital with 100% process adherence and 100% documentation/Total patients discharged in a given period * 100	specialty wise tracking can be done for any given period The Standard to achieve is >99%
output Indicator	% of in-patients discharged within the cut-off time and with 100% process adherence	Monthly Audit	IPD nursing cell + HMIS	Total patients discharged from the hospital within the cut-off time and with 100% process adherence and 100% documentation/Total patients discharged in a given period * 100	Specialty wise tracking can be done for any given period The Standard to achieve is >90%

Source: Author's owner.

As discussed in the methodology, a similar indicator designing and implementation plan was adopted for the following departments or processes:

- Scheduled Operation Theatre (OT) time management
- Critical patient tracking management
- Referral patient management
- Out Patient Department (OPD) management

16.4 CONCLUSION

The current research has created a structured monitoring tool through an effective performance management system. The current article deals with an effective review system for better management and leadership in a hospital organization (Misra et al., 2023).

A review system with a set of effective indicators is the prerequisite for optimal operation in the hospital. This chapter provides a step-by-step approach for the designing and implementation of the same.

The current article has a detailed methodology that will help practicing managers and leaders implement the performance management system in a given organization.

A real-time performance monitoring tool is designed and developed that can be implemented across all healthcare organizations of different sizes for tracking and improving the delivery of clinical services (Khang et al., 2023b).

Since the tool is based on real-time indicators defining the level of performance, the tool will be providing support to the administration team to address more than 80% of issues on spot. The analytical framework designed along with the tool will also help in understanding the gray areas and thus provides a provision for continual improvement and thus the overall performance (Tailor et al., 2022).

The authors are also researchers in the areas of the performance management system of the organization. The authors may be consulted for the establishment of the performance management system either in a particular department or at the organizational level.

REFERENCES

Aguinis, H. Performance management (3rd edition). *Boston, MA: Pearson.* (2013). https://www.sciencedirect.com/science/article/pii/S0007681312000869

Armstrong, M. Armstrong's handbook of performance management: An evidence-based guide to delivering high performance (5th edition). *Kogan Page* (2015). https://books.google.com/books?hl=en&lr=&id=wtwS9VG-p4IC

Babasaheb, J., Sphurti, B., Khang, A. Industry Revolution 4.0: Workforce Competency Models and Designs. *Designing Workforce Management Systems for Industry 4.0: Data-Centric and AI-Enabled Approaches*, (1st ed.), 14–31, (2023). CRC Press. 10.1201/9781003357070-2

Baek, H., Cho, M., Kim, S., Hwang, H., Song, M., Yoo, S. Analysis of the length of hospital stay using electronic health records: A statistical and data mining approach. *PLoS One* 13(4), e0195901 (2018 Apr 13). 10.1371/journal.pone.0195901. PMID: 29652932; PMCID: PMC5898738.

Bauer, M., Fitzgerald, L., Haesler, E., Manfrin, M. Hospital discharge planning for frail older people and their families. Are we delivering best practices? A review of the evidence. *Journal of Clinical Nursing* 18, 2539–2546 (2009). https://onlinelibrary.wiley.com/doi/abs/10.1111/j.1365-2702.2008.02685.x

Beyan, O. D., Baykal, N. A knowledge-based search tool for performance measures in health care systems. *Journal of Medicine Systems* 36, 201–221 (2012). 10.1007/ s10916-010-9459-2

Bhambri, P., Rani, S., Gupta, G., Khang, A. *Cloud and Fog Computing Platforms for Internet of Things*, ISBN: 978-1-032-101507, (2022). CRC Press. 10.1201/9781003213888

Carini, E., Gabutti, I., Frisicale, E. M. et al. Assessing hospital performance indicators. What dimensions? Evidence from an umbrella review. *BMC Health Surveillance Research* 20, 1038 (2020). 10.1186/s12913-020-05879-y

Cornell, B., Hagger, V., Wilson, S. G., Evans, S. M., Sprivulis, P. C., Cameron, P. A. Measuring the quality of hospital care: An inventory of indicators. *Internal Medicine Journal* 39(6), 352–360 (June 2009). https://onlinelibrary.wiley.com/doi/abs/10.1111/j.1445-5994.2009.01961.x

Delloite; the value of patient experience Hospitals with better patient-reported experience perform better financially, (2018). https://scholar.google.com/scholar?cites=14628141446309628975&as_sdt=2005&sciodt=0,5&hl=en

Feijter, J. M. D., de Grave, W. S., Muijtjens, A. M., Scherpbier, A. J. J. A., Koopmans, R. P. A comprehensive overview of medical error in hospitals using incident-reporting systems, patient complaints, and chart review of inpatient deaths. *PLoS One* 7(2), e31125 (2012). https://journals.plos.org/plosone/article?id=10.1371/journal.pone.0031125

Flink, M., Ekstedt, M. Planning for the discharge, not for patient self-management at home - an observational and interview study of hospital discharge. *International Journal of Integrated Care* 17(6), 1 (2017 Nov 13). 10.5334/ijic.3003. PMID: 29588634; PMCID: PMC5854016.

Fried, B. J. Performance management. Human Resources in Healthcare: Managing for Success. Chicago 111 (2002). http://196.190.117.157:8080/jspui/bitstream/123456789/38920/1/12%202008.pdf

Friele, R. D., Sluijs, E. M., Legemaate, J. Complaints handling in hospitals: An empirical study of discrepancies between patients' expectations and their experiences. *BMC Health Surveillance Resilience* 8, 199 (2008). https://research.vumc.nl/ws/files/145120/219032.pdf

Gandjour, A., Kleinschmit, F., Littmann, V., Lauterbach, K. W. An evidence-based evaluation of quality and efficiency indicators. *Quality Management in Health Care: Summer* 10(4), 41–52 (2002). https://journals.lww.com/qmhcjournal/Fulltext/2002/10040/An_Evidence_Based_Evaluation_of_Quality_and.8.aspx

Groene, O., Skau, J. K. H., Frølich, A. An international review of projects on hospital performance assessment. *International Journal for Quality in Health Care* 20(3), 162–171 (June 2008), 10.1093/intqhc/mzn008

Hajimahmud, V. A., Khang, A., Hahanov, V., Litvinova, E., Chumachenko, S., Alyar, A. V. Autonomous Robots for Smart City: Closer to Augmented Humanity. *AI-Centric Smart City Ecosystems: Technologies, Design and Implementation*, (1st ed.), (2022). CRC Press. 10.1201/9781003252542-7

Jadhav, B. Psychological resilience- A conceptual framework. *Nova Science Publisher, USA*, 223–240. (2022). (ISBN 979-8-88697-316-7). doi: 10.52305/KRLL5890

Khang, A., Gupta, S. K., Hajimahmud, V. A., Babasaheb, J., Morris, G. *AI-Centric Modelling and Analytics: Concepts, Designs, Technologies, and Applications*, (1st ed.), (2023a). CRC Press. 10.1201/9781003400110

Khang, A., Hahanov, V., Litvinova, E., Chumachenko, S., Triwiyanto, Hajimahmud, V. A., Ali, R. N., Alyar, A. V., Anh, P. T. N. The Analytics of Hospitality of Hospitals in

Healthcare Ecosystem. *Data-Centric AI Solutions and Emerging Technologies in the Healthcare Ecosystem*, (1st ed.), (2023b), P (4). CRC Press. 10.1201/9781003356189

Khang A., Rani, S., Gujrati, R., Uygun, H., Gupta, S. K., (Eds.). *Designing Workforce Management Systems for Industry 4.0: Data-Centric and AI-Enabled Approaches*, (1st ed.), (2023c). CRC Press. 10.1201/99781003357070

Khang, A., Hahanov, V., Abbas, G. L., Hajimahmud, V. A. Cyber-Physical-Social System and İncident Management. *AI-Centric Smart City Ecosystems: Technologies, Design and Implementation*, (1st ed.), (2022a). CRC Press. 10.1201/9781003252542-2

Khang, A., Hahanov, V., Litvinova, E., Chumachenko, S., Hajimahmud, V. A., Alyar, A. V. The Key Assistant of Smart City - Sensors and Tools. *AI-Centric Smart City Ecosystems: Technologies, Design and Implementation*, (1st ed.), (2022b). CRC Press. 10.1201/9781003252542-17

Khang, A., Ragimova, N. A., Hajimahmud, V. A., Alyar, A. V. Advanced Technologies and Data Management in the Smart Healthcare System. *AI-Centric Smart City Ecosystems: Technologies, Design and Implementation*, (1st ed.), (2022c). CRC Press. 10.1201/9781003252542-16

Misra A., Shah V., Khang A., Gupta, S. K., (Eds.). *AI-Aided IoT Technologies and Applications in the Smart Business and Production*, (1st ed.), (2023). CRC Press. 10.1201/9781003392224

Rana, G., Khang, A., Sharma, R., Goel, A. K., Dubey, A. K. *Reinventing Manufacturing and Business Processes through Artificial Intelligence*, (2021). CRC Press. 10.1201/9781003145011

Rani, S., Chauhan, M., Kataria, A., Khang, A. IoT Equipped Intelligent Distributed Framework for Smart Healthcare Systems. *Networking and Internet Architecture*, (2021). CRC Press. 10.48550/arXiv.2110.04997

Reader, T. W., Gillespie, A., Roberts, J. Patient complaints in healthcare systems: A systematic review and coding taxonomy. *BMJ Quality & Safety* 23(8), 678–689 (2014). Epub 2014 May 29. PMID: 24876289; PMCID: PMC4112446. 10.1136/bmjqs-2013-002437

Tailor, R. K., Pareek, R., Khang, A., (Eds.). Robot Process Automation in Blockchain. *The Data-Driven Blockchain Ecosystem: Fundamentals, Applications, and Emerging Technologies*, (1st ed.), 149–164, (2022). CRC Press. 10.1201/9781003269281-8

Vrushank, S., Vidhi, T., Khang, A., 2023. Electronic Health Records Security and Privacy Enhancement Using Blockchain Technology. *Data-Centric AI Solutions and Emerging Technologies in the Healthcare Ecosystem*, (1st ed.), (2023), P (1). CRC Press. 10.1201/9781003356189

17 Simplified Hospital Management System
Robotic Process Automation (RPA) to Rescue

*Arpita Nayak, Ipseeta Satpathy, B.C.M. Patnaik,
Rashmi Gujrati, and Hayri Uygun*

CONTENTS

17.1 INTRODUCTION

In the current world, technology is growing more significant and crucial in the lives of numerous individuals and institutions. The usage of technology, for instance, may be noted as being greatly utilized in important fields such as education, entertainment, advertising, finance, warehousing, and health. This leads to the conclusion that automation is essential and required for firms to flourish in the current environment.

Organizational automation is seen as having a significant impact on how efficiently an organization operates while also assuring the delivery of high-quality services due to the birth and development of automation systems, which are playing an increasingly significant role within society; all these activities have become feasible. It has developed to be useful for carrying out tasks including gathering, processing, storing, retrieving, and suitably presenting information as needed.

Automation systems also play a crucial role in the organization's implementation of diverse technologies by integrating resource flows, organizational management activities, and departmental working processes. Automation systems are now so essential to an organization that it would be impossible for it to run efficiently without them. To ensure outstanding performance in the 21st century, especially for companies, they must have better systems that can combine their operations more successfully.

DOI: 10.1201/9781003356189-17

A hospital management system enables hospitals to manage data and information regarding all aspects of healthcare, encompassing protocols, providers, patients, and more, enabling the efficient and effective completion of operations. When one examines all of the features and divisions of a hospital, it becomes evident that a hospital management system (HMS) is vital.

The hospital database management system has advanced significantly since its debut in 1960, allowing it to be connected with the hospital's existing hardware, assets, technology, and systems (Khang et al., 2023).

Patients may now begin their health treatment in the palm of their hands, due to mobile equipment and applications. The method is then expanded to include hospitals and medical experts.

- HMS was developed to address the challenges involved with handling the entire patient paperwork related to each of the many departments of a hospital while protecting patient privacy.
- Employees are freed from having to compile and evaluate all patient paperwork in one area thanks to HMS.

A hospital is unquestionably a great option for the adaption of RPA given the vast volumes of data, the number of participants, and the numerous activities involved. Without efficient hospital management system software, hospitals cannot hope to function smoothly, deliver top-notch treatment, secure patient and other confidentiality of data, or run efficiently.

Less human participation in paperwork and other administrative tasks, lower employee headcount for tasks that can be completed easily inside the HMS, faster operations, lower mistake rates, and data protection and safety are some advantages of a hospital management system (Babasaheb et al., 2023).

Some of the major areas where robotic process automation (RPA) aids as a helping tool for HMS are inventory management, data management, and account man RPA uses a business rules engine to often automate choices based on established rules and circumstances. It also automates operations that involve structured data and logic.

RPA can handle unorganized datasets as well, but only after a bot harvests the data and utilizes tools like optical character recognition (OCR) and natural language processing (NLP) to turn it into structured data.

When an RPA system is combined with AI, it produces intelligent automation (IA), also known as cognitive automation, which seeks to closely resemble human talent and activities, frequently with the use of bot management, supply management, and much more. Healthcare organizations run without any slack and in real time.

Processes are slowed down by laborious, error-prone tasks that can have an impact on patient care, compliance, and cost structures. By automating operations that enhance data and reporting quality and speed up decision making, RPA software generates efficiency, as shown in figure 17.1. Costs will be reduced as a result, and resources will eventually be used where they are most needed (Khang et al., 2022d).

Because of the $1.1 trillion in administrative spending that happens each year, the healthcare business stands to profit substantially from automation technologies.

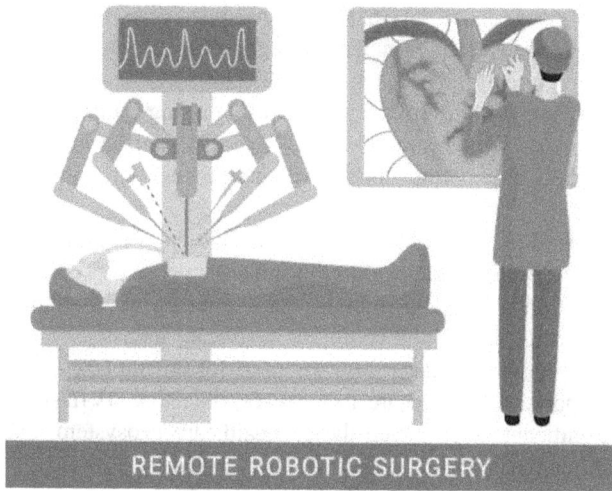

FIGURE 17.1   Illustration of RPA surgery in healthcare sector.

Source: iStock.

Pranay Kapadia, the CEO, stated according to Noteworthy, a healthcare process automation business, the healthcare industry demands eight times as much technology. Every other industry in the world uses as many materials per $1 billion in revenue. Even though given the human-centric nature of the health industry, we naturally think of RPA.

The healthcare business is one of the most technologically advanced. This is because of the vast number of data and manual, rule-based procedures that RPA is capable of handling. Complicated processes consume precious human capital and impede operations. This is especially relevant in light of the COVID-19 epidemic, which has put an enormous burden on the healthcare system and has made resource allocation a primary priority for hospitals.

Delays in diagnosis induced by COVID-19 caused and will continue to generate backlog and strain on the healthcare system, emphasizing the necessity for physicians and nurses to spend more time with patients rather than administrative, manual activities.

According to a 2021 survey, 92% of doctors spend some time on administrative chores that lead to burnout, and 64% believe there aren't enough employees to handle the massive amounts of patient data.

Healthcare RPA and IA firms offer to boost the ROI and output per hour of labor for physicians and employees in healthcare systems, resulting in increased productivity, fewer mistakes, and reduced burnout. Identifying methods that will make physicians' work less stressful is especially important in light of the "Great Resignation" (Thaler, 2022).

Organizations are using digitization for a growing number of various organizational processes. The HMS is the healthcare industry's primary priority, and it is also developing aggressively investigating innovative methods to improve performance, particularly in the private sector.

Processing organizational data has lately become more difficult due to its expanding amount, necessitating increased organizational resources to efficiently complete essential operations (Khang et al., 2022a).

Organizations are using digitization for an increasing number of various organizational activities. As a result of this demand, organizations are increasingly turning to workflow automation, such as robotic process automation (RPA) (Ratia et al., 2018).

There are several procedures associated with running a healthcare firm, ranging from paperwork to patient interactions to customer support to procuring supplies. In 2016, the U.S. Census Bureau warned that an aging population will cause a "demographic earthquake" in the country's healthcare industry.

The pandemic has only exacerbated the need for emergency medical treatment for the elderly population, who are more susceptible to COVID-19 issues. It has also shown significant holes inside the IT healthcare ecosystem, which must be filled to avoid healthcare systems from failing.

With a rising patient population, healthcare professionals will need to maintain large-scale inventories, billing, and claim to process, as well as massive amounts of digitization of patient records and patient registration. The challenge would be to ensure that all processes are flawless while also addressing patient pain points regularly.

The advantages of automation are numerous. It streamlines insurance approval processes, resulting in improved patient results. It also results in cost savings, which may then be utilized for front-line healthcare activities.

There are also fewer errors in the patient-care processes. According to Gartner, 50% of U.S. healthcare professionals anticipate investing in RPA technology over the next three years as a result of COVID-19.

Just 5% of them now use RPA technology. By a recent Accenture study, artificial intelligence might save the U.S. healthcare industry $150 billion each year by 2026. Some real-world examples of RPA application to simplify the HMS in the hospital unit are mentioned, to enhance engagement, Johns Hopkins Medicine, a renowned U.S. health institution, released AI-powered solutions to address clinician and caretaker burnout and assist them in achieving professional objectives.

The healthcare provider's conversation AI-powered documentation solutions seek to improve physician satisfaction and productivity increase quality measures for reporting and improve physician-patient relationships by reducing the load of paperwork on clinicians. Another example is a group of 50 Norwegian public hospitals and institutions that opted to automate a variety of time-consuming but routine tasks and create a centralized RPA system.

Maternity wards, monitoring and sending electronic epi crisis (the document that highlights patients' health case files) from hospitals to medical doctors, and access control were among the areas that saw significant workflow disruption (Khang & Hajimahmud, 2022b). These healthcare organizations saw several benefits, including time savings, elimination of unnecessary documentation, improved quality of the data, privacy, and greater staff engagement RPA adoption is critical for the success of healthcare systems.

It is critical that while using RPA, you have KPIs to measure its effectiveness as well as defined objectives and deployment road maps. Organizations must

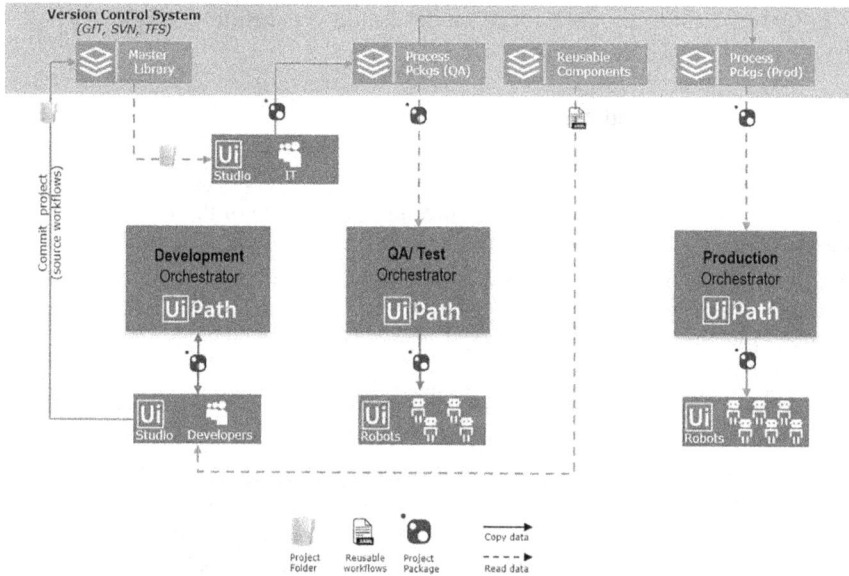

FIGURE 17.2 The model also contains a repository of reusable components (UiPath Automation Lifecycle, 2022).

Source: UiPath portal.

continually enhance their technologies this implementation makes the HMS process simpler. McKinsey & Company named RPA (in May 2019).

One of the transformative technologies that will alter healthcare and generate between $350 and $410 million in yearly value by 2025 have been discovered. RPA has already been utilized to speed up operations in healthcare as the world's scenario rapidly switched from life as normal to preparing for an epidemic in 2020, supporting organizations and professionals in coping with the COVID-19 overload. Over 30 COVID-19 usage instances have been gathered by UiPath (shows in figure 17.2).

1. Developers build the process, test, and debug pieces of it locally (Studio).
2. Once the automation development is completed, the process is published to the Development Orchestrator and tested again end-to-end.
3. The project folder is committed (not packaged) to a Master Library folder (on VCS).
4. The IT/RPA Operations team creates the project package for QA. This step is intended to be an additional safety measure: the automation source code is inspected (by a different entity) before being packaged and run by robots. For example, the packaged process is stored in the Process Packages (QA) folder on VCS, from which it is deployed to the QA robots and executed.
5. If any issue is revealed during the tests, the steps above are repeated.

6. Once all QA tests are passed, the package is pushed to a production environment, Process Pckgs (Prod).
7. When the process goes live, the process package is deployed to the production robots and executed.

A hospital in Dublin, for example, uses the company's RPA bots to analyze testing kit findings in seconds, saving the nursing staff an average of three hours each day. Another example is a Cleveland clinic that employs RPA for patient intake duties like as enrolling a patient. When the activities were conducted manually, the results were delivered in seconds rather than minutes. According to 2016 McKinsey research, the healthcare industry has a 36% technological automation potential (Vrushank et al., 2023a).

According to the authors of a 2019 study published in JMIR Research Protocols, routine procedures will surely be computerized in the future healthcare system. The most significant force behind future automation is anticipated to be healthcare robotic process automation. This is not hard to comprehend if you are conscious of both the increased productivity of human workers caused by technology and the reality that some kinds of automation indirectly raise jobs in addition to work for humans. RPA in healthcare will be made possible, which will advance and improve the HMS.

A computer system that aids in the administration of health data and the successful implementation of healthcare personnel's tasks is known as hospital management. RPA allows the HMS to process faster and reduces time consumption and result delivery.

Reduce the cost of healthcare administration, improving the speed of operations like triage, increasing the precision of data, tasks, and reporting in healthcare settings, increasing the efficiency of healthcare workers, and enhancing the patient experience are some of the benefits of enablement of RPA in the healthcare system improving the HMS system as stated in a study by IBM (Williams, 2021).

17.2 IMPACT OF RPA ON APPOINTMENT MANAGEMENT

The most common problem for hospitals, their management, and their personnel is to save operating expenses and achieve efficiency goals. In the meantime, most hospitals have insufficient resources. Their efforts to streamline the organization have made it harder for patients to move about freely during appointments and re-visits. Instead, during their stay, patients are routinely placed in long lines with little data.

More investments and installation of RPA in the appointment system is a tiny solution to this problem. All through the years, technological improvements in hospitals have enabled patients to arrange appointments in advance. The main compelling reason for the adoption of RPA in appointment management is the sudden exposure of humankind to COVID-19 scenario (Tailor, 2022).

Though appointment scheduling is almost entirely computerized in healthcare these days, it is still a mostly manual process for the majority of enterprises. Even when done online, it is the responsibility of an individual to process, arrange, input, amend, and reschedule meetings as they occur. Instead, RPA may automate calendar administration, scheduling appointments, cancellations, appointment revisions, and reminders to patients for forthcoming appointments and confirmations for patients, physicians, and administrators (Dunlap, 2022).

Because of its repetitive, step-oriented character, appointment booking is one of the best RPA processes. RPA may look at both patient and doctor calendars to help with appointment scheduling, assess how frequently a patient needs to visit a doctor, and pass the accessibility of both the clinician and the patient. RPA allows patients to make appointments without interacting with hospital personnel. This speed-up triage increases appointment turnout and improves the patient experience (Thaler, 2022).

Software robots called RPAs automate repetitive human work. The initial stages in integrating a RPA into the system is to understand the attributes, deconstruct each operation into a process flow, and then build and test a robot for each task. An RPA-ML-based eye examination was offered as a rough idea. We used RPA to help us build new roles within the screening program, such as registration, medical calendar management, and payment systems (Thainimit et al., 2022).

The healthcare system comprises a slew of time-consuming operations, such as claim processing, that need significant resource allocation. This leads to higher operating expenses and slower procedures. When it comes to the hospital or healthcare industry, the doctor is more concerned with data management than with addressing the patient, especially when they are amid several chores. The only way to retain the effort and time spent by healthcare professionals on patient care instead of other responsibilities is to automate that process.

Robotic process automation (RPA) automates procedures like appointment scheduling, medication booking, and claim management by sending bills on the computer. Employees might unshackle themselves and relax as a result of the weight of several complicated jobs. Healthcare practitioners will be able to handle patient difficulties by using the potential of technology and RPA, resulting in faster healthcare procedures, more efficient healthcare systems, and more patient satisfaction.

With the use of RPA technology in the health sector, patients will be able to arrange appointments without the involvement of hospital workers. The program also helps to improve customer interactions by allowing patients to swiftly arrange appointments at their leisure, reducing the amount of allocation of resources in appointment scheduling.

RPA bots are built to follow predefined rules. Individuals can make mistakes willingly or inadvertently, but bots cannot make mistakes when they take the position of humans. When there are no problems in the code, the rule-based tasks are completely error-free (Nallasivam, 2022).

On December 30, 2019, the first case of COVID-19 was identified in Wuhan Jinyintan Hospital in Hubei, China, followed by the lockdown implemented in the city at 10 AM on January 23, 2020, and instructed citizens to stay in the city if they got specific permission motives for departing.

Hospitals got redesigned the physical structure of outpatient services, established designated spaces for inpatient care for suspected or confirmed patients, and implemented new rules and guidelines for hospital administration in response to the COVID-19 epidemic.

RPA helped manage the HMS during this crucial period. Hospitals are finding it difficult to document and organize the appointment scheduling procedure because of the social distance. RPA has made it possible for systems to arrange appointments online while ensuring people's security in instances like these and upholding the social distance norm (Yan et al., 2020).

The management and processing of patient information is the main issue facing the healthcare industry. Employees in the healthcare sector spend a lot of time completing manual and rule-based tasks across several platforms. Applications for enrolment, scheduling appointments, invoicing, and clinical data extraction are a few of these tasks (Kim, 2014). Patient services take longer as a result, which lowers productivity and lengthens wait times.

A RPA technology can automate these time-consuming tasks, freeing up staff to concentrate on patient care. The objectives are to identify moment hospital jobs and evaluate their RPA potential to develop RPA applications (Khang et al., 2022e), where a software robot may autonomously complete the creation stronger than a person, enhancing workflow efficiency, as shown in figure 17.3.

In the period from 2017 to 2018, ESNEFT missed over 8 million healthcare appointments, excluding canceled ones. Patient appointments worth £1 billion were missed yearly due to missing appointments, which was the main problem.

There was no systematic way to keep track of and report missed appointments. Within eight weeks of deployment, ESNEFT was able to avoid missing 1365 appointments valued at £216,960, thanks to intelligent automation technologies. Thus, it is predicted that eliminating missed appointments will result in yearly savings of about £2.1 million.

Appointment cancellations are now routinely communicated to digital staff members so that the time may be transferred to new patients. Additionally, freeing up medical professionals from front desk duties can allow them to focus on patient care and other value-added tasks (Rajkhowa & Joshi, 2020).

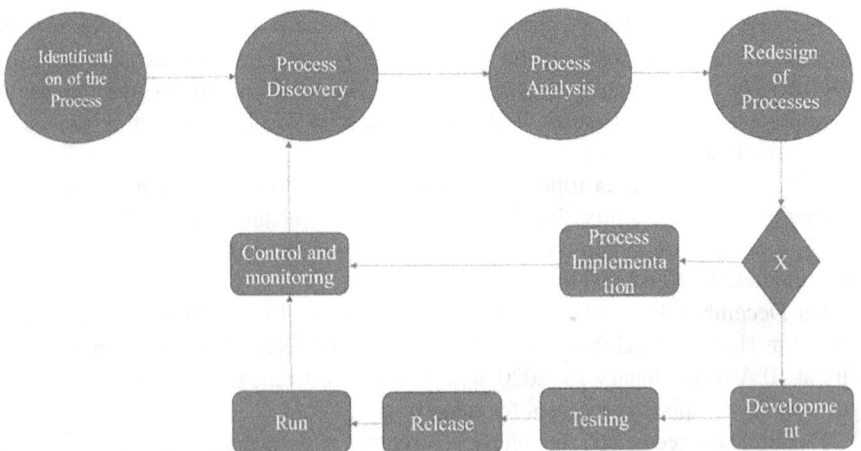

FIGURE 17.3   RPA life cycle.

Source: Author's owner.

The fast advancement of medical research has allowed for a rise in life expectancy worldwide, but as people live longer, healthcare systems must deal with escalating service demands, growing expenditures, and a workforce that cannot adequately serve patient requirements. The amount spent on healthcare is just not keeping up.

Without substantial structural and technological reforms, the healthcare system won't be able to maintain itself. Health systems require a greater workforce, however, even if the economy will add 40 million new employments to the health sector by 2030. According to the World Health Organization, there might be a 9.9 million medical, nurse, and midwife shortage in the global medical sector over that time. Therefore, we must make sure that they spend their time on patient care, where it brings the greatest value.

Professionals with high levels of expertise oversee the healthcare sector. Highly qualified individuals run the healthcare sector, and their time is incredibly precious. However, over 40% of the time spent by specialists is wasted on non-value-added tasks. Here comes healthcare robotic process automation.

The majority of these repetitive, low-value duties may be automated with RPA in healthcare, freeing up your healthcare staff to focus on more crucial responsibilities. With RPA, processes in the healthcare industry may be automated quickly, with high quality, and accuracy.

Globally, life expectancy has increased due to significant medical science advancements, but as people live longer, healthcare systems must deal with escalating service needs, growing expenditures, and a workforce that is unable to satisfy patient expectations. "By 2050, one in four persons in North America and Europe will be above the age of, according to McKinsey & Company. This implies that the healthcare systems will have to cope with more patients who have complicated demands. It is expensive to manage these patients, and systems must change from a philosophy of episodic care toward one that is considerably more pro-active and centered on long-term patient care."

RPA in healthcare can facilitate one-click installations of sophisticated software systems in addition to simple activities like auto-generating email answers and much more. Online appointment scheduling is common.

Healthcare facilities must gather personal data, diagnoses, and insurance information as part of the registration procedure. It might be laborious to make appointments using patient data (Rani et al., 2021).

Additionally, a patient's visit needs to be planned around the availability of doctors at hospitals and their various schedules. If the patient has to be diagnosed, the pediatrician's visit schedule must be modified. Additionally, if any doctors are unable to see their patients, the hospital personnel must let their patients know ahead of time. Therefore, making patient appointments might be difficult.

RPA in healthcare can allay any worries regarding patient appointment scheduling. RPA bots can automate the gathering and processing of data. Using this method, RPA bots may optimize patient appointments depending on their diagnosis, location, and the availability of their doctors.

17.3   RPA'S EFFECT ON ACCOUNT MANAGEMENT

Any institution that manages money may be said to have a strong accounting department. As a result, it has a big impact on the healthcare sector and helps it reach its full potential.

Any firm that wants to be financially cost-effective must have an accounting department. Processing claims and billing is frequently highly repetitive. RPA may automate these procedures, allowing bots to handle claim administration tasks including initial inquiries or follow-up. Processing claims and billing is frequently highly repetitive.

RPA may automate these procedures, allowing bots to handle claim administration tasks including initial inquiries or follow-up. The cost of RPA software is a pittance of what healthcare organizations pay staff members to perform manual operations. The healthcare sector may save $13.3 billion, per the CAQH report, if administrative duties are mechanized in the revenue cycle.

The time-consuming and repetitive process involved in claiming administration, including entering, processing, and evaluating documents and data, may result in a delay in billing after a health service has been delivered. In addition to automating time consuming tasks, a RPA-led claim management system may eliminate human errors during offers a systematic.

Given that Medicare loses over $60 billion a year due to fraud, mistakes, and misuse, according to the U.S. Center for Elder Justice, this is advantageous for healthcare providers. We can understand by taking the example of one of the biggest healthcare organizations Max Healthcare Institute, which is situated in New Delhi, India.

Every day, they focus on the process of processing patient transaction data. They regularly need to automate routine procedures including collecting client information, handling claims, and data rebalancing for government health programs. The institute planned to start small and expand as needed, but the major aim was to make existing procedures more efficient to assure higher accuracy and faster turnaround times.

They collaborated with a RPA consulting company to determine the best places to employ robotic automation and where the greatest effect might be made. To manage the following processes more effectively, the institute deployed a RPA platform: to deal with the smooth process of accounting systems like Filing Claims, Reconciliation of Data for the Central Government Health Program (CGHS, Data Reconciliation for the Contributory Health Program for Ex-Servicemen (ECHS).

Max Healthcare was able to cut turnaround time with this approach (TAT). For the billing process, the TAT was cut by at least 50%, and CGHS and ECHS had time reductions of between 65% and 75% (Dilmegani, 2020). RPA enables us to operate more efficiently.

In the long run, automation is inexpensive to deploy and doesn't require extensive system integration. It provides seamless integration with workflows and digital assets. In a study, Neeta Mehta Cofounder of Automation Anywhere stated that technology has only one function, which is to enable people. It can automate data digitization and accounts payable operations, increasing the efficiency of billing.

Healthcare organizations may save a lot of money and labor by modernizing their administrative procedures. RPA + AI delivers on the promise of bringing the experiences of patients and front-line employees into sharp focus (Rani et al., 2022). Time is saved, process accuracy is increased, and the impossible is made attainable for everyone thanks to technology. This is crucial since it has the biggest effects on the healthcare industry (Seuwou, 2021).

Reducing total costs and boosting efficiency are two of the top financial goals, say three out of four CEOs of hospitals and health systems, according to research by Healthcare Leaders. Automation of manual operations may be a significant component of the overall plan for performance improvement in the healthcare sector, which is always seeking ways to increase efficiency, reduce costs, and enhance quality (Khang et al., 2022b).

The volume of data that is received and processed in the finance and accounting sector has increased during the past ten years. The processing of these transactions might occasionally take longer than expected for physical teams. Bring in RPA. For audits, reporting, and compliance, automation software has made it possible for response times to be sped up.

The repetitive labor that was previously performed by human employees has also been eliminated, freeing them up to work on duties that have a more immediate effect on the organization's bottom line.

The smooth functioning of accounts with help of RPA helps in achieving a simplified process in HMS. The numerous benefits that Period-end closure benefits from RPA include reconciling low-risk accounts, closing sub-ledgers, confirming journal entries, and combining the general ledger (Khang et al., 2022d).

In fact, managers need process for making monthly, half-yearly close, internal efficiency and management reporting (collecting and analyzing operating and economic data), outside regulatory and statutory reporting, maintaining (updating, vetting) client data, creating receipts, simplifying authorizations, confirming and recording payments, collecting, billing, and correlating receipts with sales and purchase orders; money management (Tailor et al., 2022).

A study in qbotica suggested RPA helps in making the HMS system simpler by handling difficult tasks like scanning papers for important information, switching between computer programs, generating reports, and creating permission requests, it is useful to configure a robot with data capture tools.

RPA helps in making complex works like more accurate financial reporting, processing of purchase orders and invoices, reconciliation of accounts, report data aggregation, client information management, preparing tax reports, and submitting payments and Income audits more streamlined and precise.

Companies are increasingly looking to automation and robotics automation (RPA) technologies that can imitate human behavior and handle repetitive activities to be nimbler, process data more quickly, and boost productivity. More than 52.8% of professional accountants who participated in a recent Deloitte poll (bit.ly/2Vm8aGp) said that their companies want to use automation processes, analytics, and other technology in the upcoming years.

The need for business graduates with these talents has skyrocketed as a result of the growing usage of automation technologies in enterprises data entry personnel insert information from supplier invoices into the system for accounts payable operations that utilize human coding. The duties of reproducing data from an invoice, comparing that data with other data sets kept in a database, and creating reports and alarms may all be carried out swiftly by RPA.

The bot scans an email account for invoices from suppliers in the form of PDF attachments. The bot transmits critical data about that supplier into an Excel worksheet once every day. When the bot identifies an exception, it flags the transaction for human inspection (Tietz et al., 2020).

Financial institutions (FIs) were among the first to recognize the advantages of RPA and incorporate it into many of their applications. One of the procedures that have been RPA-adapted is account reconciliation. Other processes include reporting and tax planning. RPA has been a buzzword in the business for a while now, but it has only just begun to develop into a technology that is affordable to the majority of enterprises.

The RPA market has roughly tripled each year, and it is expected to expand by more than 50% by 2020. The Turkish market has experienced significant growth as well; between 2018 and 2020, more than 130 leading enterprises integrated RPA robots into their infrastructure.

Turkey's banks and IT firms use RPA 50% quicker than other industries do (Doguc, 2021). RPA has several advantages in the accounting sector. Accounting that is automated streamlines processes, lower mistake rates, and increases cash flow.

Furthermore, businesses are better positioned to generate important insights for better judgment and long-term stability with reliable financial data obtained through automated operations (Rana et al., 2021).

Automated accounting uses machine learning (ML) and artificial intelligence (AI) to carry out conventional accounting tasks like documenting transactions and compiling them into financial statements. It automates repetitive operations that would otherwise be laborious and time-consuming to complete manually, freeing up time for financial experts to concentrate on the main business (Khanh & Khang, 2021).

Organizations may guarantee data accuracy and regularly complete their books on time with the help of the correct accounting software. Data input tasks are highly accurate with automated accounting, especially when documenting transactions. The processing of transactional procedures like billing and payments is possible with the press of a button.

By doing this, businesses may run more effectively while gathering insightful financial data. Accounts receivable-related chores are replaced by automation. Companies can quickly create and distribute invoices, reconcile bills, and remind clients to make payments on time. Furthermore, automated accounting systems refresh data in real time, enhancing invoice accuracy, and facilitating speedier payment and cash flow for organizations (Achettu, 2022).

Healthcare organizations are required to keep track of, calculate, and evaluate the costs associated with diagnosing and treating each patient. This kind of data processing manually might be time-consuming.

For the correct bill computation for each patient, keeping track of numerous tests, prescriptions, doctor fees, wardroom prices, and other services is also essential. As a result, the entire procedure may become quite difficult for the hospital personnel.

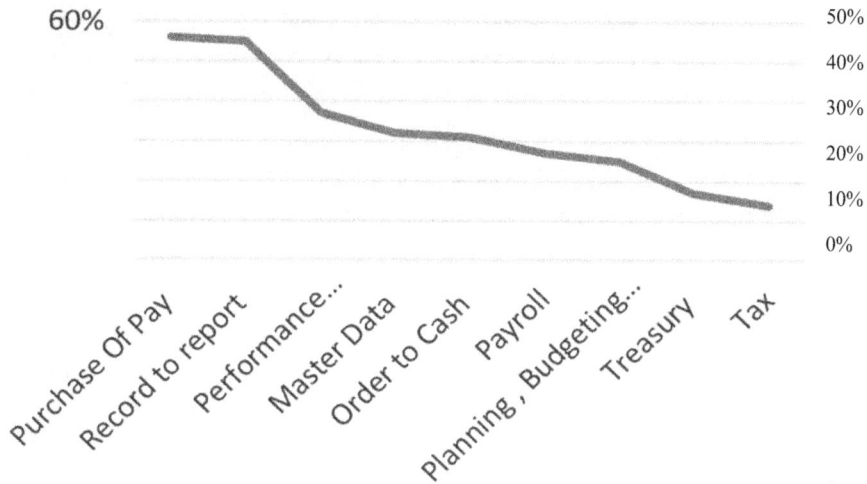

FIGURE 17.4 The utilization percentage for several functions.

Source: Author's owner.

By taking into account the cost of tests, medications, wardroom, meals, and doctor fees, RPA bots can accurately calculate the bill's total. By deploying RPA in the sector, healthcare providers may end payment delays and billing calculation errors. RPA can therefore greatly speed up account settlements in the healthcare industry. The finance function of a business is a fantastic example of where RPA may be applied and used effectively.

The most common uses for RPA are in the purchase-to-pay and record report processes. RPA has also been used to master data, which makes it possible to manage organization data more quickly and effectively (ACCA et al., 2018) (figure 17.4).

17.4 THE COMPELLING IMPACT OF RPA ON DATA MANAGEMENT

Satya Nadella, Microsoft CEO, has stated that "Everything is going to be connected to cloud and data … all of this will be mediated by software." The process of storing, maintaining, and analyzing data obtained from various sources are referred to as healthcare data management.

By managing the abundance of readily accessible healthcare data, health systems may create complete pictures of individuals, modify treatments, foster engagement, and enhance health outcomes.

All digital endeavors rely on data in some way, whether it is through key performance indicators (KPI) displays, optimization algorithms, or predictive modeling, which are now categorized as descriptive, predictive, and prescriptive data analysis.

Data management is a critical part of the area of industries. Many businesses subject master data generation to tight control methods, such as the four-eye concept, several gateways, and a predilection for drop-down options. This is done to decrease the incidence of errors with master data. However, several elements contribute to the process of sustaining data quality. Users must manually move data across unconnected systems since there are no direct connections between them.

Business processes that deal with data quality are created in a Greenfield environment without taking other business objectives or competing for operational imperatives into account. Business processes lack consistency, consistency in onboarding, training, and retraining, which quickly deteriorates process adherence.

Good data quality advantages are only noticeable at very diverse points in the value generation process, creating an issue. RPA is viewed by many enterprises as a typically affordable option that helps to reduce compliance risk and save time.

RPA has developed beyond simple screen-scraping to aid firms in maximizing efficiency and fostering commercial expansion in more intricate and crucial activities. Master data generation is one of many everyday tasks carried out manually in businesses that are currently thought to be too little or unimportant to be automated. Such regular tasks can be carried out by RPA by running across systems. Routine tasks that are done every day thousands of times and don't vary over time have been the major focus of RPA.

One of the many different forms of data that may be found in a healthcare environment is administrative data. Although administrative data entry frequently doesn't need specialist expertise, it may be an extremely monotonous process.

RPA may gather data inputs from several sources using language processing, voice recognition, and image recognition, some of which might need bots to translate into structured data. After that, the organization must use the data by entering it into a database or other repository.

(Williams, 2021; Radke et al., 2020). Before the pandemic, research predicted that by 2025, RPA in the healthcare sector will create an annual value of $350 billion to $410 billion. The healthcare sector saw a profound transformation as a result of the development of RPA (robotic process automation). RPA may be used to implement individualized care while lowering overall expenses and raising the standard of care.

Additionally, this guarantees complete compliance with rules and regulations, minimizes errors, and blunders, and ultimately boosts operational effectiveness. Automated methods increase the security of data flow (Khang et al., 2022c).

The reports area is handled by people, thus yet another employee or an unauthorized individual may gain access to the reports. The paper documents are straightforward to retrieve even if this wasn't the aim. However, automatic procedures restrict access to those who are permitted, keeping it secure.

The deployment of RPA in the healthcare sector also makes it possible to save data electronically, extract it, and migrate it for a variety of uses, including research and second opinions. The program can identify the data in source documents, emails, or attachments. For data recognition, bots search for patterns. For instance, the bot may search the document for information that matches the pattern MM/DD/YYYY, month, day, or year, to get the date. Even though patterns might be challenging, bots can detect a wide range of forms.

Adding to this some noted benefits of RPA in data management is a 360-degree amalgamation of all available resources, increase patient involvement, by monitoring existing health trends and anticipating forthcoming ones, improved health outcomes in certain geographic areas, and enhance population health outcomes in certain geographic regions by monitoring existing health trends and anticipating new ones (Gupta, 2022).

Access to and transfer of patient data must be automated. RPA is used in many healthcare institutions, speeding up the procedure. Additionally, it enables them to add the patient's information after it is gathered, allowing the hospital to share the data with other facilities and departments as needed.

Data exchange across healthcare institutions is beneficial, and implementing RPA has made it simple because the facility can do so much more readily than before RPA wasn't in place. If the patient's diagnosis includes another department, data transfer reduces the amount of effort required for therapy. It enables the connection of every device in a building to a single network, enabling data from one device to be accessed by another.

Time is saved since less administrative work is required, making the process of saving more lives easier and quicker.

To improve security standards, the institution must constantly be staffed with technological professionals and properly certified in security (Badnakhe, 2022). Robots are programmed to perform processes and data flow equal to those of a human user, and they understand applications from third parties.

RPA solutions, on the other hand, may be used by quasi-business users while traditional automated solutions frequently demand a greater level of programming knowledge.

The administration and configuration of the underlying data are crucial components in allowing RPA implementation (Vishnu et al., 2017). Because of its capacity to automate simple rule-based processes, robotic process automation has spread across various industry sectors' repetitive and laborious operations, extending the usage scenarios and will continue to expand in response to corporate needs. RPA denotes robotic process automation, and it provides cost-effective benefits with increased efficiency and accuracy.

RPA could be utilized to automate hospital administrative tasks such as maintaining patient records, medical history, and complaints system such as complaints, review process, and other data gathering tasks. From the bulk of data, RPA helps in finding out employment history verification, candidate sourcing, onboarding process, payroll processing, employee data management, cost management, and absence management, and makes sure the availability of those information quickly.

An elaborate study has highlighted that patient health data, billing, purchasing, vital statistics, monitoring, health records, and insurance are all datasets that the healthcare business interacts with. The data varies greatly, making it difficult to keep both processes and resources simplified. Low efficiency, sluggish reaction times, and reliability are other key factors that contribute to financial losses. One of the most important tasks for any hospital is ensuring a seamless patient care path.

Private details, diagnoses and problems, treatment statuses, medication descriptions, and other information comprise the patient's health data. Maintaining and evaluating a vast volume of data manually is beyond the capability of humans over time. Enterprises and hospitals can collect and optimize large amounts of data considerably faster with robotic process automation software.

Furthermore, data collected at a single location may be transferred between departments. Thus, by arranging surgeries and other medical treatments till follow-ups, the treatment path is synchronized. Aside from the treatment path, other advantages of robotic process automation include faster detection and response times to cyber-attacks, data corruption of data prevention, tracking errors, and fraud prevention in the system. It keeps records and provides data-driven judgment and forecasts to help with revenue cycle management. All of the tools can assist with financial difficulties and concealed revenue losses.

Overall, RPA is an excellent tool for effective hospital management, guaranteeing simple administrative operations, sound financial decision making, and healthcare delivery system synchronization (Morris et al., 2023).

The load on hospitals is expanding at an alarming rate as the demand for healthcare grows. Physically operating hospitals and clinics in every region are getting increasingly challenging. Similarly, maintaining appointment scheduling and medical record systems are getting increasingly complicated.

Without a doubt, due to its numerous advantages, robotic process automation can handle the issue and ensures a smooth HMS flow. Healthcare firms are increasingly concerned with lowering costs while enhancing consumer service quality.

In India, one of the most significant challenges that companies confront is maintaining and processing data that they now have in the form of physical papers or paper trails. This comprises internal and external information, billings, claims administration, patient enrolment, reporting, and so forth.

Integrating this data can assist healthcare businesses in identifying current gaps throughout all processes as well as automating dull, repetitive procedures. Several top healthcare companies across the world are now exploring RPA in healthcare programs while striving to integrate RPA solutions into their existing IT platforms (Misra et al., 2023).

The key RPA use applications in healthcare are focused on increasing throughput, decreasing manual labor, and increasing the efficacy of standardized, large-scale procedures. For example, employing chatbots to speed up claims data analysis and claims administration for insurers, reduce FWA (fraud, waste, and abuse) in claims management and communicating information with patients, make appointments, and improve patient involvement.

RPA in healthcare, in conjunction with cognitive automation, can assist expediting patient support in a variety of channels, including clinical support, monitoring health lapses, and providing information to patients.

In less than a year, a hospital in Texas was anticipated to increase its employment from 350 to even more than 1,100 experts. They employed RPA to automate their monthly basis load, which was gaffe, time consuming, and expensive.

The implementation also allowed them to confirm payment correctness on test complaints, manage and track day-to-day activities, and process the block based task, which represents the bulk of claims gathered, as well as adjust it to handle numerous typical controls.

The statistics in the healthcare industry are the most significant components of what happens in hospitals. The data contains a wealth of information on patients and other areas of hospital operations.

The manual labor of streamlining data becomes a frantic duty for the working employees and, of course, is time consuming. RPA enables the duties in an easier flow and is less time-consuming, which all contribute to the efficient operation of HMS (Khang et al., 2022e).

17.5 ROLE OF RPA IN INVENTORY MANAGEMENT

SCM (supply chain management) is another term for hospital or healthcare inventory management. It is a procedure that manages your health system's stock, operations, bookings, payments, and other data.

A stock control system is essential in healthcare organizations that handle medical supplies, order and deliver prescriptions, or sell healthcare products to consumers. Inventory management systems assist major firms in reducing both financial and product waste by maintaining a complete and up-to-date inventory of items and resources.

The major challenge that hospital inventory management handles are difficulty tracking the stored listed items, and pharmaceutical expiry date monitoring.

RPA assists in tracking the usage of all commodities within the healthcare facility. This system software allows the healthcare firm or organization to keep track of revenues and expenses. It also recognizes and accounts for both edible and non-consumable medications and products.

Hospitals and other healthcare organizations can use hospital inventory management systems to replace antiquated and inefficient inventory monitoring techniques. Controlling their inventories and tracking assets is also not a problem here.

Everything is simple and manageable. You are well aware that having a comprehensive, secure, virtualized system on hand may provide several advantages. Inventories can be classified in a variety of ways, such as distributing pharmaceuticals based on their expiration dates or registering the equipment with its maintenance data, among others.

According to recent research, around 72% of firms today have implemented RPA to automate monotonous tasks and simplify inventory management.

By implementing a focused and streamlined supply chain strategy using a healthcare inventory management system, healthcare firms can save 17.7% or $11 million per site per year. According to IBM BPM research, any hospital may accurately track up-to-date stock information with the aid of inventory management software.

The most commonly used items/things at the hospital are pharmaceuticals and surgical equipment. Every hospital should maintain a sufficient supply of medicines. It should also include vaccinations and biodegradable materials for use during an operation or surgery, such as masks, syringes, gloves, and so on.

Technology advancement has resulted in the employment of smart technologies to carry out activities and occupations via automated procedures. As the world grows increasingly mechanized and industrialized, it becomes more important to automate jobs and processes for more efficiency, lower costs, and higher product quality.

There should be adequate pharmaceuticals in hospitals; however, it has been discovered that many hospitals have a shortfall of medicines owing to a lack of efficient stock management. This issue is readily remedied by implementing RPA technology in the delivery, storage, and stock of medications, and automatically scheduling the drugs first before stock runs out.

The study conducted by Dasu and Radhakumari highlighted the before and after effects of the implementation of RPA in the system for easy handling of inventory management. Inventory management is one such crucial company operation that must be efficiently handled for the effective functioning of HMS. Underestimation of inventory raw materials frequently leads to incorrect orders, affecting customer satisfaction.

Maintaining an excess inventory level, on the other hand, results in raw material depletion. Inefficient inventory management costs are both high and unneeded. The authors have considered the adaption of UiPath (RPA Company) for the implementation of RPA in their inventory management system.

An effective RPA execution provides the management with a text-to-speech digital assistant bot that analyses transaction records and tells him or her of available inventory items, prepares a file of things that must be reordered, and, following gaining the manager's authorization, orders the products, and sends a message to the supplier.

ata entry done manually into warehouse management systems has several drawbacks, including high mistake rates; slow turnaround time; and a lack of consistency. Additional workers are being hired to double-check the correctness of manually inputted data. Increased mistake rates as a result of unanticipated increases in manual data input. Attention is diverted from cognitive work to rule-based tasks, resulting in lower employee productivity.

This study uses robotic process automation, a ground-breaking, novel machine learning technology, was utilized to automate the business operations conducted in a warehouse management system's stock control and management module (Mungla, 2019).

A shortage of medical supplies might have significant consequences, both monetarily and in terms of patient care. Inventory control for such items is a hard and time-consuming task, especially when numerous departments or locations are involved.

The use of a robotic process automation and artificial intelligence (RPA + AI) system results in better, more efficient ordering decisions.

In any domain of industry let it be inventory management is a very peculiar and minute task that needs a lot of manpower and is also time-consuming; hence, automation could find the solution for the same as shown in figure 17.5.

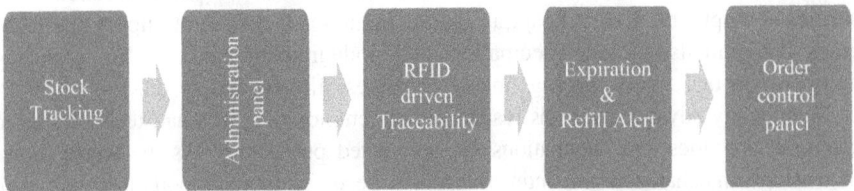

FIGURE 17.5   Illustration of inventory software features that will benefit the healthcare industry.

Source: Author's owner and adapted context from Sugalo, 2022.

Medical items range from simple syringes to pricey implants and surgical gear. Since these greater consumables make up the majority of the hospital's budget, monitoring medical inventory is crucial for good financial management.

A good inventory control system can not only enhance patient care but also avoid or mitigate the following difficulties. A hospital inventory control system is a multi-tiered software solution that assists physicians in keeping track of medications, medical items, equipment, and processes (Tailor et al., 2022).

A useful inventory management system provides five fundamental elements that enhance the hospital management system, as shown in figure 4, that aid in the administration of hospital goods.

Goods locators can assist to avoid potentially harmful circumstances, such as when a drug is needed immediately but neither the personnel nor the doctor in authority knows where it is (Vrushank et al., 2023b).

Expiration warnings notify users of pharmaceuticals that are about to expire before it's too late. Surplus medical supplies ordering is a widespread practice in healthcare institutions. Doctors and nurses can use medical inventory software to produce a list of items to buy in the amounts needed (Sugalo, 2022).

The enablement of RPA has been taken up by The University Hospital Birmingham (UHB) National Health Service Foundation Trust used RPA technology to speed up patient registration (Hajimahmud et al., 2022).

The project's purpose was to integrate registration kiosks to establish an efficient, simple, and transparent patient registration experience. In compliance with the NPfIT security policy, these kiosks are required to connect to the National Program of IT Patient Administration System (NPfIT or PAS). This technology would also have to be operational in a relatively short period before the launch of a new hospital.

Robotic process automation technology, on the other hand, has the capacity (without this deep link) to quickly access the system while adhering to the security rules, and did so within the needed period. The hospital's usage of patient identification kiosks had positive outcomes.

More than half of the patients enrolled in these kiosks, healthcare through reception was twice as fast, and personnel was 50% more productive.

The kiosks were well received by patients, who said they were simple and quick to use. The patient identification kiosks were simply the beginning of University Hospitals Birmingham's robotics process automation. After the success of RPA technology in kiosks, the hospital expanded its use to other corporate functions (Primer, 2015).

17.6 CONCLUSION

Automation is the need of the hour! RPA has the potential to change the healthcare business due to its shown impacts on time-saving, effort, and money. By implementing robotic process automation, healthcare workers will be able to concentrate on improving patient outcomes and it provides a very effective hand for the hospital management system.

RPA has proven time and again that it only helps the successful running of hospitals by assisting with crucial parts of HMS like inventory, data, accounts, and appointment scheduling. When it comes to entering, organizing, and analyzing large volumes of medical data, the digital workforce's ability to offer rapid and reliable findings will significantly contribute to expanding access to treatment. Maximizing the use of RPA adoption in health is a potential strategy for tackling industry-specific challenges.

RPA (robotic process automation) is simple and allows for rapid deployment of solutions, allowing the healthcare industry to improve every procedure and process from patient registration through claim administration. Human tasks are time consuming and error-prone, whereas RPA can readily imitate prescribed work procedures.

Healthcare providers may avoid costly and lengthy digital conversion programs by utilizing RPA-enabled automation and rapid execution plans. RPA has transformed the healthcare sector by saving time, energy, and money, decreasing paperwork, increasing working efficiency, and eventually enhancing patient care, which is where the main value of the healthcare industry lies (Khang et al., 2023).

REFERENCES

ACCA, CA ANZ, KPMG Australia. (2018). Embracing robotic automation during the evolution on finance. *The Association of Chartered Certified Accountants*. https://www.ifac.org/system/files/publications/files/Audit-Quality-in-a-Multidisciplinary-Firm.pdf

Achettu, B. (2022, January 18). Top 8 benefits of automated accounting for entrepreneurial organizations. *AGA*. Retrieved January 18, 2022, from https://acceleratedgrowth.com/blog-details/the-top-8-benefits-of-automatedaccounting-for-entrepreneurial-organizations

Babasaheb, J., Sphurti, B., Khang, A. (2023). Industry Revolution 4.0: Workforce Competency Models and Designs. *Designing Workforce Management Systems for Industry 4.0: Data-Centric and AI-Enabled Approaches* (1st ed.), 14–31. CRC Press. 10.1201/9781003357070-2

Badnakhe, R. (2022, September 9). RPA in healthcare- use cases and benefits. *Product Engineering Services*. Retrieved September 9, 2022, from https://www.einfochips.com/blog/rpa-in-healthcare-use-cases-and-benefits/

Dilmegani, C. (2020, October 8). RPA in healthcare: Benefits, use cases & case studies in 2022. *AIMultiple*. Retrieved October 8, 2020, from https://research.aimultiple.com/rpa-healthcare/

Doguc, O. (2021). Applications of robotic process automation in finance and accounting. *Beykent Üniversitesi Fen ve Mühendislik Bilimleri Dergisi*, 14(1), 51–59. https://dergipark.org.tr/en/pub/bujse/article/906795

Dunlap, S. (2022, April 12). What is the role of RPA in healthcare? *Impact. Impact Networking*. Retrieved April 12, 2022, from https://www.impactmybiz.com/blog/rpain-healthcare

Gupta, D. (2022, September 9). Top 5 applications of RPA in healthcare. Appinventiv. Retrieved September 9, 2022, from https://appinventiv.com/blog/rpa-inhealthcare/

Hajimahmud, V. A., Khang, A., Hahanov, V., Litvinova, E., Chumachenko, S., Alyar, A. V. (2022). Autonomous Robots for Smart City: Closer to Augmented Humanity. *AI-Centric Smart City Ecosystems: Technologies, Design and Implementation* (1st ed.). CRC Press. 10.1201/9781003252542-7

Khang, A., Hahanov, V., Abbas, G. L., Hajimahmud, V. A. (2022a). Cyber-Physical-Social System and İncident Management. *AI-Centric Smart City Ecosystems: Technologies, Design and Implementation* (1st ed.). CRC Press. 10.1201/9781003252542-2

Khang, A., Chowdhury, S., Sharma, S., (Eds.). (2022b). *The Data-Driven Blockchain*

Ecosystem: Fundamentals, Applications, and Emerging Technologies (1st ed.). CRC Press. 10.1201/9781003269281

Khang, A., Hahanov, V., Litvinova, E., Chumachenko, S., Hajimahmud, V. A., Alyar, A. V. (2022c). The Key Assistant of Smart City - Sensors and Tools. *AI-Centric Smart City Ecosystems: Technologies, Design and Implementation* (1st ed.). CRC Press. 10.1201/9781003252542-17

Khang, A., Ragimova, N. A., Hajimahmud, V. A., Alyar, A. V. (2022d). Advanced Technologies and Data Management in the Smart Healthcare System. *AI-Centric Smart City Ecosystems: Technologies, Design and Implementation* (1st ed.). CRC Press. 10.1201/9781003252542-16

Khang, A., Rani, S., Sivaraman, A. K. (2022e). *AI-Centric Smart City Ecosystems: Technologies, Design and Implementation* (1st ed.). CRC Press. 10.1201/9781003252542

Khang A., Rani, S., Gujrati, R., Uygun, H., Gupta, S. K., (Eds.). (2023). *Designing Workforce Management Systems for Industry 4.0: Data-Centric and AI-Enabled Approaches* (1st ed.). CRC Press. 10.1201/99781003357070

Khanh, H. H., Khang, A. (2021). The Role of Artificial Intelligence in Blockchain Applications. *Reinventing Manufacturing and Business Processes through Artificial Intelligence* 20–40. CRC Press. 10.1201/9781003145011-2

Kim, Y. (2014). Convolutional neural networks for sentence classification. CoRR, vol. abs/1408.5882. [Online]. Available: http://arxiv.org/abs/1408.5882

Misra, A., Shah, V., Khang, A., Gupta, S. K., (Eds.). (2023). *AI-Aided IoT Technologies and Applications in the Smart Business and Production* (1st ed.). CRC Press. 10.1201/9781003392224

Morris, G., Babasaheb, J., Khang, A., Gupta, S. K., Hajimahmud, V. A. (2023). *AI-Centric Modelling and Analytics: Concepts, Designs, Technologies, and Applications* (1st ed.). CRC Press. 10.1201/9781003400110

Mungla, B. O. (2019). Robotic process automation for inventory control and management: A case of Freight forwarders solutions (Doctoral dissertation, Strathmore University). https://su-plus.strathmore.edu/handle/11071/6763

Nallasivam, A. (2022, January 28). RPA in healthcare industry: Use cases and benefits. ClaySys Technologies. Retrieved January 28, 2022, from https://www.claysys.com/blog/rpa-in-healthcare-industry/

Primer, A. (2015). Introduction to robotic process automation. *Institute for Robotic Process Automation*, 1–35. https://www.irpaai.com/wp-content/uploads/2015/05/Robotic-Process-Automation-June2015.pdf

Radke, A. M., Dang, M. T., Tan, A. (2020). Using robotic process automation (RPA) to enhance item master data maintenance process. *LogForum*, 16(1). https://yadda.icm.edu.pl/baztech/element/bwmeta1.element.baztech-2bd2b0dc-5717-4bc5-8840-669b3c19d8d7

Rajkhowa, B., Joshi, S. (2020). Intelligent automation-uses, benefits, and impact. *PalArch's Journal of Archaeology of Egypt/Egyptology*, 17(6), 4610–4619. https://archives.palarch.nl/index.php/jae/article/download/1710/1704

Rana, G., Khang, A., Sharma, R., Goel, A. K., Dubey, A. K. (2021). *Reinventing Manufacturing and Business Processes through Artificial Intelligence*. CRC Press. 10.1201/9781003145011

Rani, S., Bhambri, P., Kataria, A., Khang, A. (2022). Smart City Ecosystem: Concept, Sustainability, Design Principles and Technologies. *AI-Centric Smart City Ecosystems: Technologies, Design and Implementation* (1st ed.). CRC Press. 10.1201/9781003252542-1

Rani, S., Chauhan, M., Kataria, A., Khang, A. (2021). IoT Equipped Intelligent Distributed Framework for Smart Healthcare Systems. *Networking and Internet Architecture*. CRC Press. 10.48550/arXiv.2110.04997

Ratia, M., Myllärniemi, J., Helander, N. (2018, October). Robotic process automation-creating value by digitalizing work in private healthcare. *22nd International Academic Mindtrek Conference* (pp. 222–227). https://dl.acm.org/doi/abs/10.1145/3275116.3275129

Serey, J., Quezada, L., Alfaro, M., Fuertes, G., Vargas, M., Ternero, R., Gutierrez, S. (2021). Artificial intelligence methodologies for data management. *Symmetry*, 13(11), 2040. https://www.mdpi.com/1335580

Seuwou, P. (2021). RPA: A force for good in healthcare. http://nectar.northampton.ac.uk/16068/1/Hewitt_etal_Automation_anywhere_2021_RPA_force_for_good_in_healthcare.pdf

Sreekrishna, M., Prem Jacob, T. Improving effectiveness and efficiency of cancer registry management using robotic process automation. https://scholars.ln.edu.hk/en/publications/how-hospitals-in-mainland-china-responded-to-the-outbreak-of-covi

Sugalo, I. (2022, July 26). Hospital inventory management: Architecture, features & benefits. *Hospital Inventory Management: Architecture, Features & Benefits*. Retrieved July 26, 2022, from https://www.itransition.com/blog/hospital-inventorymanagement

Tailor, R. K., Pareek, R., Khang, A., (Eds.). (2022). Robot Process Automation in Blockchain. *The Data-Driven Blockchain Ecosystem: Fundamentals, Applications, and Emerging Technologies* (1st ed.), 149–164. CRC Press. 10.1201/9781003269281-8

Thainimit, S., Chaipayom, P., Sa-arnwong, N., Gansawat, D., Petchyim, S., Pongrujikorn, S. (2022). Robotic process automation support in telemedicine: Glaucoma screening usage case. *Informatics in Medicine Unlocked*, 31, 101001. 10.1145/3275116.3275129

Thaler, E. (2022). Dr. robot or Dr. efficiency? *The Impact of Robotic Process Automation on Jobs in Healthcare*. https://repository.upenn.edu/joseph_wharton_scholars/120/

Tietz, W., Cainas, J. M., Miller-Nobles, T. L. (2020). The bots are coming … to intro accounting. *Strategic Finance*, 102(2), 24–29. https://search.proquest.com/openview/7b8ff73b7774106e403b2ac843f30dab/1?pq-origsite=gscholar&cbl=48426

UiPath Automation Lifecycle. (2022). Retrieved on Jan 2023 from https://docs.uipath.com/studio/docs/automation-lifecycle

Vishnu, S., Agochiya, V., Palkar, R. (2017). Data-centered dependencies and opportunities for robotics process automation in banking. *Journal of Financial Transformation*, 45(1), 68–76. https://www.mdpi.com/1335580https://files.openpdfs.org/jE1d4GBZ5Ob.pdf#page=68

Vrushank, S., Khang, A., Rani, S. (2023a). *AI-Based Technologies and Applications in the Era of the Metaverse* (1st ed.). IGI Global Press. 10.4018/9781668488515

Vrushank, S., Vidhi, T., Khang, A. (2023b). Electronic Health Records Security and Privacy Enhancement using Blockchain Technology. *Data-Centric AI Solutions and Emerging Technologies in the Healthcare Ecosystem* (1st ed.), P (1). CRC Press. 10.1201/9781003356189

Williams, P. (2021, September 21). Amazing ways that RPA can be used in healthcare. *IBM*. Retrieved September 21, 2021, from https://www.ibm.com/cloud/blog/amazing-ways-that-rpa-can-be-used-in-healthcare

Yan, A., Zou, Y., Mirchandani, D. A. (2020). How hospitals in mainland China responded to the outbreak of COVID-19 using information technology–enabled services: An analysis of hospital news webpages. *Journal of the American Medical Informatics Association*, 27(7), 991–999.

18 Methodological and Analytical Considerations for Development and Implementation of an Audit System for Telemedicine

Biranchi Jena, Babasaheb Jadhav, Satish Khalikar, and Apeksha Nagawade

CONTENTS

DOI: 10.1201/9781003356189-18

18.1 INTRODUCTION

Healthcare access is the most important component of any health system. The World Health Organization (WHO) has well defined the importance of universal healthcare, which ensures access to healthcare. Strengthening any given healthcare system needs a substantial improvement in healthcare access.

Healthcare access covers four dimensions of healthcare service delivery namely physical reach to the healthcare units, availability or capacity of the unit to serve the patient, quality of the care providers, and the affordability of the service including consumables. These four dimensions define the degree of healthcare access in a given geography.

As per a survey of IMS Health, it was revealed that 20% of people travel more than 5 km to avail of Out Patient Department (OPD) service, while this proportion is 32% for rural areas.

Assurance of capacity and availability of service is important for the trust of the people in any health system when people travel a considerable distance for availing of the same. As more people are depending on private sector service providers, 61% of people have opined that the assurance of the availability of the doctor in the facility is the main reason for availing services from the private sector care provider.

Quick response (56%), less waiting time (50%), and lack of specialization in the government system (14%) is the other consideration of patients showing trust in the private sector. Affordability to the service provider is also impacting the degree of healthcare access, as medicine constitutes around 65% of the total out of pocket (OOP) expenses and the amount spent on consultation contributes to 15% of the total OOP expenses.

More than 32% (IMS Health, 2016) of the patients travel more than 5 kilometers to avail themselves of OPD services in rural India. Most of the services remain unattended when it pertains either to the specialty healthcare OPD services or the physician is not available. Such a situation adds a further challenge to improving healthcare access. This is an emerging issue in the healthcare sector and thus needs a quick solution by providing access to the services.

Since more than 50% (IMS Health, 2016) of the position of specialty doctors are vacant in Community Health Centres (CHCs) across India, an innovative approach would address the challenge. "Telemedicine" could be one of the solutions.

More than 60% of the patients in the rural area prefer to take healthcare services from private providers. As per the IMS study on access to care, the lack of specialist doctors in government facilities and quick response to the medical issues of the patients are the major reasons the patients in rural India go to private service providers, even if there is an additional financial burden on the patients.

However, the need for specialist doctors remains unattended as the distance to reach out to specialist doctors is a challenge for patients in rural areas. While the goal is to improve the healthcare service access for a majority of the population, it is important to develop capabilities around non-communicable disease (NCD) management.

Management of NCD requires continuous touch with the doctor and lack of accessibility will be the biggest impediment in the same. The burden of NCD is estimated to be more than 90% by 2025 and managing this long-term nature of the diseases under NCD needs an innovative solution in terms of accessing healthcare services.

Extensive use of the internet and the use of technology in the healthcare sector has created an opportunity for innovating new processes to make healthcare access better for the citizens.

However, it is important to create appropriate prerequisites like electronic health records (EHRs) of the citizens at sub-centers (Vrushank et al., 2023), primary health centres (PHCs), and community health centres (CHCs) in the public sector and also the small clinics managed by the private clinicians. This will enable technology to create an ecosystem for facilitating healthcare service delivery (Mathad & Khang, 2023).

The internet and mobile technology-driven telemedicine can be game changers to address the challenges related to healthcare access. Although the usage of tele-medicine has increased quite significantly, its effectiveness and sustainability need to be established. The current article deals with the mechanism to establish a structured quality control on telemedicine usage and its effectiveness.

The main purpose of the current research work is to provide a broad framework of methodological and analytical support for the development and implementation of an audit system for telemedicine practices across different healthcare facilities including referrals. Thus, a structured audit with appropriate methodology would resolve the major challenges being faced by telemedicine practices across different organizations and different specialties.

18.2   METHODOLOGY AND FRAMEWORK

The authors of the current research have designed and contributed to a telemedicine assessment project for the government of Telangana, where a structured approach was used to evaluate the functionalities of telemedicine and its effectiveness.

The government of Telangana has established telemedicine in the government health centers in the network of primary health centres (PHCs), community health centres (CHCs), district hospitals (DH), and medical college hospitals. While patients in PHCs and CHCs were the receivers of telemedicine, specialist doctors in DHs and medical college hospitals were providing consulting services through telemedicine.

The authors have assessed the functioning of telemedicine in eight PHCs or CHCs and eight district hospitals or medical colleges. An audit tool was designed to assess the functioning of telemedicine-based standard guidelines. The audit tool is presented in the current research article for the benefit of audit and quality assurance of telemedicine facilities.

The assessment of the telemedicine system from the patient's perspective is important. Therefore, the current research article has also used some of the data collected through a primary survey of patients who had used the telemedicine services provided in the health facilities of the government of Telangana.

The data was collected by using a sampling frame based on the PPS (probability proportion to size) principle for the selection of beneficiaries (Bhambri et al., 2022). Before applying the PPS, the total sample size for the study was calculated by using the following formula:

$$s = \frac{x^2 * N * P(1 - P)}{d^2(N - 1) + x^2 * P(1 - P)}$$

Where

- S = sample size
- X^2 = chi-square value for alpha (3.84 for 95% of CI)
- N = population size (total number of consultations completed in the project which is ~ 170,000)
- P = population proportion (estimated proportion of patients are satisfied with the service delivery. it is assumed to be 75%; it is assumed that the probability of a patient is happy from all aspects)
- D = degree of accepting error in the proportion (usually taken as 5% or 0.05)

Thus, the total sample size is estimated to be 288 for the study. To round off, a sample of 300 was fixed for the study.

Now the sample size would be distributed among all 33 districts through the PPS principle. In other words, the sample size would be more for the districts where the patient turnover is high and vice versa.

$$S_i = S * (p_i/P * 100)$$

Where

- S_i = sample for the district
- p_i = total consultation in the district (or the total population)
- P = total consultation in the project (or total population in the project area)

Based on the above calculation, data was collected across all 33 districts of Telangana. The data was presented in the current research through bi-variate tables and insight was generated accordingly (Rani et al., 2021).

Further, the Medical Council of India (MCI, 2021) came up with Telemedicine Practice Guidelines in 2021 to facilitate adherence to basic safety practices. The guidelines suggest seven elements that can improve the functionality of telemedicine along with ensuring the quality of care through telemedicine practices. These seven components include the following;

- Context of the telemedicine
- Identification of beneficiaries and care providers
- Communication platform
- Patient consent
- Exchange of information during the service delivery
- Type of consultation and patient evaluation
- Patient management

These seven elements were further analyzed and sub-elements have been developed for evaluating the quality and outcome of the online clinical services through teleconsultation. Each sub-element has been assigned a different scoring mechanism based on its importance in achieving patient safety. Apart from the designing of the audit system for telemedicine, various statistical analysis tools are used for developing an analytical dashboard for telemedicine practices.

18.3   RESULTS AND DISCUSSIONS

The patients of the telemedicine user are primarily patients who need specialty consultation in a health facility where the specialty doctor is not available in person. Therefore, it is very important to understand the experience of the patients using the telemedicine system available to provide the services, as shown in table 18.1.

More than 89% of the patients believe that the specialty service available to them through telemedicine (TLM) is as effective as an in-person consultation. Around 10% of the patients feel that the system is either less effective or not at all effective when compared to the in-person consultation. On the other hand, around 1% of the patients feel that the system created in their facility is even better than in-person consultation (Rana et al., 2021).

During the assessment, two major aspects were covered while interacting with the beneficiaries. The first aspect is the availability of medicines in the facility prescribed by the specialty doctor and the second aspect is the availability of diagnostic services as advised by the specialist in table 18.2.

Around 81% of patients said that all the diagnostic services were available to them in the facility as advised by the specialty doctor during the teleconsultation and 13% of the patients informed that the suggested test was not available to them. The overall satisfaction regarding the diagnostic test was found to be 8.4 on a scale of 10, as shown in table 18.3.

Around 77% of patients said that all the medicines were available to them in the facility, as prescribed by the specialty doctor during the teleconsultation and 16% of the patients informed that the prescribed medicine was not available to them. The overall satisfaction regarding the availability of medicine was found to be 8.2 on a scale of 10.

TABLE 18.1

Distribution of Patients by Their Experience of the Telemedicine Services

The Efficiency Level of the System as Perceived by Patients	Total Patients	% of Patients
As effective as the in-person consultation	268	89.6%
Good but a little less effective than the in-person consultation	24	8.0%
Not effective as the in-person consultation	5	1.7%
More-effective than the in-person consultation	2	0.7%
Total	**299**	**100.0%**

Source: Author's owner.

TABLE 18.2

Distribution of Patients by Their Experience of Availing the Diagnostic Services as Advised During the Teleconsultation

Availability of diagnostic Tests Advised by the Doctor	No of Patients	%
Yes, it is available	242	81%
No, It is not available	40	13%
Not sure	18	6%
Grand Total	**300**	**100%**

Source: Author's owner.

TABLE 18.3

Distribution of Patients by Their Experience of Availing the Medicines as Prescribed During the Teleconsultation

Availability of Medicines Prescribed by the Doctor	No of patients	%
Yes, it is available	232	77%
No, It is not available	47	16%
Not sure	21	7%
Grand Total	**300**	**100%**

Source: Author's owner.

Apart from the availability of prescribed medicine and diagnosis in the health facility during the telemedicine services, other aspects of the telemedicine service were assessed from the patient's perspective; these aspects provide a better insight (Khanh & Khang, 2021).

18.4   PROCESS CHANGES AND ADHERENCE

The introduction of telemedicine needs either introduction of new processes or modification in the existing process for the delivery of services through telemedicine (Tailor et al., 2022).

The patients have to go through such changes to avail of the services that may create issues in the convenience, safety, and rights of the patients. Patients' experience towards accessing the specialty services was measured by a set of five statements with a five-point Likert scale, as shown in table 18.4.

As far as the assurance for availing the health services from the facility and ease of accessing the specialist service is concerned, around 98% of patients were found to have a positive experience.

TABLE 18.4

Response of the Patients for the Access-Related Changes in the Process Due to the Implementation of Telemedicine

Statements Measuring Attitude for Better Access	Strongly Agree	Agree	Uncertain	Disagree	Strongly Disagree
With the system in place, I am assured of getting the health consultation service	68%	29%	2%	—	—
Through the new system, I have easy access to the medical specialists I need	69%	28%	2%	—	—
I can get specialist medical consultation at my convenience	67%	29%	4%	—	—
Although the consultation is done through the telemedicine setup, necessary prescribed drugs are available at the PHC	64%	22%	7%	4%	3%
Although the consultation is done through the telemedicine setup, necessary prescribed diagnostic tests are available at the center	64%	26%	7%	3%	1%

Source: Author's owner.

Only around 2% of the patients have had some negative experience. There was also a positive experience among the beneficiaries regarding their convenience of accessing the service as almost 96% of patients feel that the system helps to match their convenience.

However, more than 10% of the patients were either uncertain or disagreed regarding the availability of medicine and diagnostic tests in the facility after having the specialty consultations done.

18.5 PROCESS FOLLOWED FOR ONLINE CONSULTATION

For evaluation of the experience towards the new processes introduced at the health centers, we have taken three statements, as shown in table 18.5.

Around 7% of the patients feel that the telemedicine system introduced in the health facility lacks some of the apparatus which could improve the outcome of telemedicine. Patient experience was quite positive towards the process during the consultation with specialty doctors at the hub.

However, around 5% of patients were still uncertain regarding the processes. Four percent of patients felt that the appointment process needs further improvement as they were not comfortable with the current process of booking the appointment.

TABLE 18.5

Response of the Patients to the Process Followed for Accessing Telemedicine

Statements Measuring Attitude for Better Access	Strongly Agree	Agree	Uncertain	Disagree	Strongly Disagree
I think the telemedicine unit has everything needed to provide complete medical care in a remote area	68%	25%	5%	1%	1%
Through the new system, the process is easy and swift for consultation with doctors from remote places	69%	26%	5%	—	—
It's easy to get an appointment for medical care right away through the new system in place	64%	32%	3%	1%	—

Source: Author's owner.

18.5.1 COMMUNICATION DURING SERVICE DELIVERY THROUGH TELEMEDICINE

Communication is an important aspect of healthcare delivery. The healthcare delivery system is already experiencing challenges in communication between healthcare professionals and patients even an in-person consultation.

When it comes to online consultation the challenges related to communication are expected to multiply. It is therefore critical to understand the beneficiaries' experience towards various aspects of teleconsultation where communication plays a role. We have taken four statements to assess the experience of patients for effective communication in online consultation, as shown in table 18.6.

The current system of telemedicine seems to have taken care of the communication-related issues effectively as the majority of the beneficiaries have had a good experience of easy and swift communication between the doctor and the patients. However, around 20% of the patients feel that doctors need to improve further while explaining the prescription and diagnostic tests during the consultation process (Khang et al., 2023a).

18.5.2 QUALITY OF CARE

Irrespective of in-person or online consultation, quality of care is crucial for having long-term trust in the health system. Patients' perceptions and attitudes toward quality of care define the sustainability of a given healthcare service. In the current assessment study, we have assessed the quality of care by taking two statements, as shown in table 18.7.

A small portion of patients either disagreed or strongly disagreed with the quality of medical care provided through telemedicine facilities.

TABLE 18.6

Experience of the Patients Regarding the Effective Communication Practiced in Telemedicine

Statements measuring attitude for better access	Strongly agree	Agree	Uncertain	Disagree	Strongly disagree
Doctors are good about explaining the reason for medical tests, even if the consultation is done online	56%	27%	8%	5%	4%
Doctors are very attentive when I explain my health issues through the online consultation mode	73%	26%	1%	—	—
Even if the doctor is available remotely, there is no issue to explain my problems to the doctors	70%	27%	3%	—	—
I do not have any problem understanding the doctor's advice and other treatment-related explanation	70%	28%	2%	—	—

Source: Author's owner.

TABLE 18.7

Experience of the Patients Regarding Quality of Care Through Telemedicine Practices

Statements Measuring Attitude for Quality of Care	Strongly agree	Agree	Uncertain	Disagree	Strongly Disagree
The medical care I have received through the telemedicine system is apt and perfect	67%	29%	2%	1%	1%
When I go for medical care from the facility having the telemedicine set up, the team is extremely careful in treating and examining including the privacy	70%	30%	—	—	—

Source: Author's owner.

The overall experience of the patients using telemedicine indicates that telemedicine services for specialty services are highly efficient in serving the needs of the patients. From the needs aspects of the patients, the assessment of the telemedicine system was found to be great. However, adherence to the basic service delivery protocol in telemedicine is of utmost critical for the safety and the individual rights of the patients.

From the system perspective, the authors have designed a criteria-based audit tool for the evaluation of the telemedicine system for the provision of healthcare services. The criteria-based audit tool is based on the seven principles defined by the Medical Council of India.

18.5.2.1 Criteria 1. Context

Telemedicine by definition deals with the delivery of healthcare services, where distance is a critical factor, by all healthcare professionals using information and communications technologies for the exchange of valid information for the diagnosis, treatment, and prevention of disease and injuries, research and evaluation, and the continuing education of healthcare workers, to advance the health of individuals and communities.

Telemedicine may be used for several purposes, including medical care, teaching, research, administration, and public health. People in rural and distant places across the world struggle to get timely, high-quality specialist medical treatment. Irrespective of the purpose of telemedicine, it is important to have a strong base for the services to be delivered under telemedicine, as shown in table 18.8.

18.5.2.2 Criteria 2: Identification of Registered Medical Practitioner (RMP) and Patient

The telemedicine consultation should not be anonymous: both the patient and the RMP must be aware of each other's identities, as shown in table 18.9.

As far as patient identification is concerned, the following are the criteria and score, as shown in table 18.10.

18.5.2.3 Criteria 3: Mode of Communication

Telemedicine consultations can be delivered using a variety of technologies. All of these technological systems have their own set of strengths and shortcomings, as well as circumstances in which they may be appropriate or insufficient for providing effective care. The major mode of telemedicine is classified into audio, video, and text by chats, images, or real-time video consulting, as shown in table 18.11.

TABLE 18.8

The criteria for the Context and the Score Defined for the Audit

1	Category of Context	Score
A	Processes for all necessary diagnosis is defined and followed and the severity of the case is less	03
B	Processes for all necessary diagnosis is defined and followed and the severity of the case is moderate or critical	02
C	None of the processes for necessary diagnosis is defined	01

Source: Author's owner.

TABLE 18.9

The criteria for the Identification of RMP/Patients and the Score Defined for Audit

2A	Identification of Registered Medical Practitioner	Score
A	RMP information including Name, Reg. No., Qualification and Specialization are displayed in the telemedicine system during the consultation	03
B	Only Name and Qualification are displayed in the telemedicine system	02
C	None of the RMP information is displayed in the telemedicine system	01

Source: Author's owner.

TABLE 18.10

Identification of Patient

2B	Identification of Patient	Score
A	Patient identification includes Patient Name, Age, Gender, Email, and Phone Number, which is available and reflected in the telemedicine platform for the viewing of the RMP	03
B	Patient Name, Age, and Gender are available and reflected in the telemedicine platform for the viewing of the RMP	02
C	None of the patient information is available and reflected in the telemedicine platform for the viewing of the RMP	01

Source: Author's owner.

TABLE 18.11

The Criteria for the mode of Communication and the Score Defined for the Audit

3	Mode of communication	Score
A	The telemedicine system provides all possible communication modes and can be toggled with one another; audio, video, and text by chat, image, or real video	03
B	The telemedicine system provides at least audio and video modes of communication together	02
C	The telemedicine system only provides an audio mode of communication equivalent to a telephonic call	01

Source: Author's owner.

18.5.2.4   Criteria 4: Patient Consent

Healthcare service provision is governed by a systematic procedure of consent from the patient. While informed consent is a common practice in the provision of healthcare services, explicit consent is critical in the case of the telemedicine system (Morris et al., 2023).

Informed consent is the process of providing crucial information regarding a medical procedure or therapy, genetic testing, or a clinical study, including potential risks and benefits. This is to assist people in deciding whether they wish to be treated, tested, or participate in the medical service provision.

Explicit consent is a process in which any type of explicit permission can be recorded. The patient may send an email, text message, or audio/video communication. The patient can express his/her purpose to the RMP through phone/video (e.g., "Yes, I consent to avail consultation via telemedicine" or any other similar communication in simple terms). This must be documented in the RMP's patient records, as shown in table 18.12.

18.5.2.5   Criteria 5: Patient Consultation

In the provision of healthcare consultative services, the service may be of the FIRST consultation or it can be of FOLLOW-UP consultation. First and follow-up consultation need a different strategy to manage the patients. Various strategies also carry a different amount of risks and benefits. When there has been no prior in-person consultation, an RMP may have only a limited grasp of the patient requesting teleconsultation for the first time, as shown in table 18.13.

However, if the initial consultation is conducted through video, RMP can make a far better judgment and hence give much better advice, including extra medications, as shown in table 18.14, if necessary.

18.5.2.6   Criteria 6: Exchange of Information for Patient Evaluation

Consultation and effective management of diseases need a reference to multiple current and previous medical records of the patients. Telemedicine systems should provide the support of accessing such medical records of patients effortlessly, as shown in table 18.15.

TABLE 18.12

The Criteria for the Patient Consent and the Score Defined for the Audit

4	Patient Consent	Score
A	The telemedicine system provides a recording of both informed and explicit consent and is accessible for reference at any point in time	03
B	The telemedicine system provides only provision of the explicit consent and is available for reference in the system	02
C	The telemedicine system does not have a provision for recording the consent	01

Source: Author's owner.

TABLE 18.13

The criteria for the Mode of Communication and the Score Defined for the Audit First Consultation

5A	First Consultation	Score
A	The patient has consulted with the same RMP earlier in person and the RMP has a better understanding and access to the patient's medication and diagnosis reports on the telemedicine platform	03
B	The patient has consulted with the other RMP earlier in person and the RMP has limited or no access to the patient's medication and diagnosis reports on the telemedicine platform	02
C	The patient is consulting with the RMP for the first time	01

Source: Author's owner.

TABLE 18.14

The Criteria for the Mode of Communication and the Score Defined for Follow Up Consultation

5B	Follow Up Consultation	Score
A	The patient is having a follow-up consultation with the same RMP	03
B	The patient is having a follow-up consultation with another RMP of the same specialization	02
C	Follow up with other RMP of other specialization	01

Source: Author's owner.

TABLE 18.15

The Criteria for the Exchange of Information for Patient Evaluation and the Score Defined for Audit

6	Exchange of Information for Patient Evaluation	Score
A	The patient's record, case history, investigation report, images, and previous prescription is available in documented format in the telemedicine platform.	03
B	Some of the patient's medical history and documents are available for view and reference	02
C	No previous patient history is available in the system	01

Source: Author's owner.

TABLE 18.16

The Criteria for Patient Management and the Score Defined for the Audit

7	Patient Management	Score
A	The system is well-balanced for health education, counselling and medication	03
B	Only appropriate for health education and counselling	02
C	Only consultation of medication	01

Source: Author's owner.

18.5.2.7   Criteria 7: Patient Management

Patient management includes a wide range of services including patient education, counseling, dietetics, consultation, and others. The technology-driven telemedicine system can be effective for some users while it may be a limitation for some services (Misra et al., 2023).

An RMP may convey lessons about health promotion and illness prevention. These might be connected to food, physical exercise, smoking cessation, infectious diseases, and other factors (Khang et al., 2023b).

Similarly, he or she may provide recommendations on vaccines, exercises, hygiene habits, mosquito control, and so on. It may also include food restrictions, do's and don'ts for a patient on anticancer medications, appropriate use of a hearing aid, home physiotherapy, and other measures to ameliorate the underlying ailment. This may also contain recommendations for new investigations that must be completed before the next consult, as shown in table 18.16.

18.6   CONCLUSION

The audit system developed by the researchers in this paper has nine criteria-based categories for the seven principles of the telemedicine system (Khang et al., 2023d). The maximum score of all the categories would be 27, whereas the minimum score would be 9.

TABLE 18.17

The Final Score of the Audit May be Interpreted

Score	Interpretation
A score between 22 and 27	The telemedicine system is excellent and provides the most appropriate healthcare services
A score between 16 and 21	The telemedicine system is comparatively better and provides moderately better healthcare services
A score between 9 and 15	The telemedicine system needs improvement

Source: Author's owner.

Any telemedicine unit may be audited and assessed through the above criteria-based method and the scores obtained are to be added to get the final score, as shown in table 18.17.

REFERENCES

Bhambri, P., Rani, S., Gupta, G., Khang, A. (2022). *Cloud and Fog Computing Platforms for Internet of Things* ISBN: 978-1-032-101507. CRC Press. 10.1201/9781003213888

Hajimahmud, V. A., Khang, A., Hahanov, V., Litvinova, E., Chumachenko, S., Alyar, A. V. (2022). Autonomous Robots for Smart City: Closer to Augmented Humanity. *AI-Centric Smart City Ecosystems: Technologies, Design and Implementation* (1st ed.). CRC Press. 10.1201/9781003252542-7

IMS Healthcare (2016). Understanding Healthcare Access in India, IMS, 2016. https://www.scribd.com/document/255552955/Understanding-Healthcare-Access-in-India

Khang, A., Ragimova, N. A., Hajimahmud, V. A., Alyar, A. V. (2022). Advanced Technologies and Data Management in the Smart Healthcare System. *AI-Centric Smart City Ecosystems: Technologies, Design and Implementation* (1st ed.). CRC Press. 10.1201/9781003252542-16

Khang, A., Gupta, S. K., Rani, S., Karras, D. A., (Eds.). (2023a). *Smart Cities: IoT Technologies, Big Data Solutions, Cloud Platforms, and Cybersecurity Techniques* (1st ed.). CRC Press. 10.1201/9781003376064

Khang, A., Hahanov, V., Litvinova, E., Chumachenko, S., Triwiyanto, Hajimahmud, V. A., Ali, R. N., Alyar, A. V., Anh, P. T. N. (2023b). The Analytics of Hospitality of Hospitals in Healthcare Ecosystem. *Data-Centric AI Solutions and Emerging Technologies in the Healthcare Ecosystem* (1st ed.), P (4). CRC Press. 10.1201/9781003356189

Khang, A., Rana, G., Tailor, R. K., Hajimahmud, V. A., (Eds.). (2023c). *Data-Centric AI Solutions and Emerging Technologies in the Healthcare Ecosystem* (1st ed.). CRC Press. 10.1201/9781003356189

Khang, A., Rani, S., Vrushank, S. (2023d). *AI-Based Technologies and Applications in the Era of the Metaverse* (1st ed.). IGI Global Press. 10.1201/9781668488515

Khanh, H. H., Khang, A. (2021). The Role of Artificial Intelligence in Blockchain Applications. *Reinventing Manufacturing and Business Processes through Artificial Intelligence* 20–40. CRC Press. 10.1201/9781003145011-2

Mathad, K., Khang, A. (2023). Hospital 4.0: Capitalization of Health and Healthcare in Industry 4.0 Economy. *Data-Centric AI Solutions and Emerging Technologies in the Healthcare Ecosystem* (1st ed.), P (14). CRC Press. 10.1201/9781003356189

MCI (2021). Telemedicine Practice Guidelines, Medical Council of India, 2021. https://www.ncbi.nlm.nih.gov/pmc/articles/PMC9111269/

Misra, A., Shah, V., Khang, A., Gupta, S. K., (Eds.). (2023). *AI-Aided IoT Technologies and Applications in the Smart Business and Production* (1st ed.). CRC Press. 10.1201/9781003392224

Morris, G., Babasaheb, J., Khang, A., Gupta, S. K., Hajimahmud, V. A. (2023). *AI-Centric Modelling and Analytics: Concepts, Designs, Technologies, and Applications* (1st ed.). CRC Press. 10.1201/9781003400110

Rana, G., Khang, A., Sharma, R., Goel, A. K., Dubey, A. K. (2021). *Reinventing Manufacturing and Business Processes through Artificial Intelligence*. CRC Press. 10.1201/9781003145011

Rani, S., Chauhan, M., Kataria, A., Khang, A. (2021). IoT Equipped Intelligent Distributed Framework for Smart Healthcare Systems. *Networking and Internet Architecture*. CRC Press. 10.48550/arXiv.2110.04997

Tailor, G., Pareek, R., Khang A., (Eds.). (2022). Robot Process Automation in Blockchain. *The Data-Driven Blockchain Ecosystem: Fundamentals, Applications, and Emerging Technologies* (1st ed.), 149–164. CRC Press. 10.1201/9781003269281-8

Vrushank, S., Vidhi, T., Khang, A. (2023). Electronic Health Records Security and Privacy Enhancement using Blockchain Technology. *Data-Centric AI Solutions and Emerging Technologies in the Healthcare Ecosystem* (1st ed.), P (1). CRC Press. 10.1201/9781003356189

19 Hospital 4.0

Capitalization of Health and Healthcare in Industry 4.0 Economy

Kavita Mathad and Alex Khang

CONTENTS

19.1   INTRODUCTION

Industry 4.0 brings in powerful and sharply defined forms of digital transformation to get into yet another Industrial Revolution. Organizations and firms look for the apt deployment of resources to help accelerate the digital transformation of practices and processes involved.

However, it has not been an easy route to incorporate digital transformation. Companies had to encounter perennial challenges to integrate the information and communications technology (ICT) and the business process as each of the business dimensions is unique (Martinez Caro et al., 2020)

Digital transformation is all about aligning the best technology suitable to the best business practices of the firm incorporated majorly to optimally utilize the resources and gain more returns with the least cost combinations through achieving greater results. It's about disrupting the way business operations are run by using

DOI: 10.1201/9781003356189-19

newer technologies or techniques that would further catalyst increased opportunities for success and growth.

Digital technologies mainly deal with information computation and communication, including computing, communication, and the connectivity technologies like cloud computing, information technology (IT), artificial intelligence (AI), and blockchain technologies to name a few (Bhardwaj et al., 2013). Most of the early adopters' firms realized that digital transformation is inevitable and is here to grow not just to stay updated, but to excel at a faster space (Khang et al., 2023a).

Digital technologies have advanced exponentially, the imperative for all organizations including service-based and B2B as well, wherein digital transformation has become a universal go-to irrespective of the size or the nature of the companies.

For these companies to adapt technologies for resultants, they evolved from digitization to digitalization to digital transformation. Digitization is moving from analog to digital so that it can be stored, processed, and or transmitted.

Digitalization is about using digitized data to perform roles, processes, and workflows meticulously using digital technologies for greater efficiency and productivity of resources, including the time consumed.

The digitalization helps to manage business faster and more efficiently as the data required is instantly accessible and not trapped in a file cabinet. A compatible combination of digitization and digitalization would lead to a digital transformation journey with a clear-set destination that aligns with the company's strategic plan and modernization strategy prioritizing the solutions.

The solutions that are required recognize the process that requires agility and flexibility of resources, be it the IT infrastructure or the human capital.

While digital transformation utilizes a hub-and-spoke model, it delivers out-of-the-box capabilities to allow businesses to create and manage integrations centrally to streamline communication and make employees more efficient and boost their productivity (Chowdhury et al., 2022).

Innovations in science are coming up with rosy predictions of expanding longevity and improving healthcare and the health system for increasing the bandwidth of accessibility and delivery. Businesses on the other hand are experiencing gloomy reports of galloping health insurance with high premiums and less insurance coverage making affordability of medical care difficult.

Not surprisingly, there is ambiguity as to whether these trends in outcomes and expenditure are a cause for celebration or concern. The think tanks and the economists point towards technological advancements as a source for both the advancement in the outcomes and expenditure of healthcare.

Many developed countries have witnessed that the expenditure on healthcare has been increasing year on year, resulting in very little push towards the maturity phase of development.

In medicine advancement, there has been impressive development in the area of precision medicine, immunotherapy, microbiology, and genetic engineering to mention a few. The research and development in these areas are trying consciously to reduce the cost of the procedures in order to make them accessible to more people; for example, genome mapping, a relatively new procedure, is now costing less than USD$1000.

Similarly, in the case of the pharmaceutical sector, more than 15,000 drugs are identified to be effective in curing cancer. Parallel to the advancements in science and medicine, technological advancements have been very strategically used to leverage health and healthcare by addressing the three major concerns:

    i. an increase in the older population,
    ii. an increase in higher cost, and
    iii. an inequality of access to various healthcare services.

This culmination of scientific advancements and technology has led to the digitalization of health and healthcare. Currently, 318,000 health apps are available on top app stores and an additional 200 health apps join the league every day (Insight Report, 2019). From an optimistic view, it can be understood that the integration of data will enable a system biology app to prevent disease surveillance, early detection, and intervention (Bhambri et al., 2022).

The current frontiers of science, technology, and infrastructure worlds are dispersing fast with the advent of new technologies such as artificial intelligence (AI), the Internet of Things (IoT), 4G and 5G telecommunications, big data, advanced robotics, 3D printing, cloud platforms, etc. (Rana et al., 2021).

These technological developments have concreted their way to Industry 4.0, bringing fundamental changes in production, distribution, and consumption in almost all sectors including the healthcare sector (Khang et al., 2023a).

The countries and firms today have realized that these technologies are here to stay and have identified the compulsion to absorb and leverage technological advancements to eliminate production inefficiencies and improve outcomes.

Industry 4.0, originally proposed by the German government, is based on the methods of self-optimization, self-configuration, self-diagnosis, cognition, and intelligent support of intellectual capital. This autonomous decision making of machines, a real disruptive element of Industry 4.0, has naturally made its way to capitalize on the health and healthcare services, resulting in Hospital 4.0.

As Industry 4.0 assures effectiveness, efficiency, and accuracy, it is a proven requisite incorporation in the healthcare sector wherein inefficiencies can be a matter of life and death.

Technological advancements would integrate clinics, hospitals, laboratories, pharmacies, and healthcare providers, thereby minimizing the time lost in coordinating between them and increasing efficiency and reducing healthcare costs (Tyagi, 2018). Healthcare can thus be a significant beneficiary of the current wave of technological advancements, which would go a long way toward humanity.

Technological innovations and rising healthcare demand are rapidly changing the way healthcare products are developed and healthcare services are delivered. Hospital 4.0 is mainly based on the Internet of Things (IoT), artificial intelligence, 3D printing, big data, and analytics and is a technology merge of real and virtual that performs valuable services to facilitate health and healthcare service (Rani et al., 2021).

For example, drug manufacturers are using robotic processes, AI, and blockchain (Khanh & Khang, 2021) to build efficient and automated supply chains on the one hand and on the other hand, technology is empowering patients to track their health conditions and make informed treatment choices (Ernst & Young, 2019).

The beneficiaries of Hospital 4.0 are not only the healthcare providers but also the patients who gain access to better quality and timely diagnosis through the help of data science-based predictive analytics diagnosis.

19.2   OPPORTUNITIES

Hospital 4.0 deals with designing better health systems, medical devices, and wearables through the application of various aspects of Industry 4.0 like AI, blockchain (Tailor et al., 2022), and virtual reality/augmented reality (VR/AR).

19.2.1   MEDICAL DEVICES

Medical devices include point-of-care and diagnostic devices that use technology to provide quick diagnosis and new innovative devices like smart bandages, 3D printers for organs, Bluetooth-enabled inhalers, etc.

19.2.2   MOBILE HEALTH (mHEALTH)

Mobile Health includes the use of mobile and wireless technologies to support the achievement of health objectives. It can improve the performance of front-line health workers as it allows the use of automated management of beneficiaries, audio-visual self-learning, and counseling tools (Sittig & Singh, 2014).

19.2.3   ARTIFICIAL INTELLIGENCE (AI)

In artificial intelligence, machines are programmed to develop cognitive functions for learning and problem solving, which is the reason why it is aptly used for supporting diagnostics for the highest level of accuracy and avoiding misdiagnosis (Jain et al., 2023).

19.2.4   BLOCKCHAIN TECHNOLOGY

Blockchain is defined as a distributed, decentralized data ledger but can be simply described as a shared database. The technology enables the creation of digital records and their sharing among the network of stakeholders (Sayles, 2012).

The database is updated in real time, which enables data exchange while safeguarding security, integrity, provenance, transparency, and control of the data (Khang et al., 2022c).

19.2.5   WEARABLES

Wearables include products like smartwatches, fitness trackers, and devices that may be linked to mobile applications for following a post-operative care regime and medicine alerts, movement analytics and blood pressure monitoring, emergency dialing to present numbers, etc.

These devices result in user-generated data and personal data such as phone numbers used or credit card transactions, which would be a great source of data for powerful analytical and predictive capabilities for healthcare providers and policymakers (Khang et al., 2022b).

19.2.6 ROBOTICS AND AUTOMATION

Robotics includes their use to provide healthcare services, including the use of virtual reality devices for surgeries; electronic ICUs; and drones to deliver drugs, vaccines, and medical aid faster to distant places, especially during disasters or medical emergencies (Hajimahmud et al., 2022).

19.2.7 VIRTUAL REALITY (VR)/AUGMENTED REALITY (AR)

Virtual reality (VR) is an artificial, computer-generated simulation or re-creation of a real-life environment or situation. Augmented reality (AR) is a technology that layers computer-generated enhancements on top of existing reality to make it more meaningful through the ability to interact with it.

Both have great potential in changing the medical landscape, more so in the case of treatment protocols for mental health conditions that enable direct active learning and coaching in real-world situations without therapists having to make time for sessions outside the clinic.

19.2.8 3D PRINTING

3D printing is an additive manufacturing process, in which a three-dimensional physical object is created from a digital design by printing material layer by layer. This technology plays a major role in the tailoring of drug dosage and size form or allowing for a combination of multiple drugs into one pill helps meet the needs of users with unique challenges.

19.3 APPROACHES

Hospital 4.0 is also leading to inter-linkages with other sectors. For example, in the case of designing medical devices and mobile applications, the engineers and product designers are collaborating with doctors and healthcare professionals.

Data science and data analytics and geo-locations are extensively used for predictive diagnosis, drug availability, and faster response time for patients; these complex functions are made simple (Rani et al., 2023).

The World Health Organization (WHO) came up with a resolution and directed its member nations to incorporate it for better healthcare facilitation in the respective countries.

The WHO Resolution on Digital Health that passed in May 2018 championed countries embrace the rapid adoption of technology to strengthen health systems and achieve universal health coverage (UHC). The adoption of the Digital Health Resolution and aligning it with the Sustainable Development Goals (SDGs) viz., SDG 3: Good Health and Wellbeing is one of the striking milestones of WHO.

Resolution on Digital Health when executed would ensure equity on health priorities on both the public and the private front, and dissemination and replication of the well-established best practices through empowering digital health workforce development (Snehal et al., 2023).

While every country's digital health ecosystem is unique in terms of the value chain and scalable digital health solutions, each rests on facilitating compatible infrastructure, appropriate opportunities for financing, and supportive policies in order to have a sustainable local capacity.

Currently, the literature says that most countries do not have the enablers in place to maximize the benefits of digital health to improve health outcomes and health systems.

The Global Digital Health Index (GDHI), Maturity Model, 2019 to start with considers 20 select countries from six regions as participants in developing this index, which depicts that average digital health ecosystem maturity is in phase three out of five (based on the seven selected dimensions of measures).

Among these countries, the majority of them ranked high on the leadership and governance among other parameters of digital GDHI; refer to figure 19.1.

Among the select regions for the index, Southeast Asia and Western Pacific Regions have more mature digital health ecosystems (in phase 4 in comparison of 5) than the other regions. European, Southeast Asia, and Western Pacific Regions scored 4 out of 5 on the GDHI's maturity model, and all other regions are just behind with 3 out of 5 in overall digital health maturity; refer to figure 19.2.

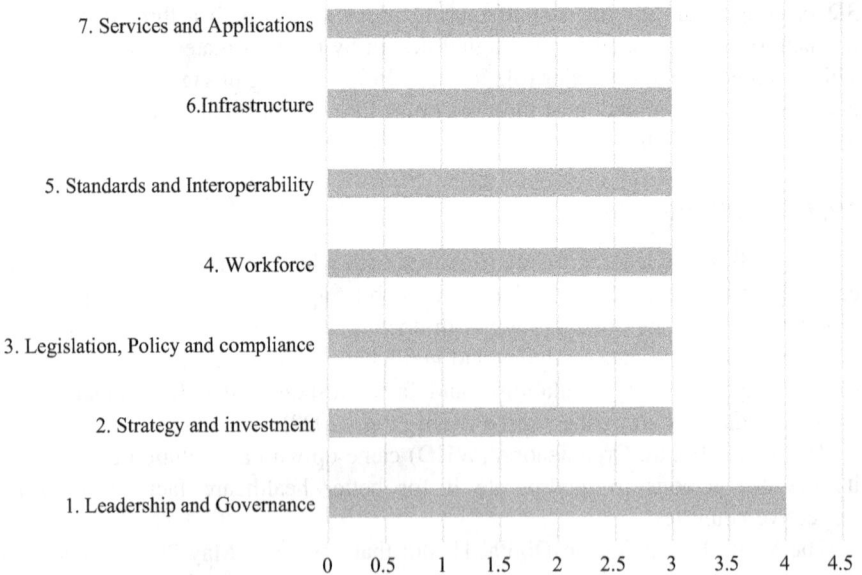

FIGURE 19.1   Digital health maturity phase.

Source: The state of Digital Health Report, 2019, Global Development Incubator.

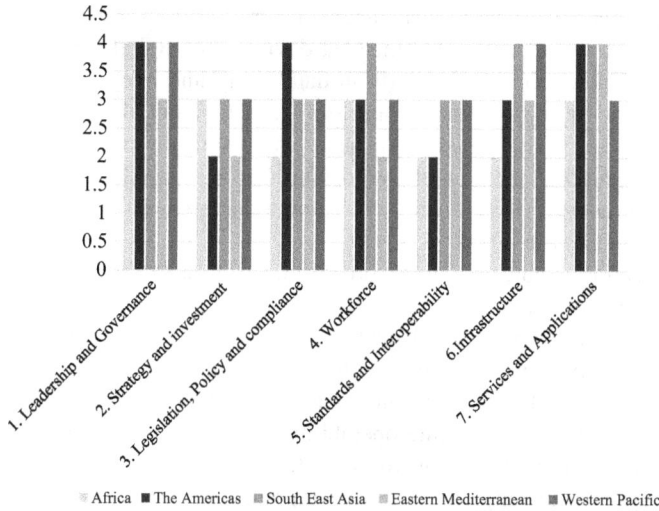

FIGURE 19.2   Digital health maturity phase by region.

Source: The state of Digital Health Report, 2019, Global Development Incubator.

According to the Digital Health Report, 2019, it is estimated that by 2040 the world will annually spend around USD 25 trillion on healthcare, implying that there could be tangible outcomes. However, the results of these expenditures on healthcare are not seen in a few cases as in the case of the United States, which spends more than five times as much per person as Estonia, yet both countries have similar life expectations.

Though the overall healthcare expenditures are increasing, there seems to be a constraint in receiving reasonable healthcare service across the world. Records say 800 million people spend at least 10% of the household budget on health expenditures.

According to the Digital Health Report, 2019, countries across the world are prioritizing digital health planning at their national level, although the institutional structures lag behind the IT infrastructure and the relevant regulation for institutionalized digital health governance. Countries are putting in their baby steps toward the digitalization of health and healthcare.

The majority of the countries considered in the index see themselves in the fourth phase of development out of the five phases on the scale. However, the success of the planning depends upon strategic investment; while a few of the countries have designed investment plans, many of the countries lag in this front.

Malaysia reported 3–5% of the national spending on health is committed to digitalization; however, in major cases, the investments in digitalization of healthcare are not keeping pace with the aspiration of the respective countries.

19.4   CHALLENGES

The investment in digitalization is very crucial for the countries not just for making healthcare affordable or/and accessible but to protecting individuals' privacy of health data. This calls for a robust framework on processes governing the clinical and patient care use of connected medical devices and digital health services like telemedicine applications, particularly in data safety and integrity; more so in the case of cross-border data exchange and storage (Cranen et al., 2011).

Building Hospital 4.0 investment is never complete with just the development of infrastructure and digitalization of the hospital, but there needs to be a convergence of digitization as well. A compatible workforce matters a lot in driving the digital health system in any country.

Digital health training for health professionals through specific programs as a part of their pre-service training requirements or in-service training is a must to get tangible results from the established digital health, health informatics health information systems, and biomedical informatics degree programs.

However, there is still a significant amount of work to be done and improvement in the areas of standards and interoperability and digital health workforce development. With a strong push towards investment in and deployment of effective healthcare systems undertaking elaborate training in new e-healthcare systems is very critical for operations, organization expectations, and interaction between various stakeholders in the healthcare systems.

A longitudinal study was done on the efficiency e-healthcare system in connecting the various stakeholders like doctors, patients, para medicine, nurses, administration team, etc., in the U.S. economy resulting in tracing a highly significant role in connecting the doctors and the patients rather than any other interpersonal connection between the other stakeholders (Uygun & Gujrati, 2020).

Interoperability is a persistent challenge in most of countries, with more digital health devices and services advancing in scale and magnitude; there is a need to transit from siloes to integration in the value chain by fully leveraging the information and communication technologies (ICTs) (Uygun & Gujrati, 2022).

Incorporating this in India would have variability among states, having fully scaled digital health platforms and electronic registries that have scaled nationally, particularly for births and immunizations that have a national digital health architectural framework and/or health information exchange established.

The full potential of digital health will only be achieved through its effective integration into the curricula and training of the health professionals that are meant to use them. In addition, as technology advances, new skillsets are needed to harness the benefits of technology.

In the case of national strategy development, specific skills are required, including project and change management, technology and public health technical expertise, health economics costing, political savviness, and skills in facilitating collaboration and coordination since digital health is multi-sectoral and multi-disciplinary.

Regarding infrastructure, some of the key needs identified are skills required to deploy and maintain hardware, software, and connectivity alongside infrastructure and architecture as well as the ability to build foundational and reusable infrastructure that generates economies of scale. This has pushed the job markets to come up with new roles and profiles like data scientists, business intelligence, visualization analysts, enterprise architects, data architects and modelers, machine learning and natural language processing specialists, and systems networking and communications experts, including human to machine interaction, security, and cryptography experts (Hussain et al., 2022).

While data science is not new, there is an increasing availability of data, and the need to improve its effective use is increasing the demand in health for new data modeling and integration skills.

In addition, with increased adoption and use of technology for health by individuals, new approaches to data ownership and use are necessary. Similar new approaches are required regarding AI, especially regarding new responsibilities related to ethical considerations.

India, being proud of its recent initiation of Ayushman Bharat the world's largest government-funded healthcare launched on September 23, 2018 (Ayushman Bharat, 2018), has a huge potential and a competitive advantage over other similar-looking markets.

The highly appreciable IT and Information Technology Enabled Services (ITeS) sectors and skilled and rising manpower show high potential for a better healthcare system that is affordable and accessible to the people of India, as shown in table 19.1.

On the demand side, the Indian healthcare market is expected to reach USD 372 billion in the year 2022. The rising income of the people and greater health awareness, lifestyle diseases, and increasing access to insurance among Indian consumers is leading to a surge in the demand.

On the supply side, the most important facilitator is the manpower in healthcare that is seen increasing; the number of doctors has increased to 841,104 in 2017 from 827,006 in 2010.

The hospital industry is expected to grow at a CAGR of 16–17% to reach Rs. 8.6 trillion (USD 132.84 billion) by Fiscal Year (FY) 2022 from 4 trillion (USD 61.79 billion) in FY 2017 (ibef.org).

As witnessed in table 19.1, the overall increase in the general government expenditure as percent of GDP is too insignificant to cope with and compete with the other countries in the discussion. As in the case of the above discussion, India too has similar constraints.

The key challenge in applying AI to healthcare is translating technical success into meaningful clinical impact coupled with the ethical and legal challenges in data sharing and management. Blockchain technology's ability to record digital events and information of patients, and enable peer-to-peer sharing between parties, on a robust system is a challenge (Khang et al., 2022).

TABLE 19.1

Domestic General Government Health Expenditure as a % of GDP (%)

Year	2000	2005	2010	2015	2020
India	0.83	0.8	0.86	0.92	0.99

Source: WHO.org, https://www.who.int/gho/health_financing/public_exp_health/en/

19.5 CONCLUSION

The above deliberation can be summed up by mentioning that for a successful implementation of Hospital 4.0 across the globe there could be majorly two constraints; one is the increasing costs with the increase in the innovative methods of treatment and procedure, which would eventually hamper the affordability to people.

The second is the suitably skilled workforce required to run these innovative products and services in the healthcare industry wherein the perfection of execution is zero defect. This calls for customized training and development workshops to be conducted at intervals and/or as and when the need arises (Ashwini et al., 2023).

The existing regulatory frameworks will need to be examined to ensure they are suitable for emerging technologies. Policymakers need to revisit the method evidence is collected and evaluated. It is a need of the hour that the decision makers must modernize governance frameworks and implement policy levers in order to encourage the appropriate use of health technologies, balancing the need to protect patients, spend resources wisely, and continue to promote future innovation.

While digital transformation supports scalability, agility, and cost savings, more than anything security is very crucial in that the employees possess the digital competencies to ensure proper implementation of the four important Ds of digital transformation, digital strategy, digital integrity, and digital control for achieving the aspired result in Industry 4.0 economy.

Taking forward the expertise and the digital competencies of the leadership and employees of an organization need to be in line with the digital strategy and integrity in the technical skills or the business acumen.

Most of the organizations that focus on the required knowledge and skills and ensure that the human capital of the organization has acquired the required skillset have proved to be the star performers (Khang et al., 2023d).

REFERENCES

Ashwini, Y., Sonawane, & Khang, A. 2023. Challenges Faced by Marketers in Developing and Managing Contents in Workforce Development System. *Designing Workforce Management Systems for Industry 4.0: Data-Centric and AI-Enabled Approaches*, (1st ed.), 332–359. CRC Press. 10.1201/9781003357070-18

Ayushman Bharat 2018. NHA | Official website Ayushman Bharat Digital Mission. https://abdm.gov.in/ and http://ab-hwc.nhp.gov.in/

Bhambri, P., Rani, S., Gupta, G., & Khang, A. 2022. *Cloud and Fog Computing Platforms for Internet of Things*, ISBN: 978-1-032-101507. CRC Press. 10.1201/9781003213888

Bharadwaj, A., El Sawy, O. A., Pavlou, P. A., & Venkatraman, N. 2013. Digital business strategy: Toward a next generation of insights. *MIS Quarterly*, 37(2), 471–482. https://www.jstor.org/stable/43825919

Chowdhury, S., Rodriguez-Espindola, O., Dey, P., & Budhwar, P. 2022. Blockchain technology adoption for managing risks in operations and supply chain management: Evidence from the UK. *Annals of Operations Research*, 1–36. https://link.springer.com/article/10.1007/s10479-021-04487-1

Cranen, K., Veld, R. H., Ijzerman, M., & Vollenbroek-Hutten, M. 2011. Change of patients' perceptions of telemedicine after brief use. *Telemedicine and e-Health*, 17(7), 530–535. https://www.liebertpub.com/doi/abs/10.1089/tmj.2010.0208

Ernst & Young (EY), 2019. Life sciences 4.0: Transforming health care in India, available at https://www.ey.com/Publication/vwLUAssets/ey-transforming-health-care-inindia/$File/ey-transforming-health-care-in-india.pdf (accessed on 3 July 2019).

Hajimahmud, V. A., Khang, A., Hahanov, V., Litvinova, E., Chumachenko, S., & Alyar, A. V. 2022. Autonomous Robots for Smart City: Closer to Augmented Humanity. *AI-Centric Smart City Ecosystems: Technologies, Design and Implementation*, (1st ed.). CRC Press. 10.1201/9781003252542-7

Hussain, S. H., Sivakumar, T. B., & Khang, A., (Eds.). 2022. Cryptocurrency Methodologies and Techniques. *The Data-Driven Blockchain Ecosystem: Fundamentals, Applications, and Emerging Technologies*, (1st ed.), 149–164. CRC Press. 10.1201/9781003269281-2

Insight Report, 2019. Health and healthcare in the fourth Industrial revolution. *World Economic Forum*, April 2019. https://apo.org.au/node/235506

Jain, P., Tripathi, V., Malladi, R., & Khang, A. 2023. Data-Driven AI Models in the Workforce Development Planning. *Designing Workforce Management Systems for Industry 4.0: Data-Centric and AI-Enabled Approaches*, (1st ed.), 179–198. CRC Press. 10.1201/9781003357070-10

Khang, A., Hahanov, V., Abbas, G. L., & Hajimahmud, V. A. 2022a. Cyber-Physical-Social System and İncident Management. *AI-Centric Smart City Ecosystems: Technologies, Design and Implementation*, (1st ed.). CRC Press. 10.1201/9781003252542-2

Khang, A., Hahanov, V., Litvinova, E., Chumachenko, S., Hajimahmud, V. A., & Alyar, A. V. 2022b. The Key Assistant of Smart City - Sensors and Tools. *AI-Centric Smart City Ecosystems: Technologies, Design and Implementation*, (1st ed.). CRC Press. 10.1201/9781003252542-17

Khang A., Chowdhury, S., & Sharma, S., (Eds.). 2022c. *The Data-Driven Blockchain Ecosystem: Fundamentals, Applications, and Emerging Technologies*, (1st ed.). CRC Press. 10.1201/9781003269281

Khang A., Ragimova, N. A., Hajimahmud, V. A., & Alyar, A. V. 2022d. Advanced Technologies and Data Management in the Smart Healthcare System. *AI-Centric Smart City Ecosystems: Technologies, Design and Implementation*, (1st ed.). CRC Press. 10.1201/9781003252542-16

Khang, A., Gupta, S. K., Rani, S., & Karras, D. A., (Eds.). 2023a. *Smart Cities: IoT Technologies, Big Data Solutions, Cloud Platforms, and Cybersecurity Techniques*, (1st ed.). CRC Press. 10.1201/9781003376064

Khang, A., Gupta, S. K., Shah, V., & Misra, A., (Eds.). 2023b. *AI-Aided IoT Technologies and Applications in the Smart Business and Production*, (1st ed.). CRC Press. 10.1201/9781003392224

Khang, A., Rani, S., & Vrushank, S. 2023c. *AI-Based Technologies and Applications in the Era of the Metaverse*, (1st ed.). IGI Global Press. 10.4018/9781668488515

Khang, A., Rani, S., Gujrati, R., Uygun, H., & Gupta, S. K., (Eds.). 2023d. *Designing Workforce Management Systems for Industry 4.0: Data-Centric and AI-Enabled Approaches*, (1st ed.). CRC Press. 10.1201/99781003357070

Khanh, H. H., & Khang, A. 2021. The Role of Artificial Intelligence in Blockchain Applications. *Reinventing Manufacturing and Business Processes through Artificial Intelligence*, 20–40. CRC Press. 10.1201/9781003145011-2

Martínez-C-Caro, E., Cegarra-Navarro, J. G., & Alfonso-Ruiz, F. J. 2020. Digital technologies and firm performance: The role of digital organisational culture. *Technol. Forecast. Social Change*, 154, 119962. https://www.sciencedirect.com/science/article/pii/S0040162519312193

Morris, G., Babasaheb, J., Khang, A., Gupta, S. K., & Hajimahmud, V. A. 2023. *AI-Centric Modelling and Analytics: Concepts, Designs, Technologies, and Applications*, (1st ed.). CRC Press. 10.1201/9781003400110

Rana, G., Khang, A., Sharma, R., Goel, A. K., & Dubey, A. K. 2021. *Reinventing Manufacturing and Business Processes through Artificial Intelligence.* CRC Press. 10.1201/9781003145011

Rani, S., Bhambri, P., Kataria, A., Khang, A., & Sivaraman, A. K. (Eds.). 2023. *Big Data, Cloud Computing and IoT: Tools and Applications,* (1st ed.). Chapman and Hall/CRC. 10.1201/9781003298335

Rani, S., Chauhan, M., Kataria, A., & Khang, A. 2021. IoT Equipped Intelligent Distributed Framework for Smart Healthcare Systems. *Networking and Internet Architecture.* CRC Press. 10.48550/arXiv.2110.04997

Sayles, N. B. 2012. *Health Information Management Technology: An Applied Approach.* Chicago, IL: American Health Information Management Association. https://mwcc.edu/ctl/files/2014/03/HIM101-Introduction-to-Health-Data.pdf

Sittig, D. F., & Singh, H. 2014. Defining Health Information Technology-Related Errors: New Developments Since to Err Is Human. In D. F. Sittig (Ed.), *Electronic Health Records: Challenges in Design and Implementation.* Toronto: Apple Academic Press, 27–36. https://api.taylorfrancis.com/content/chapters/edit/download?identifierName=doi&identifierValue=10.1201/b16306-10&type=chapterpdf

Snehal, M., Babasaheb, J., & Khang, A. 2023. Workforce Management System: Concepts, Definitions, Principles, and Implementation. *Designing Workforce Management Systems for Industry 4.0: Data-Centric and AI-Enabled Approaches,* (1st ed.), 1–13. CRC Press. 10.1201/9781003357070-1

Tailor, R. K., Pareek, R., & Khang, A., (Eds.). 2022. Robot Process Automation in Blockchain. *The Data-Driven Blockchain Ecosystem: Fundamentals, Applications, and Emerging Technologies,* (1st ed.), 149–164. CRC Press. 10.1201/9781003269281-8

Tyagi, H. 2018. Digital health start-ups in India: The challenge of scale. *ISB Insights.* Available at http://isbinsight.isb.edu/digital-health-start-ups-in-india-thechallenge-of-scale/ (accessed on 2 July 2019)

Uygun, H., & Gujrati, R. 2020. Digital innovation: Changing the face of businesses. *Int. J. Forensic Engineering,* 4(4), 332–342. https://www.researchgate.net/profile/Rashmi-Gujrati-2/publication/351274752_Digital_innovation_changing_the_face_of_business/links/60a9541a45851522bc0dd7a0/Digital-innovation-changing-the-face-of-business.pdf

Uygun, H., & Gujrati, R. 2022. Role of artificial intelligence & machine learning in social media. *International Journal of Mechanical Engineering,* 7(5), 494–498. https://avesis.erdogan.edu.tr/yayin/3a80288e-397c-408d-bb13-0a47128a1112/role-of-artificial-intelligence-machine-learning-in-social-media

20 Use of Technology for Monitoring the Immunization Status of Children Aged Five Years

Ankita Sharma and Monika Mathur

CONTENTS

20.1 INTRODUCTION

Immunizations are among the top ten public health accomplishments of the early 20th century because they helped reduce cases, hospitalizations, deaths, and healthcare costs related to diseases that could have been prevented with vaccines (Groom et al., 2015).

The Millennium Development Goals are also meant to improve the health of mothers, lower the death rate of children, and fight diseases like HIV/AIDS, malaria, and others (Kaewkungwal et al., 2010). At both the global and national levels, achieving universal health coverage (UHC) is now widely acknowledged as a key development agenda.

In December 2012, the United Nations (UN) General Assembly passed a resolution that shows how momentum can build (Prinja et al., 2017). The Expanded Program on Immunization (EPI) originated in the late 1970s as a result of a smallpox eradication program with the World Health Organization (WHO) support.

Due to inadequate financial and material resources, lack of epidemiologic and programmatic knowledge, and weak political commitment, the initiative made poor progress in immunizing the world's children.

The Universal Childhood Immunization (UCI) initiative aimed to immunize all children by 1990. With UCI, coverage for six EPI-preventable illnesses has increased (Brenzel et al., 1994). Even though it took India three decades to formulate its first formal policy on children's immunization, vaccination has always been an integral component of the country's Reproductive and Child Health (RCH) programs.

Under the WHO goal of "Health for All by 2000," the Indian government launched the Universal Immunization Program (UIP) in 1985 to achieve immunization coverage for children. Since the beginning of the immunization program, broad policy and funding choices have been made at the national level while being executed at the state level (Singh, 2013).

Despite the best efforts of the government and other organizations, reaching the goal of 100% universal coverage for eligible under-five children and pregnant women is still a long way off (G. S. and S. P., 2010). As of August 2018, 71 countries had not reached the goal of 90% or more DTP-3 coverage set by the Global Vaccine Action Plan. Between 2000 and 2016, the third dose of the DTP vaccine attained 85% global coverage, while the measles vaccine reduced mortality by 84%.

Despite progress, immunizations have slowed in the 20th century. In 2017, 19.9 million infants under the age of one did not receive all three doses of the DTP-3 vaccine, while 20.8 million children were refused a single dose of the measles vaccine (Khang et al., 2022).

Infectious diseases lead to global morbidity and mortality. WHO believes that an additional 1.5 million fatalities per year might be averted if worldwide vaccine coverage improved (Kim et al., 2017). A number of challenges have emerged as legitimate threats to maintaining coverage, conducting efficient surveillance, and allowing immunization programs to respond promptly to new problems (Khetrapal, 2020).

Costs associated with routine immunization vary significantly across hospitals and nations (Hajimahmud et al., 2022). Few studies have explored the cost drivers of routine immunization programs as part of the EPI Costing and Financing (EPIC) project. However, there is a lack of such research in big countries like India.

Due to variations in healthcare systems, demography, and vaccination schedules, it is essential to have national-level data on costs and cost-influencing variables (Rani et al., 2021). In 2012–13, India's vaccination program cost $718 million, according to the comprehensive multi-year plan for immunization (cMYP).

A recent study on the expenses of regular immunizations revealed substantial variation among facilities, districts, and states. During 2013–14, the weighted average cost per dose distributed at the state level ranged from $1.31 to $2.79, including the vaccination cost. While the cost per child vaccinated with the third dose of Diphteria-Tetanus-Pertussis (DPT) varied between $19.11 and $33.13 (Chatterjee et al., 2018).

20.2 ROLE OF TECHNOLOGY FOR MONITORING IMMUNIZATION STATUS

While there is widespread agreement that "people-centeredness" is crucial to healthcare delivery, the debate continues on "how to put people at the center of health systems" (Khang et al., 2023a).

As recognized by international organizations, the digitalization of healthcare offers tools for people's care, enabling individuals to manage their health, promoting prevention, and facilitating user feedback and engagement with health-care providers (Khang & Hajimahmud, 2022b).

In a time when vaccine hesitancy is one of the ten global health challenges, it's pivotal to explore how to employ digital technologies to promote vaccine preventable diseases (VPD) prevention (Balzarini et al., 2020).

Higher immunization coverage in a population requires the execution and coordination of public policy, healthcare, and community-based interventions (Groom et al., 2015).

In most developing countries, vaccination logistics are paper-based, restricting updates and information accessibility. Access to vaccination information is limited, preventing timely and complete data-driven vaccination strategies. Inaccessible data can potentially impair vaccine safety and effectiveness (Bhambri et al., 2022).

In some countries, immunization records are maintained locally, so citizens may have trouble accessing them. Paper-based dose tracking has explicit safety and timing constraints (Tozzi et al., 2016).

Using immunization data in electronic form permits the real-time identification of children who need to get vaccinated on a broader scale than individual record review. It also lays the groundwork for vaccine-oriented parental communication or clinician warnings that are flexible and personalized (Rani et al., 2023).

There is a small but expanding body of research integrating IT into vaccination treatments aimed at the family or individual children, the healthcare provider or system, or the community. These include nontraditional reminder and recall techniques, clinical decision-making support in the electronic health record, and the change of workflow by using technology and social media (Stockwell & Fiks, 2013).

Globally, 95% of the population has access to a mobile cellular network, and in emerging countries, mobile broadband subscribers have increased by double digits (Khang et al., 2022a).

e-Health may reduce human error, speed up procedures, and expand the reach of intervention, providing researchers and program administrators with the means to develop vaccination campaigns (Kim et al., 2017).

With the increasing improvement, better access, and enhanced capability of mobile technology in low- and lower-middle-income nations, it is ethical and important to use mHealth (mobile health) to expand global vaccination coverage. VPDs continue to impose a significant cost on society, but mobile technology has the potential to assist in mitigating this burden.

As the number of people with mobile phones continues to grow, so does the chance that mHealth will help improve vaccination efforts. Also, it is much easier to count the number of doses given, but it is much more important to know if children have been immunized (Berkley, 2017).

In 2015, WHO's Strategic Advisory Group of Experts came up with a number of ways to reduce gaps in coverage. These include improving the quality and use of data; getting the community involved; giving marginalized and vulnerable groups access to immunization services; and making health systems stronger (Khang et al., 2023b).

In addition, they concluded that digitalization offers new tools for immunization activities, such as digital information systems for combining data or electronic registries, decision-support tools, mobile and geospatial technologies, and predictive analytics to keep improving coverage and population estimates. But most of these tools haven't been used by many people or tested well.

National and global strategies for controlling VPD encourage the usage of digital immunization information systems (DIIS) to improve the effectiveness of vaccination programs (Khang et al., 2022c).

DIIS help healthcare professionals administer immunizations and provide policymakers with population-level data to inform routine immunization (Tailor et al., 2022). Aside from HCWs and policymakers, vaccine end users may also have access to DIIS data through their personal electronic health record (PEHR). It's a very helpful way for vaccination providers and healthcare systems to work together and coordinate interventions for a whole population (Groom et al., 2015).

Nevertheless, robust approaches for tracking individual and population vaccination numbers are required to preserve progress in the face of an increasingly complicated immunization backdrop in upper-middle and high-income countries. Individuals who are part of a population being served can have their immunization records stored in a central database called an immunization information system (IIS). IISs can identify people at greater risk for under immunization based on geographic, demographic, or behavioral features (Atkinson et al., 2020).

20.3   AVERAGE EXPENDITURE AND ITS IMPACT ON IMMUNIZATION STATUS

Immunization against VPDs is necessary for human development (Rwashana et al., 2009). In 2005, under the Global Immunization Vision and Strategy (GIVS), the World Health Organization (WHO), and the United Nations Children's Fund (UNICEF) established a target for all nations to attain 90% national vaccine coverage and 80% district vaccination coverage by 2010. The UIP has failed to accomplish these objectives.

In 2007, just 53.5% of children were fully immunized, and vaccination rates throughout the country varied substantially. Even though vaccination rates have increased over the past several years, they remain below 70% in urban areas and below 60% in rural areas.

Even in a high-quality health system, vaccination policy confronts a significant market failure: individuals have a propensity to under-vaccinate, and government action is necessary to address this problem.

Despite India's success in eradicating polio, regular vaccination has become less effective. Targeted vaccination campaigns may be easier to execute than routine immunization initiatives (Megiddo et al., 2014).

Table 20.1 illustrates that for social groups in rural areas and urban areas, the mean average expenditure on immunization in the last 365 days was higher for other social groups. Whereas the lowest mean average expenditure on immunization in the last 365 days was incurred by SC in rural areas, the lowest was incurred by ST in urban areas.

In terms of religion, the mean average expenditure on immunization in the previous 365 days for rural and urban areas was highest for Christians and lowest for Muslims. Taking into account the quintile class, mean average expenditure on

TABLE 20.1

Average Expenditure on Immunization During Last 365 Days and Number of Children Received any Type of Immunization During Last 365 Days for Socioeconomic Groups

	RURAL		URBAN	
	Mean (Std. Error)	Number of Children Receiving Any Type of Immunization	Mean (Std. Error)	Number of Children Receiving Any Type of Immunization
SOCIAL GROUP				
SC	18.00 (2.31)	8,071	138.33 (20.79)	2,279
ST	20.67 (.88)	8,939	109.67 (5.49)	3,965
OBC	43.00 (6.93)	17,198	201.00 (15.89)	11,348
Others	49.00 (.00)	9,017	389.00 (37.24)	9,441
All	35.67 (3.76)	43,225	251.33 (4.91)	27,033
RELIGION				
Hinduism	35.67 (3.76)	32,152	277.33 (7.80)	19,146
Islam	32.00 (4.62)	6,313	150.67 (7.22)	5,442
Christianity	47.33 (8.67)	3,031	388.00 (27.15)	1,595
Others[*]	46.33 (6.64)	1,729	324.67 (26.28)	850
All	35.67 (3.76)	43,225	251.33 (4.91)	27,033
QUINTILE				
1st Quintile	19.00 (1.732)	8,646	75.67 (14.449)	7,653
2nd Quintile	19.00 (.000)	7,954	109.67 (6.642)	6,277
3rd Quintile	33.00 (4.619)	8,726	228.33 (23.383)	5,244
4th Quintile	37.00 (1.732)	8,413	312.33 (21.372)	4,519
5th Quintile	91.00 (11.846)	9,486	863.00 (65.886)	3,340
All	35.67 (3.756)	43,225	251.33 (4.910)	27,033

Source: Author's calculations from NSS 75th Round Report.
[*] Sikhism, Jainism, Buddhism, Zoroastrianism, etc.

immunization during the last 365 days in rural areas was highest for the 5th quintile, representing 20% of the population with the highest consumption expenditure; the 1st and 2nd quintile represented 20% of the poorest households with the lowest consumption expenditure.

In urban areas, the 5th quintile spent the most on immunizations on average over the course of a year, while the 1st quintile spent the least.

Hence, the above Table 20.1 reveals that for social groups, the highest number of children receiving any type of immunization in rural areas and urban areas was for OBC groups as compared to SC, ST, and other social groups, while the children belonging to the SC category had the lowest number of children receiving any type of immunization in rural areas and urban areas.

Similarly, the highest number of children receiving any type of immunization in rural areas and urban areas was for the children who were Hindu, whereas the children who were Christian had the lowest number of children receiving any type of immunization in rural areas and urban areas.

In urban areas, the 5th quintile group had the lowest number of children getting any type of immunization, whereas in rural areas, the 2nd quintile group had the lowest number of children getting any type of immunization.

Therefore, incurring average expenditure on immunization doesn't significantly impact the immunization status of children as socioeconomic groups who incurred less average expenditure on immunization have a majority of children who have received any type of immunization, which was the same for socioeconomic groups who incurred more average expenditure on immunization in rural areas and urban areas. Similarly, consider table 20.2.

TABLE 20.2

Average Expenditure on Immunization During Last 365 Days and Number of Children Fully Immunized Aged 5 Years

	Rural Areas		Urban Areas	
	Average Expenditure on Immunization in Last 365 Days (Rs.)	Children Fully Immunized (0–5 Years)	Average Expenditure on Immunization in Last 365 Days (Rs.)	Children Fully Immunized (0–5 Years)
Andhra Pradesh	18	746	206	414
Arunachal Pradesh	72	234	125	137
Assam	19	595	148	177
Bihar	34	1,162	434	483
Chhattisgarh	6	665	154	339
Delhi	247	14	164	277
Goa	5	36	90	47
Gujarat	114	583	203	572
Haryana	101	721	493	505
Himachal Pradesh	41	589	203	107
Jammu & Kashmir	63	630	228	422
Jharkhand	10	786	288	256
Karnataka	37	630	354	495
Kerala	85	700	116	601
Madhya Pradesh	12	1,095	188	725
Maharashtra	56	1,197	328	1,121
Manipur	34	563	15	437
Meghalaya	79	310	134	129
Mizoram	10	310	48	286
Nagaland	19	83	90	37
Odisha	46	842	117	260

TABLE 20.2 (Continued)
Average Expenditure on Immunization During Last 365 Days and Number of Children Fully Immunized Aged 5 Years

	Rural Areas		Urban Areas	
	Average Expenditure on Immunization in Last 365 Days (Rs.)	Children Fully Immunized (0–5 Years)	Average Expenditure on Immunization in Last 365 Days (Rs.)	Children Fully Immunized (0–5 Years)
Punjab	58	444	184	408
Rajasthan	7	1,217	144	602
Sikkim	28	70	23	19
Tamil Nadu	66	848	249	652
Telangana	76	497	527	430
Tripura	9	210	5	64
Uttarakhand	29	369	64	209
Uttar Pradesh	29	2,337	210	1,355
West Bengal	26	1,201	240	565
A & N Islands	2	56	185	54
Chandigarh	4	9	113	59
Dadra & Nagar Haveli	3	42	285	31
Daman & Diu	5	25	110	7
Lakshadweep	20	23	0	48
Puducherry	1	8	26	41

Source: Author's calculations from NSS 75th Round Report.

But looking at children aged five years who are fully immunized, average expenditure incurred on immunization doesn't affect the immunization status of children in rural and urban areas, respectively. From the table and numbers below, it's clear that the states that spent the most on immunization had the lowest percentage of fully immunized aged five years compared to the states that spent less on immunization.

At the national level, it is especially important to keep track of immunization rates and outcomes related to immunization to retain political clout for India's NRHM and ensure there is enough funding to meet the government's goals for immunization coverage (Patel et al., 2009).

Several programmatic initiatives, including the Universal Immunization Program (1985), the Child Survival and Safe Motherhood Program (1992), the National Health Policy (2002), and the National Rural Health Mission (2005) have been implemented to expedite the coverage of essential health services.

The failure of both the "demand" and "supply" sides is one of the primary causes of low vaccination rates. Due to the absence of vaccination campaigns and

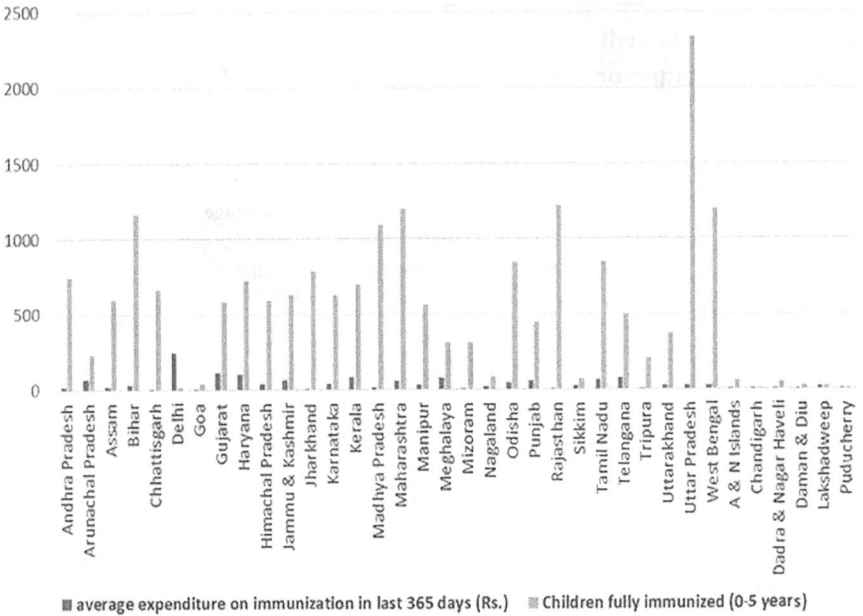

FIGURE 20.1 Children aged five years fully immunized with respect to average expenditure on immunization during last 365 days in rural areas.

Source: Author's calculations from NSS 75th Round Report.

insufficient family education, there is a knowledge gap on the benefits of vaccines, which adds to the demand failure. However, supply or system problems include health workers' absenteeism, inadequate supplies, etc.

The high-level expert group (HLEG) has suggested the "National Health Package" for all Indian citizens' primary, secondary, and tertiary healthcare requirements by 2022. Children's vaccinations should be a top priority in the proposed National Health Package, which could be a step toward getting everyone vaccinated (Singh, 2013).

Figure 20.1 and Figure 20.2 below, Delhi incurred the highest average expenditure on immunization during the last 365 days, followed by Gujarat and Haryana in rural areas. Whereas, in urban areas, Telangana incurred the highest average expenditure on immunization during the last 365 days, followed by Haryana and Bihar.

20.4 USAGE OF HEALTH FACILITIES AND ITS IMPACT ON IMMUNIZATION STATUS

The health and well-being of a country's people are hugely dependent on a developed, accessible, and efficient healthcare infrastructure (Taqi et al., 2017). To improve the overall health of a country's population, having a healthcare system that is well developed is absolutely necessary.

Recognizing the significance of health in terms of both development and the role that health infrastructure plays in the enhancement of health in India, the infrastructure for

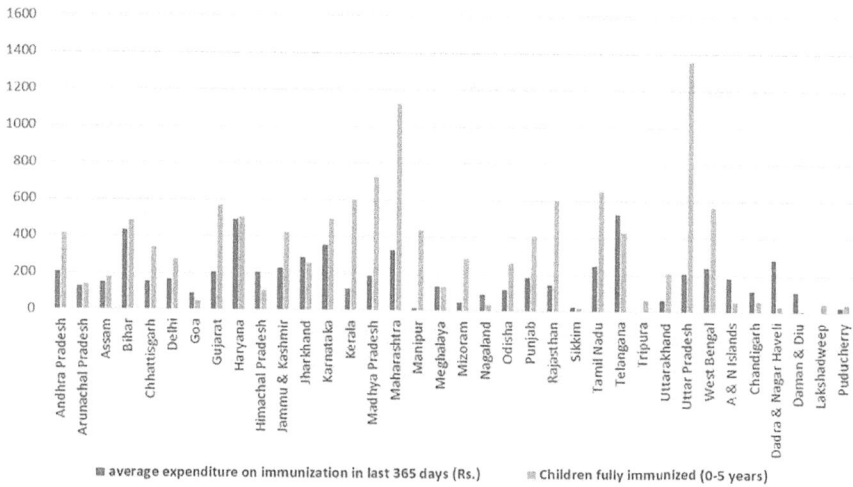

FIGURE 20.2   Children aged five years fully immunized with respect to average expenditure on immunization during last 365 days urban areas.

Source: Author's calculations from NSS 75th Round Report.

providing healthcare in rural areas has been developed as a triangular system, with the sub-center, primary health centers (PHC), and community health centers (CHC) serving as the respective pillars (Saikia, 2014).

Table 20.3 reflects that a unit increase in average expenditure on immunization during the last 365 days (in Rs.) by .159 units; visits to grassroots level centers by .465 units; private health centers by .954 units; and government centers and others by .322 units will lead to an increase in fully immunized children aged five years in rural areas.

This implies that with an increase of 15.90% in average expenditure by individuals on immunization during the last 365 days and a 46.50%, 95.40%, and 32.20% increase in the type of health facilities from which the child had received immunization i.e., grassroots level centers, private health centers, government centers, and others, will increase the rate of fully immunized children aged five years in rural areas.

Likewise, table 20.4 shows a unit increase in average expenditure on immunization during 365 days (in Rs.) by .051 units; visits to HSC/Anganwadi center/PHC/dispensary/CHC/mobile medical units by .517 units; private hospital/private doctor/clinic by .254 units; and govt./public hospital/charitable/trust/NGO run hospital by .407 units will lead to an increase in fully immunized children aged five years in urban areas (Khang et al., 2023c).

This implies that with an increase of 5.10% in average expenditure by individuals on immunization during the last 365 days and a 51.7%, 25.40%, and 40.70% increase in the types of health facilities from which the child had received immunization i.e., grassroots level centers, private health centers, government centers and others, will increase the rate of fully immunized children aged five years in urban areas.

Thus, both rural areas and urban areas state that the immunization rate is higher when children/households are visiting grassroots level centers and government

TABLE 20.3

Values of Multiple Linear Regression Model for Rural Areas

Model	Unstandardized Coefficients		Standardized Coefficients	Collinearity Statistics	
	B	Standard Error	Beta	Tolerance	VIF
(Constant)	3.400 [.133], (.895)	25.638			
Average expenditure on immunization during last 365 days (in Rs)	.159 [.491], (.627)	.324	.015	.838	1.194
Grassroots level centers	.465 [21.657], (.000)	.021	.874	.483	2.069
Private health centers	.954 [1.445], (.159)	.660	.064	.405	2.468
Government centers and others	.322 [3.150], (.004)	.102	.117	.567	1.764

Source: Author's calculations from NSS 75th Round Report; t values in [], p values in ().
Dependent Variable: Children fully immunized aged five years R Square: .976
Adjusted R Square: .972

TABLE 20.4

Values of Multiple Linear Regression Model for Urban Areas

Model	Unstandardized Coefficients		Standardized Coefficients	Collinearity Statistics	
	B	Standard Error	Beta	Tolerance	VIF
(Constant)	−5.349 [−.343], (.734)	15.610			
Average expenditure on immunization during last 365 days (in Rs)	.051 [.742], (.464)	.069	.022	.679	1.473
Grassroots level centers	.517 [17.052], (.000)	.030	.651	.391	2.558
Private health centers	.254 [1.557], (.130)	.163	.083	.199	5.019
Government centers and others	.407 [6.382], (.000)	.064	.314	.235	4.250

Source: Author's calculations from NSS 75th Round Report; t values in [], p values in ().
Dependent Variable: Children fully immunized aged five years R Square: .982
Adjusted R Square: .980

centers and others during the last 365 days, and have a positive relationship with children fully immunized aged five years.

While the average immunization expenditure incurred over 365 days and private health centers do not make a significant contribution to fully immunized children aged five years, as considering table 20.5.

The government needs to develop more grass root level centers and government health centers and others, as Anganwadi centers and Anganwadi workers play an important role due to their close and continuous contact with individual groups, especially children and women.

As it is an important function of Anganwadi workers to provide immunization services to children and pregnant women, apart from their other work. Ideally, community health workers (CHWs) can play a vital and dynamic role in overcoming community-specific obstacles to improving vaccination coverage.

CHWs offer a mechanism to reach vulnerable individuals in rural areas by virtue of their status as trusted community members. As indigenous community members, CHWs are ideally suited to assist with identification, tracking, and outreach services, as well as to provide community members with information, education, and communication.

To promote rural health, India must ensure the health system's support and adopt ways to involve the community in the implementation and oversight of the national CHW program.

Globally, and particularly in developed nations, the use of IT in healthcare has expanded substantially. In contrast, developing nations are attempting to implement technology in a sustainable manner, particularly in primary healthcare systems.

The use of information and technology in the field of maternal and child health (MCH) relates primarily to primary healthcare services, antenatal care, immunization, and disease control programs, as well as administrative issues such as reporting, inventory management, financial management, and vehicle and personnel management (Kumar et al., 2023). A robust health information management system is crucial for administering a health system (Bhati, 2015).

Most immunization takes place at grassroots level centers followed by government centers during the last 365 days, both in rural and urban areas, as shown in figure 20.3.

Private health centers are taken into least consideration for the immunization of children aged five years in both rural and urban areas, as shown in figure 20.4.

20.5   TECHNOLOGY FOR IMPROVING IMMUNIZATION STATUS IN INDIA

As in the above recommendation, this section also depicts the technology for improving immunization status in a specific nation, and we use context and data of India. India possesses several areas of achievement in the realm of e-governance, yet there are still many untouched sectors. Immunization of children is only partially investigated, although many programs have been launched by local governments and government entities to bring about the future of e-Government (Khang et al., 2023).

TABLE 20.5

Immunization Taken by Children Aged Five Years from Major Sources

	Rural Children Aged Five Years			Urban Children Aged Five Years		
	Grass Root Level Centers	Private Health Centers	Government Health Centers	Grassroot Level Centers	Private Health Centers	Government Health Centers
Andhra Pradesh	1226	14	189	579	39	165
Arunachal Pradesh	451	6	253	113	8	180
Assam	1357	22	402	259	58	181
Bihar	2460	43	352	728	119	389
Chhattisgarh	1201	5	99	317	59	322
Delhi	10	11	19	471	28	179
Goa	44	0	33	82	3	45
Gujarat	1134	26	115	789	139	335
Haryana	1025	70	104	497	124	278
Himachal Pradesh	788	24	272	94	4	123
Jammu & Kashmir	760	31	542	325	28	450
Jharkhand	1566	23	211	351	43	227
Karnataka	1131	37	296	516	240	342
Kerala	804	89	475	758	134	220
Madhya Pradesh	2160	32	263	1159	62	288
Maharashtra	2224	147	346	1159	439	1007
Manipur	676	15	253	500	9	221
Meghalaya	587	25	82	107	23	139
Mizoram	464	4	6	447	11	29
Nagaland	417	6	62	105	19	100
Odisha	1578	18	136	402	10	110
Punjab	711	27	240	381	87	487
Rajasthan	2268	26	278	571	61	623
Sikkim	168	3	44	29	0	37
Tamil Nadu	1102	62	778	568	255	660
Telangana	768	25	188	508	150	193
Tripura	539	1	127	99	0	141
Uttarakhand	628	5	107	324	21	84
Uttar Pradesh	4397	110	476	1774	326	933
West Bengal	2134	21	200	902	92	264
A & N Islands	92	0	43	40	10	72
Chandigarh	24	0	20	84	4	43
Dadra & Nagar Haveli	79	0	0	51	9	3
Daman & Diu	48	0	3	19	2	22
Lakshadweep	48	1	1	9	0	78
Puducherry	57	0	6	61	3	138

Source: Author's calculations from NSS 75th Round Report.

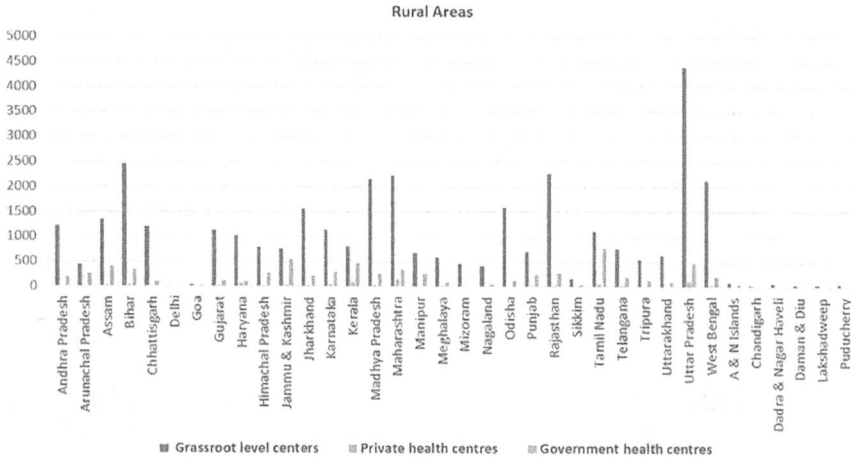

FIGURE 20.3   Sources of most immunization in rural areas.

Source: Author's calculations from NSS 75th Round Report.

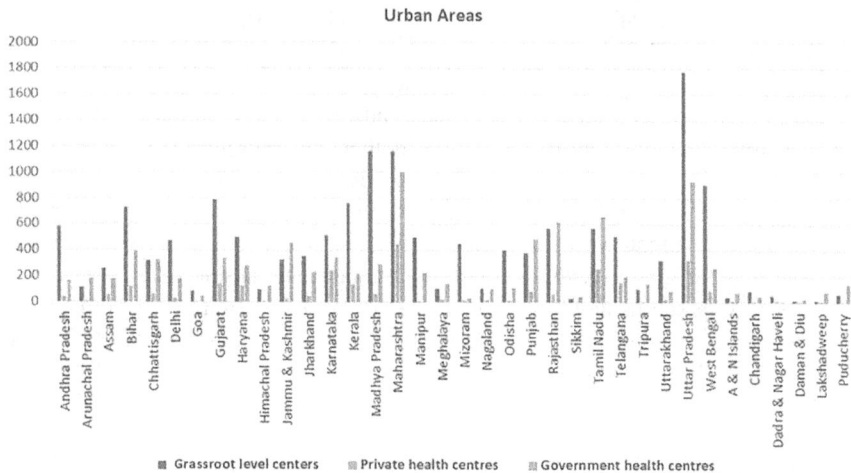

FIGURE 20.4   Sources of most immunization in urban areas.

Source: Author's calculations from NSS 75th Round Report.

Efforts have been made on several fronts to streamline the delivery of public services and make them easier to obtain. Indian e-Government has progressed from simple departmental computerization to more nuanced programs emphasizing citizen-centricity, service orientation, and openness.

The progressive e-Governance approach of the country was heavily influenced by the lessons learned from past e-Governance efforts. Although India's IT infrastructure extends to the village level, the vaccination procedure lacks an IT complement (Babasaheb et al., 2023).

The vaccination procedure is not totally electronic, and many sorts of paper records are still maintained. Due to a lack of ICT in this area, communication moves slowly. This causes a number of problems, such as problems with the demand and supply of pharmaceuticals in certain areas, drug shortages or oversupplies, etc. It has been taken into consideration that a programmatic approach, directed by a shared vision and strategy, is necessary to expedite the implementation of e-Governance across the various branches of government at the national, state, and local levels (Snehal et al., 2023).

This strategy could save a lot of money by making it easier to share core and support infrastructure, making it easier for systems to work together through standards, and giving people the same experience across all levels of government (M. of E. & I. T. IT, 2023).

Recently, ANMs in rural areas of Rajasthan utilized a mobile app called pregnancy, child tracking, and health services management system (PCTNS) to record and report real-time data on the health services they deliver to the local populations.

The program G2C (government to citizen) was deployed all over Rajasthan by the National Informatics Centre. It is a massive breakthrough in the domain of healthcare. Its primary objective is to reduce the mortality rate among mothers and children. It will improve rural and urban healthcare, particularly for the poor (Saikia et al., 2014; Bhati et al., 2015; M. of E. & I. T. IT, 2023).

There are over 17,000 ANMs using the app, who are stationed in over 167,000 government health facilities across the state. The smartphone app collects information in real time from health sub-centers and PHCs. All children's birth records are kept in conjunction with those of their mothers and siblings. The ANM's work schedule is also communicated through a mobile app (Centers, 2023).

Using PCTNS has many benefits because this app does online monitoring for every pregnant woman who enrolls at a PHC. The tracking also included prenatal care, services for giving birth, every abortion, and maternal mortality.

The system is online and has a central database, which ensures that both old and new data are always available. It also lets you check online for information about each live birth, like birth weight, hemoglobin, vaccinations, and vitamin A dosages. In addition, it tracks the area as well as district-wise sex ratios along with vaccination dropouts and absenteeism.

In addition to these benefits, there are a few downsides associated with it. Because the system is not countrywide and is thus limited to a particular state, it is not possible to utilize it for centralized planning purposes throughout the entire country. The "Aadhar" number is not being utilized by the system that is responsible for ensuring one's authenticity.

The provision of health services to pregnant women is the main focus of this initiative. If a mother or child moves out of the state, online tracking cannot be done on them since it is not possible to do so. It is not possible to generate various certifications, such as a birth certificate or a death certificate, among other certificates.

When a woman registers herself at a public health facility, only then it is possible to execute the tracking. It was made by NIC (National Informatics Centre) as an internal project, which means that no private partners were involved in making it (Kumar & Kumar, 2013).

20.6 CONCLUSION

Technology, omnipresent in today's society, offers novel and burgeoning approaches to increase immunization coverage. Because of its pervasiveness and flexibility, technology provides intriguing solutions to vaccination challenges for families, healthcare professionals, and people across the globe (Rana et al., 2021).

This widespread use of technology offers an excellent platform for administering vaccinations, one of the most important public-health initiatives. It can help parents, providers, the system, and the community deal with different problems that lead to low vaccination rates.

To vaccinate a child, the family must be aware that the child is at risk for VPDs, that the child needs an immunization, that the vaccine is safe and effective, that they know where to go to get vaccinated, and that they remember to come in for the vaccination.

In India, a model must be proposed and implemented. It will be a great addition to the government's current services. We already have a fully functional ICT (information and communication technology) infrastructure at all levels, and as part of the National eGovernance Plan, every village will soon be given a common service center (CSC), so the proposed model may be implemented without spending exorbitant costs.

Along with this, the government should also preserve electronic records by assigning numbers to the mother and child protection card (MCPC), which provides information on the immunization schedule of children. This would ensure that the records are accessible in the event that they are needed in the future. It would be helpful in keeping track of the vaccination data for children (Vrushank et al., 2023).

Moreover, the introduction of technologically advanced health tools into routine immunization leads to much-needed improvement. With the help of this strategy, India's immunization rate will definitely go up, which will be a big step toward making the country healthier (Khanh & Khang, 2021).

REFERENCES

K. M. Atkinson, S. S. Mithani, C. Bell, T. Rubens-Augustson, and K. Wilson, "The digital immunization system of the future: Imagining a patient-centric, interoperable immunization information system," *Ther. Adv. Vaccines Immunother.*, vol. 8, pp. 1–15, 2020, doi: 10.1177/2515135520967203

J. Babasaheb, B. Sphurti, and Khang, A., "Industry Revolution 4.0: Workforce Competency Models and Designs," *Designing Workforce Management Systems for Industry 4.0: Data-Centric and AI-Enabled Approaches*, (1st ed.), 2023, pp. 14–31. CRC Press. 10.1201/9781003357070-2

F. Balzarini et al., "Does the use of personal electronic health records increase vaccine uptake? A systematic review," *Vaccine*, vol. 38, no. 38, pp. 5966–5978, 2020, doi: 10.1016/j.vaccine.2020.05.083

S. Berkley, "Immunization needs a technology boost," *Nature*, vol. 551, no. 7680, pp. 273–274, 2017, doi: 10.1038/d41586-017-05923-8

P. Bhambri, S. Rani, G. Gupta, and Khang, A., *Cloud and Fog Computing Platforms for Internet of Things*, ISBN: 978-1-032-101507, 2022. CRC Press. 10.1201/9781003213888

D. K. Bhati, "Impact of Technology on Primary Healthcare Information Management: A Case of North India," *Perspect. Heal. Inf. Manag.*, no. International issue, 2015, [Online]. Available: http://bok.ahima.org/doc?oid=301177.

L. Brenzel, and P. Claquin, "Immunization programs and their costs," *Soc. Sci. Med.*, vol. 39, no. 4, pp. 527–536, 1994, doi: 10.1016/0277-9536(94)90095-7

N. I. Centers, 2023. "PCTS Awarded at eINDIA 2010 _ Informatics News." https://informatics. nic.in/news?search_kw=pcts&search_type=news&state_id=&start_date= &end_date=

S. Chatterjee, A. Ghosh, P. Das, N. A. Menzies, and R. Laxminarayan, "Determinants of cost of routine immunization programme in India," *Vaccine*, vol. 36, no. 26, pp. 3836–3841, 2018, doi: 10.1016/j.vaccine.2018.05.006

S. G., and P. S, "Vaccine hesitancy in India-the challenges: A review," *Int. J. Community Med. Public Heal.*, vol. 7, no. 11, pp. 4643–4647, 2020, doi: 10.18203/2394-6040.ijcmph 20204768

H. Groom et al., "Immunization information systems to increase vaccination rates: A community guide systematic review," *J. Public Heal. Manag. Pract.*, vol. 21, no. 3, pp. 227– 247, 2015, doi: 10.1097/PHH.0000000000000069

V. A. Hajimahmud, Khang, A., V. Hahanov, E., Litvinova, S. Chumachenko, and A. V. Alyar, "Autonomous Robots for Smart City: Closer to Augmented Humanity," *AI-Centric Smart City Ecosystems: Technologies, Design and Implementation*, (1st ed.), 2022. CRC Press. 10.1201/9781003252542-7

J. Kaewkungwal, P. Singhasivanon, A. Khamsiriwatchara, S. Sawang, P. Meankaew, and A. Wechsart, "Application of smart phone in 'better border healthcare program': A module for mother and child care," *BMC Med. Inform. Decis. Mak.*, vol. 10, no. 1, pp. 1–12, 2010, doi: 10.1186/1472-6947-10-69

A. Khang, V. Hahanov, E. Litvinova, S. Chumachenko, V. A. Hajimahmud, and A. V. Alyar, "The Key Assistant of Smart City - Sensors and Tools," *AI-Centric Smart City Ecosystems: Technologies, Design and Implementation*, (1st ed.), 2022a. CRC Press. 10.1201/9781003252542-17

A. Khang, N. A. Ragimova, V. A. Hajimahmud, and A. V. Alyar, "Advanced Technologies and Data Management in the Smart Healthcare System," *AI-Centric Smart City Ecosystems: Technologies, Design and Implementation*, (1st ed.), 2022b. CRC Press. 10.1201/9781003252542-16

A. Khang, V. Hahanov, G. L. Abbas, and V. A. Hajimahmud, "Cyber-Physical-Social System and İncident Management," *AI-Centric Smart City Ecosystems: Technologies, Design and Implementation*, (1st ed.), 2022c. CRC Press. 10.1201/9781003252542-2

A. Khang, S. Chowdhury, & S. Seema,*The Data-Driven Blockchain Ecosystem: Fundamentals, Applications, and Emerging Technologies*. (1st ed). 2022d. CRC Press. 10.1201/ 9781003269281

A. Khang, G. Rana, R. K. Tailor, and V. A. Hajimahmud, (Eds.). *Data-Centric AI Solutions and Emerging Technologies in the Healthcare Ecosystem*, (1st ed.), 2023a. CRC Press. 10.1201/9781032398570

A. Khang, S. Rani, R. Gujrati, H. Uygun, and S. K. Gupta, (Eds.). *Designing Workforce Management Systems for Industry 4.0: Data-Centric and AI-Enabled Approaches*, (1st ed.), 2023b. CRC Press. 10.1201/99781003357070

A. Khang, V. Hahanov, E. Litvinova, S. Chumachenko, Triwiyanto, V. A. Hajimahmud, R. N. Ali, A. V. Alyar, and P. T. N. Anh, "The Analytics of Hospitality of Hospitals in Healthcare Ecosystem," *Data-Centric AI Solutions and Emerging Technologies in the Healthcare Ecosystem*, (1st ed.), 2023c, P (4). CRC Press. 10.1201/9781003356189

H. H. Khanh, and Khang, A., "The Role of Artificial Intelligence in Blockchain Applications," *Reinventing Manufacturing and Business Processes Through Artificial Intelligence*, 2021, pp. 20–40. CRC Press. 10.1201/9781003145011-2

S. Khetrapal, "Going digital to boost immunization coverage," *ADB: Asian Development Bank*, 2020. https://policycommons.net/artifacts/389724/going-digital-to-boost-immunization-coverage/1354236/

S. S. Kim, M. Patel, and A. Hinman, "Use of m-health in polio eradication and other immunization activities in developing countries," *Vaccine*, vol. 35, no. 10, pp. 1373–1379, 2017. https://www.sciencedirect.com/science/article/pii/S0264410X1730124X

P. Kumar, and D. Kumar, "A conceptual e-governance framework for improving child immunization process in India," *Int. J. Comput. Appl.*, vol. 69, no. 1, pp. 39–43, 2013, doi: 10.5120/11808-7464

D. V. S. Kumar, R. Chaurasia, A. Misra, P. K. Misra, and Khang, A., "Heart Disease and Liver Disease Prediction Using Machine Learning," *Data-Centric AI Solutions and Emerging Technologies in the Healthcare Ecosystem*, (1st ed.), 2023, P (13). CRC Press. 10.1201/9781003356189

M. of E. & I. T. IT, 2023. "National e-Governance Plan (Government of India)." https://www.meity.gov.in/divisions/national-e-governance-plan#nice-menu-1.

I. Megiddo et al., "Analysis of the universal immunization programme and introduction of a rotavirus vaccine in India with IndiaSim," *Vaccine*, vol. 32, no. S1, pp. A151–A161, 2014, doi: 10.1016/j.vaccine.2014.04.080

A. R. Patel, and M. P. Nowalk, "Expanding immunization coverage in rural India: A review of evidence for the role of community health workers," *Vaccine*, vol. 28, no. 3, pp. 604–613, 2010, doi: 10.1016/j.vaccine.2009.10.108

S. Prinja et al., "A composite indicator to measure universal health care coverage in India: Way forward for post-2015 health system performance monitoring framework," *Health Policy Plan.*, vol. 32, no. 1, pp. 43–56, 2017, doi: 10.1093/heapol/czw097

G. Rana, Khang, A., R. Sharma, A. K. Goel, and A. K. Dubey. *Reinventing Manufacturing and Business Processes Through Artificial Intelligence*, 2021. CRC Press. 10.1201/9781003145011

S. Rani, P. Bhambri, A. Kataria, Khang, A., and A. K. Sivaraman (Eds.). *Big Data, Cloud Computing and IoT: Tools and Applications*, (1st ed.), 2023. Chapman and Hall/CRC. 10.1201/9781003298335

S. Rani, M. Chauhan, A. Kataria, and Khang, A., "IoT Equipped Intelligent Distributed Framework for Smart Healthcare Systems," *Networking and Internet Architecture*, 2021. CRC Press. 10.48550/arXiv.2110.04997

A. S. Rwashana, D. W. Williams, and S. Neema, "System dynamics approach to immunization healthcare issues in developing countries: A case study of Uganda," *Health Informatics J.*, vol. 15, no. 2, pp. 95–107, 2009, doi: 10.1177/1460458209102971

D. Saikia, "Health care infrastructure in the rural areas of North-East India: Current status and future challenges," *J. Econ. Soc. Dev.*, vol. 10, no. 1, pp. 83–99, 2014. https://www.researchgate.net/profile/Dilip-Saikia-3/publication/265511171_Health_Care_Infrastructure_in_the_Rural_Areas_of_North-East_India_Current_Status_and_Future_Challenges/links/54aa987e0cf2ce2df668a529/Health-Care-Infrastructure-in-the-Rural-Areas-of-North-East-India-Current-Status-and-Future-Challenges.pdf

P. K. Singh, "Trends in child immunization across geographical regions in India: Focus on urban-rural and gender differentials," *PLoS One*, vol. 8, no. 9, p. e73102, Sep. 2013, doi: 10.1371/journal.pone.0073102

M. Snehal, J. Babasaheb, and Khang, A., "Workforce Management System: Concepts, Definitions, Principles, and Implementation," *Designing Workforce Management Systems for Industry 4.0: Data-Centric and AI-Enabled Approaches*, (1st ed.), 2023, pp. 1–13. CRC Press. 10.1201/9781003357070-1

M. S. Stockwell, and A. G. Fiks, "Utilizing health information technology to improve vaccine communication and coverage," *Hum. Vaccines Immunother.*, vol. 9, no. 8, pp. 1802–1811, 2013, doi: 10.4161/hv.25031

R. K. Tailor, R. Pareek, and Khang, A., (Eds.). "Robot Process Automation in Blockchain," *The Data-Driven Blockchain Ecosystem: Fundamentals, Applications, and Emerging Technologies*, (1st ed.), 2022, pp. 149–164. CRC Press. 10.1201/9781003269281-8

M. Taqi, S. Bidhuri, S. Sarkar, W. S. Ahmad, and P. Wangchok, "Rural healthcare infra-structural disparities in India: A critical analysis of availability and accessibility," *J. Multidiscip. Res. Healthc.*, vol. 3, no. 2, pp. 125–149, 2017, doi: 10.15415/jmrh.2017.32011

A. E. Tozzi, F. Gesualdo, A. D'Ambrosio, E. Pandolfi, E. Agricola, and P. Lopalco, "Can digital tools be used for improving immunization programs?," *Front. Public Heal.* vol. 4, p. 36, 2016, doi: 10.3389/fpubh.2016.00036

S. Vrushank, and Khang, A., "Internet of Medical Things (IoMT) Driving the Digital Transformation of the Healthcare Sector," *Data-Centric AI Solutions and Emerging Technologies in the Healthcare Ecosystem*, (1st ed.), 2023, P (1). CRC Press. 10.1201/9781003356189

S. Vrushank, T. Vidhi, and Khang, A., "Electronic Health Records Security and Privacy Enhancement Using Blockchain Technology," *Data-Centric AI Solutions and Emerging Technologies in the Healthcare Ecosystem*, (1st ed.), 2023, P (1). CRC Press. 10.1201/9781003356189

21 Intelligent Handy Healthcare System in Medical Ecosystem

P Karthikeyan, Surya K, Vibishanan S, Vivek AR, and Sakthi S

CONTENTS

21.1 INTRODUCTION

When anyone is currently afflicted with an illness, they must see a doctor, which is both time consuming and depends upon their availability. It can also be difficult for the people if they are not near doctors and hospitals because the illness cannot be identified (Khang & Hajimahmud, 2022a).

As an initial step, if we predict the illness using an automated software that saves time and makes the patient get knowledge about their illness even before they visit their doctors, it could be better for the patient, making the process go more smoothly by taking some precautionary measures that can help them avoid future risks (Khang et al., 2022b).

Disease predictor is a mobile application-based system that predicts a user's disease based on the symptoms they have. Various diseases and their probability dataset have been obtained for the disease prediction system.

Related work is done to find the best possible solution to the problem. The use of machine learning algorithms in the disease predictor application paves the way for people to identify the disease with the symptoms they are suffering from.

DOI: 10.1201/9781003356189-21

21.2   PROBLEM STATEMENT

The identification of the problem was done as the initial process. The problem statement was about people being unaware about their health conditions (Snehal et al., 2023). So, patient health needs to be monitored from time to time on a regular basis in order to avoid any health risks. Hence, patients sometimes need to get information regarding their health condition in order to take primitive actions.

21.3   PROPOSED WORK

In order to promote and encourage a healthy work environment, a firm code of cooperation and focus group discussion were made and discussed by the team members. It primarily focused on keeping up a healthy communication between the team and to keep up with the recent trends so that the team members could be updated with the best solution that was available during the course of the project (Rani et al., 2021).

Once the problem was understood, we started with the literature survey. It included mostly research papers from reputed sites like Google Scholar, ScienceDirect, and ResearchGate. The surveys related to the problems were taken from research papers and more articles were referred to to propose a best suitable solution to this problem. A detailed overview of related work is provided under the related work section of this chapter (figure 21.1).

From this literature survey, we identified machine learning algorithms that were useful to predict the disease with their key as well as through the common symptoms that each disease has. These algorithms are also economically feasible to implement and proved to be easy to use (Hajimahmud et al., 2022).

This could ensure availability for the people through an android application. First, we have chosen the algorithms such as decision tree classifier, Naive-Bayes multinomial, random forest classifier, and gradient boosting. Each of these algorithms are

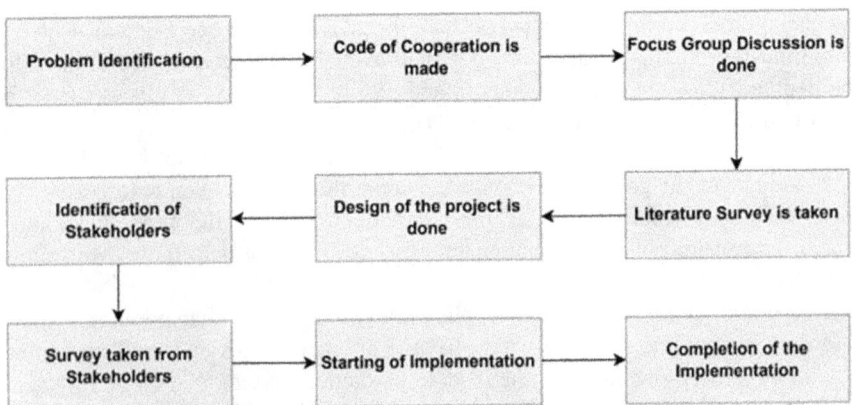

FIGURE 21.1   Project work plan.

Source: This Flowchart is designed by Surya K, Sakthi S.

tested in our case to find the algorithms having a high accuracy of prediction (Khanh & Khang, 2021).

The results obtained by comparison of algorithms have been discussed briefly in the "Usage of Machine Learning Algorithms" section of this chapter.

For the design of a low-cost model, we have used Figma, a collaborative web application for interface design. Also, stakeholder identification and survey were done. From the survey, we got results favoring development of a mobile application. So, we decided to develop a disease prediction application (Rana et al., 2021).

21.4 RELATED WORK

The content from the related work is provided as an abstract to get insight about the references. We have considered eight research articles published in international journals or articles or conference papers for this study.

Disease prediction has been done using health data taken from various sources like SCOPUS and PubMed using several keywords. Aim of the study is to understand the key trends observed in various machine learning algorithms based on their performance and usability for disease prediction, as shown in figure 21.2.

Also, several papers proposed a shared decision-making system for a particular disease prediction using a class-imbalanced electronic health record (EHR) as the dataset. This could help the physicians and the patients get a better understanding of the current health conditions (Rani et al., 2022).

In a comparative study between Naïve-Bayes, support vector machine (SVM), K-nearest neighbors (KNN), and random forest algorithms for a hepatitis disease dataset, the best performance was achieved by random forest classifier with a classification accuracy of 92.14% (Khang et al., 2023a).

Usage of random forest algorithm for disease prediction system with a dataset of 132 symptoms and classification proposal for 41 diseases. The proposed system

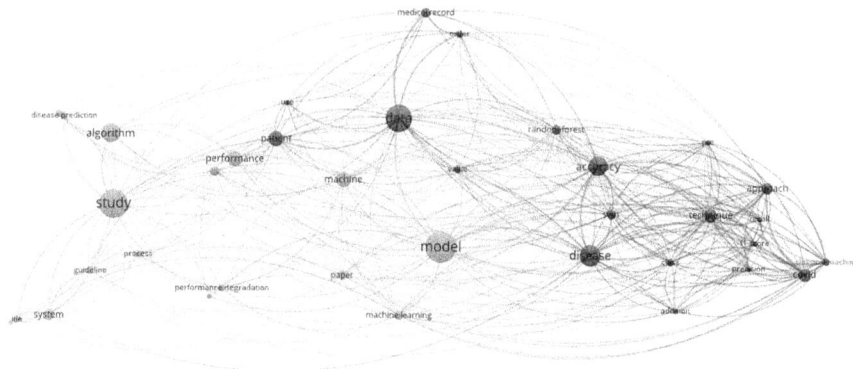

FIGURE 21.2 Keywords visualization.

Source: Made using VOSViewer Application (www.vosviewer.com) by providing data from the abstract of the research articles as input.

predicts a most probable disease based on the input given by the user in terms of the symptom (Morris et al., 2023).

With the accuracy and rejection curves, it can be observed that the algorithm is quite optimized and reduced performance degradation can be observed (Khang et al., 2022a).

21.5 USAGE OF MACHINE LEARNING ALGORITHMS

Usage of machine learning technology in the field of medicine proves to be very useful and more effective in pre-medical analysis and classification of diseases. With the evolution of ML technology, the patients and the general public can now have access to a well-defined mobile application that predicts the disease according to the combination of symptoms provided by them (Khang et al., 2022c).

In this article, we have discussed the most prominent ML algorithms that perform well in classification-related tasks. We have compared random forest, Naïve-Bayes–multinomial, decision trees, and gradient boosting algorithms. We have used pre-trained ML models from GitHub and have analyzed them based on a dataset (Khang et al., 2022d).

The dataset contains about 133 independent records with the fields being disease concerned, prognosis, and probability of occurrence. The dataset is split into a partition of 63:37 for better performance and results. Sixty-three percent of the records are partitioned as a training dataset and the remaining 37% is split for testing the model (Misra et al., 2023).

21.5.1 CLASSIFICATION FORMULAS

$$\text{Information Gain} = \text{Entropy}(S) - [(\text{Weighted Average}) * \text{Entropy}(\text{each feature})] \quad (21.1)$$

Equation 21.1: Information Gain

Source: https://medium.com/capital-one-tech/random-forest-algorithm-for-machine-learning-c4b2c8cc9feb

$$Gini = 1 - \sum_{i=1}^{C} (p_i)^2 \quad (21.2)$$

Equation 21.2: Gini Index

Source: https://medium.com/capital-one-tech/random-forest-algorithm-for-machine-learning-c4b2c8cc9feb

$$Entropy = \sum_{i=1}^{C} - p_i * \log_2(p_i) \quad (21.3)$$

Equation 21.3: Entropy

Source: https://medium.com/capital-one-tech/random-forest-algorithm-for-machine-learning-c4b2c8cc9feb
  Where S = Total Number of Samples
  P(yes) = Probability of Yes
  P(no) = Probability of No

21.5.2   BAYES RULE

$$Posterior\ Probability = \frac{Conditional\ Probability * Prior\ Probability}{Predictor\ Prior\ Probability}$$

$$P\left(\frac{A}{B}\right) = \left(\frac{P(A \cap B)}{P(B)}\right) = \frac{P(A) * P\left(\frac{B}{A}\right)}{P(B)} \tag{21.4}$$

Equation 21.4: Probability Calculation from Bayes Rule

Source: https://www.mygreatlearning.com/blog/multinomial-naive-bayes-explained/
  Where P (A) = the prior probability of occurring A
  P (B/A) = the condition probability of B given that A occurs
  P (A/B) = the condition probability of A given that B occurs
  P (B) = the probability of occurring B

21.5.3   GRADIENT BOOSTING ALGORITHM – P (ODDS)

$$P(Odds) = e * \log(odds)/(1 + e * \log(odds)) \tag{21.5}$$

Equation 21.5: Probability of Odds Occurrence

Source: https://blog.paperspace.com/gradient-boosting-for-classification/

$$\frac{\Sigma Residual}{\Sigma[PreviousProb * (1 - PreviousProb)]} \tag{21.6}$$

Equation 21.6: Transformation Formula for adding leaf nodes

$$\log(\text{Odds}) = \text{Old Tree} + \text{Learning Rate} * \text{New Tree} \qquad (21.7)$$

Source: https://blog.paperspace.com/gradient-boosting-for-classification/

Equation 21.7: Recursive formula for log (Odds) until maximum number of trees is reached

Source: https://blog.paperspace.com/gradient-boosting-for-classification/

Random forest and decision tree classifiers use the formulas for Information Gain (equation 21.1), Gini Index (equation 21.2), and Entropy (equation 21.3) to compute the predictions. Multinomial Naïve-Bayes classifier uses Bayes Rule (equation 21.4) to compute predictions. Gradient boosting algorithm uses probability of odds (equation 21.5), transformation formula for leaf nodes (equation 21.6), and log (Odds) recursive formula (equation 21.7) to make predictions.

21.6 DATA INCLUSION IN APPLICATION

We have included six diseases in the primary release of the application, namely typhoid, malaria, diarrhea, cardiovascular disease, blood pressure, and diabetes (Khang et al., 2023b). Table 21.1 refers to the symptoms and their mapping with the diseases.

21.7 RESULTS AND IMPLEMENTATION

From the observations obtained and from table 21.2, all the algorithms have a similar trend in accuracy and effectiveness. Gradient boosting and decision tree classifier

TABLE 21.1
Mapping of Symptoms with Diseases Used

Disease	Common Symptoms	Key Symptom(s)
Diarrhea	Vomiting, Fever, Nausea, Weight Loss	Stomach Ache
Blood Pressure	Nausea, Vomiting, Shortness of Breath, Dizziness, Chest Pain	Blurry or Double Vision, Headaches
Cardiovascular Disease	Shortness of Breath, Chest Pain	Fast Heartbeat, Pressure or Heaviness in Chest, Anxiety
Diabetes	Dizziness, Skin Itching, Hunger, Weight Loss	Frequent Urination, Blurry or Double Vision, More Thirsty Than Usual
Typhoid	Constipation, Dry Cough, Muscle Pain, Weakness/Fatigue	Abdominal Pain
Malaria	Fever, Sweating, Fast Heartbeat	Muscle and Body Pain, Abdominal Pain

Source: This table was prepared by Vivek Ar, Vibishanan S.

TABLE 21.2

Implementation of Machine Learning Algorithms

Criteria	Naïve-Bayes Multinomial	Gradient Boosting	Decision Tree Classifier	Random Forest Classifier
Accuracy Score (Validation)	95.70%	96.77%	96.77%	97.85%
Accuracy Score (Training)	98.21%	98.21%	98.21%	96.43%
Data Fitting Time	0.90 ms	1755.65 ms	1.58 ms	31.60 ms

Source: This table was designed by Vivek Ar, Dr P Karthikeyan.

show similar percentages in terms of accuracy score during training and validation. But they differ in the time taken for fitting data into the model (Gupta et al., 2023).

Since the dataset used for training and testing of the model remains the same, we obtain a similar accuracy score for training in Naïve-Bayes Multinomial, gradient boosting, and decision tree classifier algorithms, whereas random forest classifier shows a lesser score compared to the others (Khang et al., 2023c).

Also, we can observe that the highest and lowest accuracy scores for validation are obtained by random forest classifier and Naïve-Bayes Multinomial (Rani et al., 2021). In contrast, accuracy score for training is lowest for random forest classifier and highest for the other three algorithms, as shown in table 21.2.

From the classification report obtained, we have observed that except for random forest classifier, other algorithms produced a precision, recall, and f1-score to be the same for both macro average and weighted average individually (Bhambri et al., 2022).

The random forest classifier produced less precision, recall, and f1-score compared to the other algorithms. Table 21.3 provides the details of precision, recall, and f1-scores of the ML algorithms.

Decision tree classifier has the highest accuracy score for training and also less data fitting time with a validation accuracy score of 96.77%, which can be selected for the development of mobile application because of better performance and less time taken for the same dataset and represents an ideal/optimal machine learning algorithm for the disease predictor (Tailor et al., 2022).

The mobile application has three basic functions: Situating a nearby hospital and SOS call feature embedded, details of the doctor in case of an emergency, and the disease predictor itself (Vrushank et al., 2023) (figure 21.3.1).

The user needs to provide an input based on the symptoms list that can be accessed after providing the username and age of the person. Then the application prompts the user to finalize their selection by selecting "Know Your Disease" button. The application would predict the disease based on the input given by the user (figure 21.3.2).

As an additional feature, the application also has been provided with a hyperlink that directs the user to the search engine for letting the user know about the complete information about the disease, including its diverse effects, medications, etc (figures 21.3.3–21.3.6).

TABLE 21.3

Precision, Recall, and f1-Score for ML Algorithms

Criteria	Random Forest Classifier	Multinomial Naïve Bayes	Decision Tree Classifier	Gradient Boosting Classifier
Macro Average for Precision	0.93	0.96	0.96	0.96
Macro Average for Recall	0.93	0.96	0.96	0.96
Macro Average for f1-Score	0.93	0.96	0.96	0.96
Weighted Average for Precision	0.96	0.98	0.98	0.98
Weighted Average for Recall	0.96	0.98	0.98	0.98
Weighted Average for f1-Score	0.96	0.98	0.98	0.98

Source: This table was designed by Vivek Ar, Dr P Karthikeyan.

The mobile application consists of a list of symptoms from which the user selects and the corresponding disease is predicted by the ML algorithm in the backend. This is the main application of the mobile app. Apart from this, there are several additional features to promote security of the patient in case of any emergency.

The application also provides a facility to navigate to the nearby hospitals using Google maps. An emergency SOS call feature is also enabled for easier contact of the emergency contact number. The details of the doctor and helpline numbers are also provided within the Contact Us page of the mobile application.

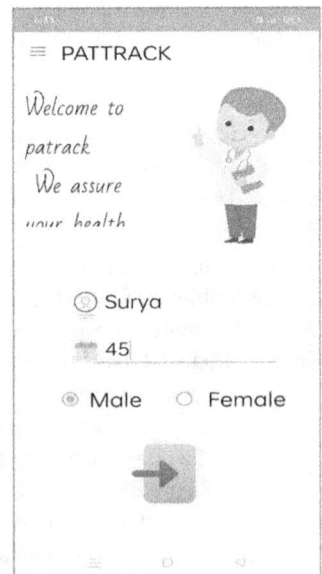

FIGURE 21.3.1 Home page.

Source: Screen Mockup of mobile application done by Surya K, Vibishanan S, Vivek Ar, Sakthi S.

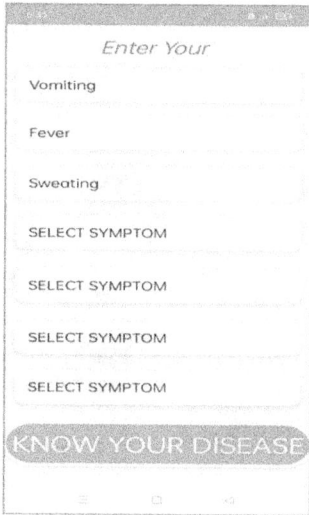

FIGURE 21.3.2   Symptoms selection page.

Source: Screen Mockup of mobile application done by Surya K, Vibishanan S, Vivek Ar, Sakthi S.

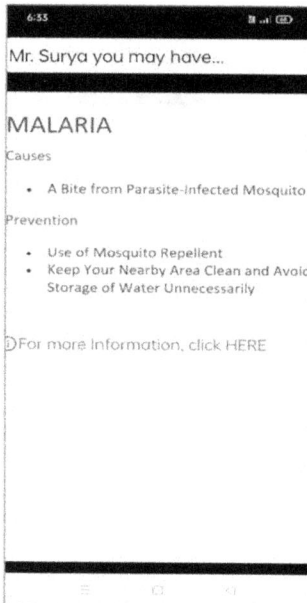

FIGURE 21.3.3   Disease predictor page.

Source: Screen Mockup of mobile application done by Surya K, Vibishanan S, Vivek Ar, Sakthi S.

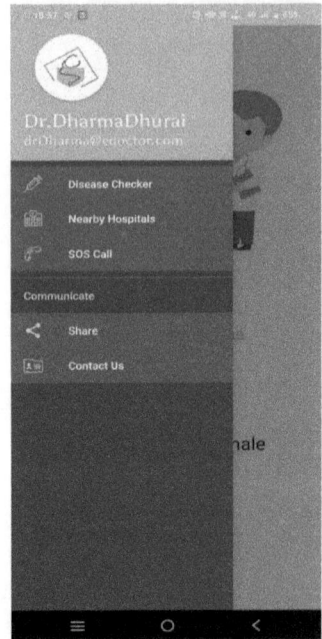

FIGURE 21.3.4 Menu bar – Other features of the app.

Source: Screen Mockup of mobile application done by Surya K, Vibishanan S, Vivek Ar, Sakthi S.

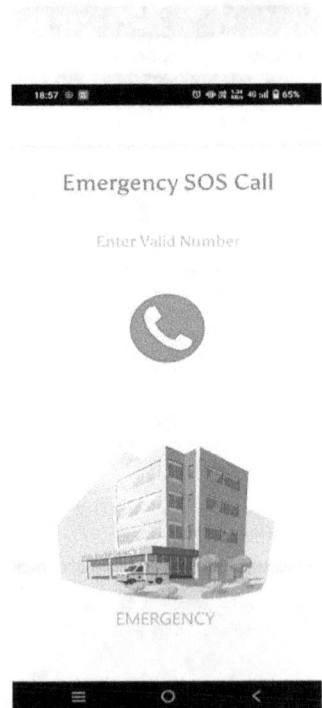

FIGURE 21.3.5 SOS emergency call page.

Source: Screen Mockup of mobile application done by Surya K, Vibishanan S, Vivek Ar, Sakthi S.

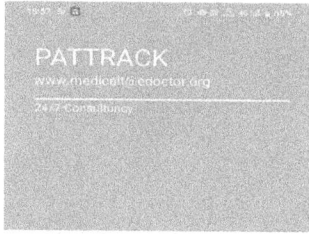

+91 8980688666

Drsharma12@gmail.com

D-11, Royal Court Road,
Near Government Hospital,
Madurai Medical College
Madurai 625-011

FIGURE 21.3.6 "About us" details page.

Source: Screen Mockup of mobile application done by Surya K, Vibishanan S, Vivek Ar, Sakthi S.

21.8 CONCLUSION

From the ML algorithms investigated in this article, the decision tree classifier algorithm is best suited for the classification-related tasks. It provided the highest accuracy and is also an optimal algorithm. Due to this reason, it has the best performance in handling the particular dataset, and it is recommended to be used in our disease predictor mobile application.

REFERENCES

F. Amato, L. Coppolino, G. Cozzolino, G. Mazzeo, F. Moscato, R. Nardone, *Enhancing random forest classification with NLP in DAMEH: A system for Data Management in eHealth Domain, Neurocomputing*, Vol. 444, (2021), pp. 79–91. https://www.sciencedirect.com/science/article/pii/S0925231221001302

P. Bhambri, S. Rani, G. Gupta, Khang, A. *Cloud and Fog Computing Platforms for Internet of Things*, ISBN: 978-1-032-101507, (2022). CRC Press. 10.1201/9781003213888

S. Goyal, R. Singh, "Detection and classification of lung diseases for pneumonia and Covid19 using machine and deep learning techniques," *J Ambient Intell Human Comput* (2021). 10.1007/s12652-021-03464-7

S. K. Gupta, Khang, A. P. Somani, C. K. Dixit, A. Pathak, "Data Mining Processes and Decision-Making Models in Personnel Management System," *Designing Workforce Management Systems for Industry 4.0: Data-Centric and AI-Enabled Approaches*, (1st ed.), 89–112. (2023). CRC Press. 10.1201/9781003357070-6

V. A. Hajimahmud, Khang, A. V. Hahanov, E. Litvinova, S. Chumachenko, A. V. Alyar, "Autonomous Robots for Smart City: Closer to Augmented Humanity," *AI-Centric Smart City Ecosystems: Technologies, Design and Implementation*, (1st ed.), (2022). CRC Press. 10.1201/9781003252542-7

A. Khang, V. Hahanov, G. L. Abbas, V. A. Hajimahmud, "Cyber-Physical-Social System and İncident Management," *AI-Centric Smart City Ecosystems: Technologies, Design and Implementation*, (1st ed.), (2022a). CRC Press. 10.1201/9781003252542-2

A. Khang, V. Hahanov, E. Litvinova, S. Chumachenko, V. A. Hajimahmud, A. V. Alyar, "The Key Assistant of Smart City - Sensors and Tools," *AI-Centric Smart City Ecosystems: Technologies, Design and Implementation*, (1st ed.), (2022b). CRC Press. 10.1201/9781003252542-17

A. Khang, N. A. Ragimova, V. A. Hajimahmud, A. V. Alyar, "Advanced Technologies and Data Management in the Smart Healthcare System," *AI-Centric Smart City Ecosystems: Technologies, Design and Implementation*, (1st ed.), (2022c). CRC Press. 10.1201/9781003252542-16

A. Khang, S. Rani, A. K. Sivaraman, *AI-Centric Smart City Ecosystems: Technologies, Design and Implementation*, (1st ed.), (2022d). CRC Press. 10.1201/9781003252542

A. Khang, S. K. Gupta, C. K. Dixit, P. Somani, "Data-Driven Application of Human Capital Management Databases, Big Data, and Data Mining," *Designing Workforce Management Systems for Industry 4.0: Data-Centric and AI-Enabled Approaches*, (1st ed.), 113–133. (2023a). CRC Press. 10.1201/9781003357070-7

A. Khang, G. Rana, R. K. Tailor, V. A. Hajimahmud, (Eds.). *Data-Centric AI Solutions and Emerging Technologies in the Healthcare Ecosystem*, (1st ed.), (2023b). CRC Press. 10.1201/9781032398570

H. H. Khanh, Khang, A. "The Role of Artificial Intelligence in Blockchain Applications," *Reinventing Manufacturing and Business Processes Through Artificial Intelligence*, 20–40. (2021). CRC Press. 10.1201/9781003145011-2

A. Misra, V. Shah, Khang, A. S. K. Gupta, (Eds.). *AI-Aided IoT Technologies and Applications in the Smart Business and Production*, (1st ed.), (2023). CRC Press. 10.1201/9781003392224

G. Morris, J. Babasaheb, Khang, A. S. K. Gupta, V. A. Hajimahmud, (1 Ed.). *AI-Centric Modelling and Analytics: Concepts, Designs, Technologies, and Applications*, (1st ed.), (2023). CRC Press. 10.1201/9781003400110

G. Rana, Khang, A. R. Sharma, A. K. Goel, A. K. Dubey. *Reinventing Manufacturing and Business Processes Through Artificial Intelligence*, (2021). CRC Press. 10.1201/9781003145011

S. Rani, P. Bhambri, A. Kataria, Khang, A. "Smart City Ecosystem: Concept, Sustainability, Design Principles and Technologies," *AI-Centric Smart City Ecosystems: Technologies, Design and Implementation*, (1st ed.), (2022). CRC Press. 10.1201/9781003252542-1

S. Rani, M. Chauhan, A. Kataria, Khang, A. "IoT Equipped Intelligent Distributed Framework for Smart Healthcare Systems," *Networking and Internet Architecture*, (2021). CRC Press. 10.48550/arXiv.2110.04997

M. Snehal, J. Babasaheb, Khang, A. "Workforce Management System: Concepts, Definitions, Principles, and Implementation," *Designing Workforce Management Systems for Industry 4.0: Data-Centric and AI-Enabled Approaches*, (1st ed.), 1–13. (2023). CRC Press. 10.1201/9781003357070-1

R. K. Tailor, R. Pareek, Khang, A. (Eds.). "Robot Process Automation in Blockchain," *The Data-Driven Blockchain Ecosystem: Fundamentals, Applications, and Emerging Technologies*, (1st ed.), 149–164. (2022). CRC Press. 10.1201/9781003269281-8

S. Vrushank, T. Vidhi, Khang, A. 2023. "Electronic Health Records Security and Privacy Enhancement Using Blockchain Technology," *Data-Centric AI Solutions and Emerging Technologies in the Healthcare Ecosystem*, (1st ed.), (2023), P (1). CRC Press. 10.1201/9781003356189

Index

For Product Safety Concerns and Information please contact our EU
representative GPSR@taylorandfrancis.com
Taylor & Francis Verlag GmbH, Kaufingerstraße 24, 80331 München, Germany